MICROSURGERY OF THE ANTERIOR SEGMENT OF THE EYE

VOLUME II
THE CORNEA: OPTICS AND SURGERY

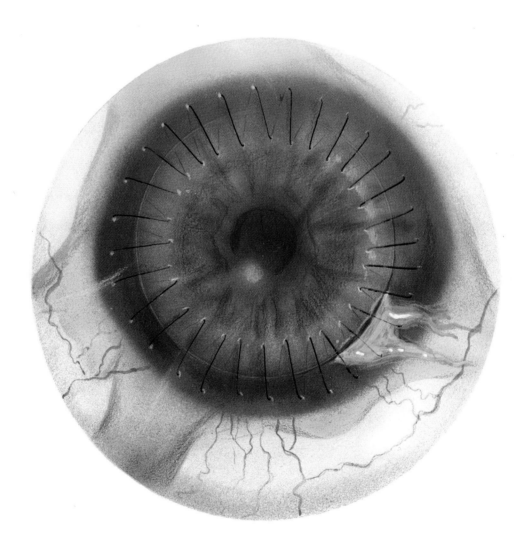

Fluorescein test to detect wound leakage.

MICROSURGERY OF THE ANTERIOR SEGMENT OF THE EYE

VOLUME II
THE CORNEA: OPTICS AND SURGERY

Richard C. Troutman, M.D., F.A.C.S.

Professor and Head, Division of Ophthalmology,
State University of New York, Downstate Medical Center,
Brooklyn, New York; Surgeon Director,
Manhattan Eye, Ear and Throat Hospital,
New York, New York

With 396 tone drawings in 136 plates by

Virginia Cantarella

The C.V. Mosby Company

Saint Louis   1977

VOLUME II

Copyright © 1977 by The C. V. Mosby Company

Volume I copyrighted 1974

Printed in the United States of America

Distributed in Great Britain by Henry Kimpton, London

The C. V. Mosby Company
11830 Westline Industrial Drive, St. Louis, Missouri 63141

Library of Congress Cataloging in Publication Data (Revised)

Troutman, Richard C
    Microsurgery of the anterior segment of the eye.

    Includes bibliographies and index.
    CONTENTS: v. 1. Introduction and basic techniques.
—v. 2. The cornea: optics and surgery.
    1. Anterior chamber (Eye)—Surgery. 2. Micro-
surgery. I. Cantarella, Virginia, illus. II. Title.
[DNLM: 1. Anterior chamber—Surgery. 2. Microsurgery. WW168 T861m]
RE80.T76   617.7'4   74-12453
ISBN 0-8016-5106-9

TS/CB/B 9 8 7 6 5 4 3 2 1

To my wife, Dr. Suzanne Véronneau-Troutman,
who has encouraged me constantly to write this as well as the previous
volume and who may yet succeed in getting me to write Volume III

I would like to acknowledge the Hartford Foundation,
whose philanthropy made the realization of this book possible by its
broad support of my research in microsurgery and corneal optics

FOREWORD

Microsurgery of the eye is not limited to refinement of surgical technique and use of more delicate instruments and suture material. The surgical microscope is not only a therapeutic but also a diagnostic instrument and, therefore, greatly facilitates instant and continuous adaptation to any newly developing situation during an ongoing surgical procedure.

Surgical textbooks in the past usually outlined, rather rigidly, sequential steps of a surgical procedure as they had proved successful in the hands of the experienced author. Such directions provided safety and avoided complications, especially in operations that could not be controlled optically in a sufficient manner. Clearly, the good results of earlier eye surgeons show that these directions were well reasoned and justified. The introduction of the surgical microscope, therefore, does not enter an underdeveloped field, and one should not necessarily expect spectacularly improved results in all types of operations. Even now, there are occasional doubts whether it is really necessary to use the microscope for all intraocular procedures, but these doubts are fading. For example, the use of the microscope in corneal surgery is no longer controversial. Here, it is obvious that the improved precision leads to better surgical results, which in turn facilitate postoperative treatment and consequently lessen the burden on the patient.

I am honored to introduce this surgical textbook and to have the opportunity to draw the attention of the reader not only to the refinements of techniques but also to those unique "procedural adaptations" that the surgical microscope not just allows but literally enforces. The author of any modern surgical text will have to make this clear, and new textbooks in ophthalmic microsurgery must be different from those of former years. They have to present the variety of technical possibilities from which the surgeon must choose while adapting to a continuously changing surgical situation during an ongoing procedure. Obviously, Richard Troutman was guided by these ideas when writing this book and when selecting the numerous and very instructive illustrations.

In this book the author also emphasizes the following aspect: the first phase in the development of keratoplasty consisted of inserting water-tight transplants and of maintaining transparency during healing. These problems have essentially been solved. The task is now to develop procedures for the improvement of optical quality. The author has made particular efforts to achieve this latter goal. He presents methods to keep regular and irregular astigmatism at a minimum by specific suturing techniques or by secondary corrective procedures. This introduces a promising second phase in the development of plastic corneal surgery. Particular attention should be paid to the numerous technical hints regarding combined procedures, such as combinations of keratoplasty with lens, iris, or tension-lowering operations.

For the last 14 years I have been aware of the author's way of thinking and working. I know how consistently and devotedly he has worked on the instrument and methodologic improvements of microsurgery of the anterior segment. I collaborated in several of his courses on microsurgery for beginners and advanced participants at the Downstate Medical Center in New York. It was there that introduction to the plurality of surgical choices was understood as a didactic and specific principle of modern microsurgery. All this is reflected in a book that is shaped by the author's rich experience and dedication. It deserves wide recognition.

Professor Dr. Gunter Mackensen
Universitats-Augenklinik
Freiburg, Germany, 1977

PREFACE

Clinical transplantation of the human cornea has become increasingly successful as a result of continuing advances both in the laboratory and in clinical sciences. The technical surgical aspects of keratoplasty presented here represent a synthesis of these advances with particular emphasis on the use of the ophthalmic surgical microscope.

The use of the surgical microscope has expanded the technical parameters of keratoplasty, not only to ensure a better anatomic result but also to make possible, for the first time, the detection and management of optical distortions of the cornea. In addition to the former, it is this latter aspect of corneal microsurgery to which I have addressed myself as a major topic of this book. To this time, corneal surgeons, in general, have been concerned only indirectly with corneal optics and have accepted astigmatic or axial errors as a matter of course. Success in penetrating keratoplasty is still measured primarily in terms of the "clear graft" often to the neglect of the final optical result.

It is my hope that emphasizing the principles and techniques of optical surgery, in particular the use of intraoperative optical measuring devices such as the Troutman surgical keratometer, will increase the extent of the knowledge in this important area and will stimulate the interest of this and future generations of corneal surgeons.

The possibilities for correction of ametropia, whether iatrogenic, traumatic, or developmental in origin, by alteration of corneal curvatures and thickness, are just beginning to be realized. New techniques and instrumentation will be required, new possibilities will emerge, and new benefits to our patients will accrue.

The technical aspects of microsurgery regarding the microscope, other instruments, sutures, and surgical techniques employed also are treated extensively. The techniques are presented from a personal rather than from a survey basis. They are meant to guide and to instruct the surgeon in the basic technical surgical aspects of keratoplasty and to initiate the surgeon in the thinking of the author. The reader is encouraged to develop his or her own technique for the individual case.

As an author, I would be remiss not to acknowledge the various individuals who have made this volume possible. First thanks go to Virginia Cantarella, whose illustrations have saved thousands of words and increased the value and meaning of each sentence of the text so concisely edited by Aurora C. Clahane and typed to perfection by Sylvia Baer and Doris Druce. Just as success in penetrating keratoplasty is not just a clear graft, success in authorship is not just a single effort.

Richard C. Troutman

CONTENTS

1 The cornea, 1

2 Optical considerations, 7

3 Corneal surgery—indications and operative plan, 34

4 The donor eye, 56

5 Instrumentation, 96

6 Common techniques, 116

7 Lamellar keratoplasty technique, 180

8 Simple penetrating keratoplasty, 200

9 Combined cataract surgery and keratoplasty, 216

10 Aphakic keratoplasty, 245

11 Troutman corneal wedge resection for correction of astigmatism, 263

12 Glaucoma surgery and keratoplasty, 287

13 Surgical management of postoperative complications, 307

14 Postoperative management of the successfully grafted eye, 321

Selected readings, 336

MICROSURGERY OF
THE ANTERIOR SEGMENT
OF THE EYE

VOLUME II
THE CORNEA: OPTICS AND SURGERY

CHAPTER 1

THE CORNEA

Introduction and general considerations
Summary

INTRODUCTION AND GENERAL CONSIDERATIONS

Modern microsurgical keratoplasty techniques would not be possible were it not for the accomplishments of those few gifted, hardy surgeons who surmounted the early, difficult days of corneal surgery. One thinks first of Dr. Ramón Castroviejo, who pioneered the development of the instrumentation and techniques that form the basis of modern penetrating keratoplasty, and of Professor Louis Paufique, who did the same for lamellar keratoplasty.

I had the good fortune to be associated closely with Dr. R. Townley Paton, who, in addition to his innovative surgical techniques, provided the means to obtain the necessary human donor material for keratoplasty by implementing the concept of the community eye bank. Dr. John McLean, my mentor, also had an interest in eye-banking and in the improvement of keratoplasty technique and was responsible, initially, for my interest in corneal surgery.

In 1957, after having worked with Dr. Paton for 7 years, I met and became a close professional collaborator with Dr. Joaquin Barraquer. His meticulous keratoplasty technique further enhanced my interest in this field. These experiences and observations added emphasis to my long (since 1953) enthusiasm for the use of the dissecting microscope for anterior segment surgery. This interest led eventually to the development of the first zoom magnification ophthalmic surgical microscope and other new and modified instrumentation outlined in *Microsurgery of the Anterior Segment of the Eye, Volume I: Introduction and Basic Techniques,* more recent developments or improvements of which are detailed in Chapter 5 of this volume.

In September 1963, I met Dr. Gunter Mackensen and Professor Heinrich Harms, who introduced me to elastic monofilament nylon suture. The improved wound apposition, which is ensured by the microsurgical use of this thread for corneal wound closure, more than any other single factor, has resulted in the markedly improved surgical prognosis and final anatomic and functional results of penetrating keratoplasty.

At the First World Congress on the Cornea held in Washington, D.C., in October 1964, I presented a systematized microsurgical approach to penetrating keratoplasty, utilizing 30-micron (9-0) monofilament elastic nylon (Perlon) suture material together with my microsurgical instruments and zoom ophthalmic surgical microscope. At that meeting, only two other brief references were made to the potential use of a surgical microscope for corneal surgery. No one else, other than Harms and Mackensen who were not present, reported the use of monofilament nylon suture. In just 12 years, by the Second World Congress on the Cornea held in Washington, D.C., in April 1976, numerous papers reported the use of the surgical microscope and of elastic monofilament suture material by a majority of corneal surgeons.

Immediately following the International Ophthalmological Congress in Munich in 1966, Harms, Mackensen, and I organized the first meeting of the Microsurgery Study Group. This was attended by less than thirty ophthalmic surgeons, from almost as many countries, who had by that time started to use the surgical microscope for anterior segment surgery, in particular for keratoplasty. This meeting, which was also attended by representatives of several major manufacturers of microscopes, instruments, and suture materials, accelerated the development of microsurgical instrumentation and the interest in microsurgery in Europe, Asia, Africa, and the Americas.

This volume will detail my personal approach to microsurgery of the cornea—especially for penetrating keratoplasty—as it has evolved through the continuing use of the surgical microscope, microsurgical instruments, and monofilament suture materials. These combined surgical modalities have made keratoplasty, formerly one of the more difficult and prognostically problematic ophthalmic surgical procedures, one of the safer, more effective ophthalmic operative interventions. Microsurgery has simplified these techniques to the point where, in my opinion, they can be used by any ophthalmic microsurgeon.

To the ophthalmic surgeon not accustomed to using the surgical microscope, keratoplasty is tedious at first. However, once the microscope, instruments, and suture techniques are mastered, the surgeon's facility in dealing with the technical aspects of corneal surgery improves greatly. Microsurgical technique is of particular value in ensuring the firm and accurate apposition of the homograft to the recipient cornea. Long-term, secure wound closure is essential to prevent devastating operative and postoperative complications. Though it has been my experience that a resident surgeon, when instructed first in the laboratory and then in the operating room, can manage well the technical aspects of corneal homografting, competent surgical technique alone does not always ensure a satisfactory postoperative result. Medical and surgical judgment and therapeutics, in addition to optimal anatomic and optical conditions, must be combined to ensure an optimal functional result.

Even if ophthalmic surgeons reading this volume do not have the immediate intention of including corneal surgery in their surgical armamentaria, they can further develop clinical microsurgical skills from careful study and practice of the techniques described. In any event, the operative techniques described should be practiced on an animal or cadaver eye before being performed in a clinical situation. Familiarity with microsurgical instrumentation should be developed sufficiently so the surgeon can devote full attention to the technical, surgical management of the pathology without having to be concerned with the details of handling instruments and sutures, tying knots, and adjusting the microscope. Residents or fellows, before performing their first keratoplasties, are required to perform practice keratoplasties in a nonsensitive laboratory situation to ensure the adequacy of their mechanical skills. Trainees usually require 15-25 laboratory operations to be able to perform well an uncomplicated phakic keratoplasty. Even with no previous anterior segment microsurgical experience, a trainee can be made technically proficient for the first clinical keratoplasty. Without exception, the more experienced trainees contend that their techniques in other anterior segment surgical procedures are improved as a result of corneal surgery practice sessions.

We can confidently recommend to the reader the use of the descriptive, illustrated surgical portions of this volume as a guide for such technical practice sessions. Surgery is an art as well as a science. Artists do not attempt recitals or concerts on which their careers may depend without days of practice. To surgeons, such practice is doubly important not just for their own sakes but more for the ultimate good of the patients to whom their skills will be addressed.

In point of fact, once mastered technically, microsurgery of the cornea often can be easier in the uncomplicated case than is microsurgery of a cataract and, thus, is more ideal as a microsurgery practice technique. To begin with, it takes place largely in a single plane and is performed within a relatively limited range of magnification. Often an accurately cut donor button fits the recipient edge better than do the less regular, shelved, apposing edges of a cataract incision. Completing the corneal incision accurately with scissors is easier when the site is not obstructed partially by a conjunctival flap. At its more centripetal position, in relation to the anterior chamber angle, the inner blade of the keratoplasty scissors is less likely to damage the iris and angle structures. Because of the direct approach to the iris and lens, sphincter surgery or midperipheral iridectomy is easier, as is the intracapsular or extracapsular removal of a cataract. An intraocular lens can be inserted in the pupil more readily directly through a central trephined opening. There is potentially less trauma to corneal endothelium from the direct approach than from the oblique approach necessary with a limbal cataract incision. Vitrectomy also is performed more readily by the direct approach. When necessary, the posterior vitreous can be resected down to the retina without the necessity of using a fundus contact lens, and the more complicated pars plana approach is avoided. Though accurate appositional suturing of a keratoplasty incision is more difficult than closing a cataract incision, surgeons are forced to develop precise and painstaking suturing techniques to the eventual benefit of their microsurgical cataract suture techniques.

In the past, a major cause of graft failure has been the use of inelastic, thick, and irritating suture material, necessitating, in turn, a fundamental error in suture technique—partial thickness, vertically incomplete wound closure. Elastic monofilament suture, when handled improperly or removed too early, can be even less forgiving to technical error than silk or absorbable suture materials. However, when elastic monofilament thread is deeply placed, the suture loops tied securely, and the knots buried in the needle tract beneath the epithelial surface, both anatomic and optical problems common to silk and absorbable suture materials are virtually eliminated.

With microsurgical instrumentation and techniques and viable donor material, in the relatively uncomplicated case of penetrating keratoplasty, an optically clear graft is now virtually assured to the meticulous anterior segment microsurgeon. However, most ophthalmic surgeons, including many specialized in corneal surgery, have ignored the corneal ametropia—in particular, astigmatism—which occurs often in otherwise successful, optically clear grafts. It is my contention that severe, vision-compromising, optical aberrations are preventable and, should they occur in spite of every surgical precaution, are correctable postkeratoplasty. The causes and management of these neglected spherical and meridional errors, uncorrected by or induced by corneal surgery, will comprise an important part of the technical and surgical discussions to follow.

Therefore, before beginning a discussion of microsurgical keratoplasty techniques, there must be an understanding of the anatomic and optical bases for and theoretic considerations of the existing or residual ametropia that will be encountered during surgical management of corneal disease. In Chapter 2, the ocular globe and cornea are discussed with particular emphasis on how the corneal optics can be altered by disease or by surgical intervention, and by what means such pathologic aberrations or surgically induced aberrations may be controlled and modified.

Chapter 3 gives the indications for keratoplasty based on corneal topographic, anatomic, and optical aberrations rather than by specific disease states. An operative plan is developed, insofar as possible, not only to normalize the anatomy of the anterior segment and to provide an optically clear cornea but also to reduce to a minimum the spherical and meridional ametropia. Specular microscopy is introduced as a new method to refine the diagnosis and surgical indications to improve the prognosis of a given procedure.

Chapter 4 is a detailed account of the current methods used to obtain and to process human eye donor material, beginning with a discussion of the history of eye-banking and including the most recent techniques for tissue preservation. Eye-bank techniques—from the acquisition and processing of

4

donor material to the cutting of the donor button—are discussed in detail. This detailed approach, though elementary for the ophthalmologist reading this volume, was designed as a potential aid to the surgeon in the training of technical personnel in day-to-day eye-bank procedures. The quality as well as the viability of the donor is stressed as of prime importance. Not only should a donor button demonstrate a viable endothelium but also it must be clear and regular optically. The technique I prefer for accurately cutting the donor button from the endothelial surface of a previously prepared corneo-scleral segment is discussed.

My surgical zoom microscope and many of the microsurgical instruments used for keratoplasty have been described in Volume I. In Chapter 5, modifications or improvements of the microscope and instruments are discussed. The instrument set used for keratoplasty is presented in detail. Later chapters on technique detail the intraoperative use of the microscope and instrumentation.

Chapter 6, on technical considerations, describes individual points of operative technique, with particular reference to placement of deep-to-Descemet's membrane or through-and-through sutures, indications for and application of finer threads, and a new elastic monofilament suture material, polypropylene (Prolene).

In Chapter 7, the lamellar techniques described in Chapter 6 of Volume I are expanded to include tectonic total lamellar and composite lamellar-penetrating techniques.

Chapter 8 describes the technique of simple penetrating keratoplasty to replace an opaque or diseased cornea in an eye with an otherwise normal anterior segment. In such favorable cases, often the result is compromised only by an optical failure. Therefore techniques presented will apply not only to correction of the anatomic pathology but also to correction of coexisting optical deformities. The use of a donor button of a diameter different from that of the recipient opening and the fixation of the graft by different suture patterns are explained not only in relation to their anatomic importance but also according to the final optical result.

When cataract occurs in combination with sight-compromising corneal pathology or when cataract develops following successful simple penetrating keratoplasty, some special techniques or variations in technique are required. Chapter 9 describes the technique for combined cataract extraction and keratoplasty. Removal of the cataractous lens by simple intracapsular or extracapsular lens extraction and, when indicated and surgically feasible, the insertion of one of several types of intraocular lenses are discussed. Damage to the endothelium of the graft can be caused by an excessively traumatic cataract procedure, by disruption of the vitreous, or both, and especially by the insertion of an intraocular lens. An infusion-aspiration technique for extracapsular extraction, especially when combined with ultrasonic lens disruption, should be utilized carefully. The use and limitations of both extracapsular cataract extraction and intraocular lens implantation are discussed. The specular microscope is considered as an aid to developing the most advantageous surgical plan.

The success of keratoplasty in the aphakic eye has been increased markedly by the use of the surgical microscope and microsurgical suture materials and techniques. Concomitant reconstruction of the anterior segment with anterior vitrectomy using sponges and, more recently, vitreous suction-cutting instruments, and iris surgery (coreoplasty) have combined to improve further the prognosis of aphakic keratoplasty, especially in cases with severe corneal and anterior segment pathology. These techniques, together with variations of procedure necessary in the more complicated cases, are described in detail in Chapter 10. Some special considerations in the use of the intraocular lens in aphakic keratoplasty will be discussed.

In Chapter 11 material on corneal optics, presented in Chapter 2, is reviewed and amplified in relation to the use of my wedge-resection technique for correction of high astigmatism following keratoplasty. The management of graft edge elevation or wound separation is considered separately.

In aphakic keratoplasty in particular, glaucoma can complicate the postoperative course and nullify an otherwise successful surgical result. Techniques for trabeculotomy, trabeculectomy, and cyclocryothermy are presented in Chapter 12. It is emphasized that glaucoma surgery should be done only when medical treatment fails to control the increased ocular pressure.

Following keratoplasty there may occur postoperative complications, other than glaucoma, which can compromise a technically successful procedure. When these complications occur, they may be successfully managed medically or surgically, as outlined in Chapter 13.

Chapter 14 presents chronologically the routine postoperative management of the successfully grafted eye. Management of some minor complications not discussed in Chapter 13 that may occur during the postoperative course from keratoplasty until the sutures are removed and the patient is discharged is presented as well.

SUMMARY

This book presents primarily my personal techniques. In no way does it imply that there are not other surgical techniques that can produce the same or similar results. However, emphasis has been placed on areas not ordinarily covered in textbooks on corneal surgery, especially those having to do with the use of the surgical microscope, the detailed use of microsurgical instruments, and the use of elastic monofilament suture materials, with particular emphasis on optical as well as anatomic considerations in keratoplasty. Even with these refinements, it can be recognized that surgical keratoplasty is far from an exact science. Careful surgical judgment and, above all, the constant application of the art of medicine are required in addition to microsurgical keratoplasty to bring to the patient, as well as to the patient's eye, an optimal therapeutic and functional result.

CHAPTER 2

OPTICAL CONSIDERATIONS

General considerations
Mechanisms of corneal-induced ametropia
   in keratoconus
Optical effects of disparate-sized graft and
   recipient opening
Mechanisms of corneal-induced astigmatic
   ametropia

Effect of corneal optics on corneal
   ametropia
Other ocular structures of secondary optical
   importance
Effect of anatomic and optical diameters on
   corneal ametropia
Measurement of the cornea — clinical and
   surgical keratometry
Summary

GENERAL CONSIDERATIONS

When keratoplasty has been successful from the anatomic standpoint and the pathology has been controlled or eliminated, there remains often an excessive astigmatic band or axial ametropia that can limit severely the vision result. At best, it is necessary for the patient to wear either a strong correction spectacle lens or an uncomfortable or difficult to retain contact lens. In an attempt to minimize or to control such defects, I have developed special corneal graft cutting techniques, suturing techniques, and the "wedge-resection" procedure. These procedures have been shown consistently to reduce, to within acceptable limits, myopia or hyperopia and astigmatic bands. I have developed also an instrument, the surgical keratometer, to monitor and to aid in the correction of optical defects induced by surgery. The causes and the principles governing the correction of surgical ametropia are explained in this chapter. The optical, as well as the anatomic or reconstructive, indications for keratoplasty are discussed in Chapter 3. Later chapters deal with the corrective or compensating operative techniques and postoperative management, as they relate to both anatomic and optical final results. Let us examine first the mechanisms of corneal-induced axial and curvature ametropia.

MECHANISMS OF CORNEAL-INDUCED AMETROPIA IN KERATOCONUS

At the time when surgery finally becomes necessary from the vision standpoint, the cornea almost always has a spherical equivalent power greater than 55 diopters. If one is able to refract such an eye, despite the irregularity of the corneal optical surfaces, a high minus cylinder and sphere will be required to correct partially the ametropia. A graft smaller than 8 mm in diameter will not correct fully either the pathologic deformity or the optical defect. Though the graft that is smaller than 8 mm may be clear and the astigmatism regularized, a spherical equivalent myopic error, in inverse proportion to the diameter of the graft, remains postoperatively. A graft 8 mm or more in diameter, healed in a recipient opening of the same diameter, compensates almost entirely this spherical equivalent myopia when microsurgical technique and a double continuous monofilament suture closure (see Chapter 8) are used (Plate 2-1). Of course, if such an eye is axially myopic, a spherical equivalent axial myopia is retained, even when there is full surgical compensation of the corneal myopia. However, a predetermined axial myopia can be compensated partially by inducing deliberately a flatter, more hyperopic corneal curvature (approximately in the 40-diopter range), by using a graft slightly smaller in diameter than the recipient opening.

Plate 2-1

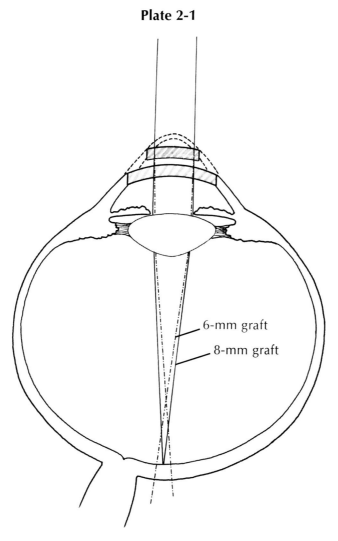

6-mm graft

8-mm graft

In the keratoconic cornea, the smaller (6-mm)
graft induces myopia; the larger (8-mm) graft
restores emmetropia. Cross section.

OPTICAL EFFECTS OF DISPARATE-SIZED GRAFT AND RECIPIENT OPENING

Let us examine in detail some optical effects that may be induced by mating disparate-sized graft and recipient opening in a schematic eye. The surgical keratometer projection, explained in detail later in this chapter, is essential to the intraoperative evaluation and the surgical correction of such corneal optical aberrations. From the center of the cornea of the emmetropic anastigmatic schematic eye with an average K of 43 diopters, a circular button, 8 mm in diameter, is cut (Plate 2-2). The recipient opening (the excised button) is cut so as to be centered at the visual axis. This circular button is put aside.

Plate 2-2

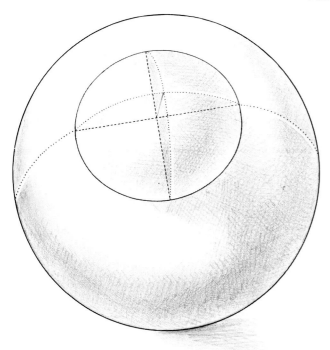

A. Schema of an anastigmatic cornea in an emmetropic eye.

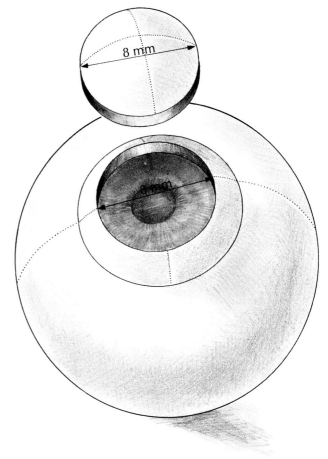

8 mm

B. 8-mm circular button excised from an emmetropic anastigmatic cornea.

A second eye of identical dimensions is selected and another circular corneal button is excised; this time, however, the button is 7.5 mm in diameter. This 7.5-mm diameter button is sutured precisely into the 8-mm diameter recipient opening of the first eye (Plate 2-3, *A* and *B*). The effect optically is twofold. First, the curvature both of the button and of the recipient cornea is flattened equally in all meridians (Plate 2-3, *C*). Second, the axial length of the eye is shortened. The shortened axial length, combined with the decreased power of the cornea, results in hyperopia.

Plate 2-3

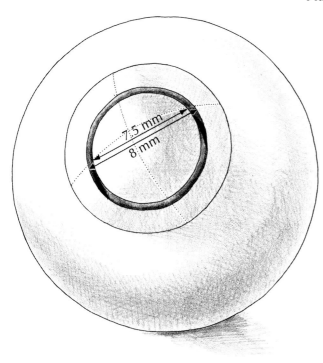

A. 7.5-mm button in 8-mm recipient opening.

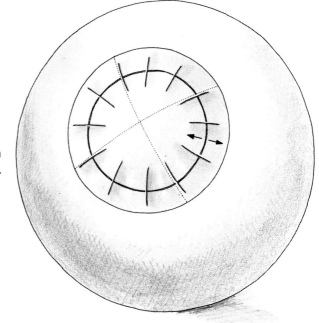

B. 7.5-mm button sutured into 8-mm recipient opening.

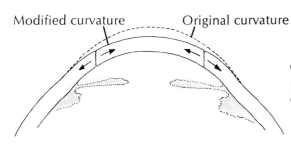

C. The corneal curvatures are flattened (axial length shortened). Cross section.

Conversely, if the larger, 8-mm diameter, corneal button is sutured into the 7.5-mm recipient opening of the second schematic eye, the optical effect is to steepen equally the curvatures of the larger button in all meridians (Plate 2-4, *A* and *B*). This steepening increases both the axial length and the dioptric power of the cornea, each of which contributes to an increase in myopia (Plate 2-4, *C*). While these perfect examples rarely are encountered clinically, they do demonstrate the optical errors that can be induced by using a circular donor button and a recipient opening of disparate diameters (or curvatures). These examples demonstrate also how optical errors can be compensated or minimized by the selection of equal- or disparate-sized diameters of recipient opening and graft, individualized to the optical requirements of the case.

For example, though the central corneal curvatures of a keratoconic cornea steepen markedly, the peripheral curvatures may be normal. If the excised portion of the recipient cornea includes all the steeper central zone, the resultant graft-recipient curvatures approximate normal, and the usual postoperative refraction is a spherical equivalent emmetropia, unless there is a concomitant posterior axial myopia or hyperopia. However, if some of the steeper portion of the recipient cornea is not excised, though the graft button may retain initially its normal curvature, eventually it will steepen as it protrudes on the thinner periphery of the pathologic cone (Plate 2-1). This steepening of the graft curvature and lengthening of the visual axis produce a corneal myopia, often seen following penetrating keratoplasty for keratoconus. Though this error could be compensated by using a donor button slightly smaller in size than the recipient opening (Plate 2-3), a more permanent correction can be obtained if all the pathology can be excised and the donor button cut to the same size as the recipient opening.

The converse is true of an excessively flat recipient cornea, such as is encountered in some familial or acquired dystrophies. Here, a smaller-diameter recipient opening is fitted with a larger-diameter button, resulting in a steeper, less hyperopic cornea (Plate 2-4). This approach has the added advantage of providing a deeper anterior chamber and a more open angle.

A third clinical application of the use of disparate-sized diameters of recipient opening and donor button is in aphakic keratoplasty or in combined cataract and keratoplasty. In this instance, the use of a donor button larger than the recipient opening reduces the aphakic hypermetropia. This has the advantage also of deepening the anterior chamber, thus reducing the possibility of iris or vitreous contacting or adhering to the posterior aspect of the incision and the graft endothelium.

Plate 2-4

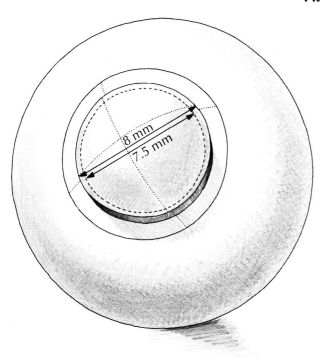

A. 8-mm button over 7.5-mm recipient opening.

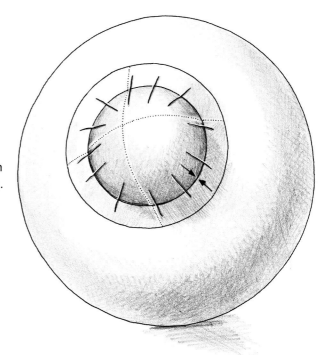

B. 8-mm button sutured into 7.5-mm recipient opening.

Modified curvature   Original curvature

C. The corneal curvatures are steepened (axial length increased). Cross section.

MECHANISMS OF CORNEAL-INDUCED ASTIGMATIC AMETROPIA

Let us now examine some of the mechanisms of corneal-induced astigmatism. An oval button is cut from a cornea of the same curvature and diameter as the schematic eye in the first example (see Plate 2-2, *A*). The oval button will have the same circumference (therefore, the same area) as the 8-mm circular recipient opening. Consequently, it is approximately 7.5 mm in the shorter meridian and 8.5 mm in the meridian at right angles (Plate 2-5, *A*). This oval button, with a difference of 1 mm between perpendicular meridians, when compressed into the 8-mm circular recipient opening, induces an astigmatic distortion. The cornea is steepened across the shorter, 7.5-mm, meridian of the button and flattened across the longer meridian at right angles (Plate 2-5, *B*). The astigmatism induced is mixed, the steeper meridian being myopic, the flatter being hyperopic (Plate 2-5, *C*). This graft-recipient disparity effect differs from that of the previous examples in that the curvature of the shorter, 7.5-mm diameter, meridian is steepened, whereas the curvature of the meridian at a 90° angle to the first, on the longer diameter of 8.5 mm, is flattened. We have seen that when a larger, 8-mm diameter, graft, is used in a smaller, 7.5-mm, recipient opening, the cornea steepens in *all* meridians, whereas it flattens in *all* meridians when a 7.5-mm button is used in a larger, 8-mm, recipient opening. In the first instance, the circumferences are disparate and the meridians are equal, whereas in the second, the circumferences are the same and the meridians are disparate.

These graft-recipient disparity effects, either singly or in combination, induce the optical ametropia and astigmatism seen clinically. An understanding of these effects is essential to an understanding of the causes of corneal-induced astigmatism and of myopia or hyperopia and the rationale behind the various corrective surgical procedures to be described.

Plate 2-5

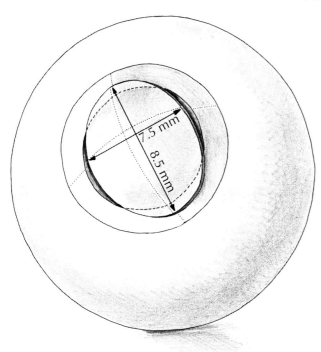

A. 7.5-mm x 8.5-mm oval button over an 8-mm round recipient opening.

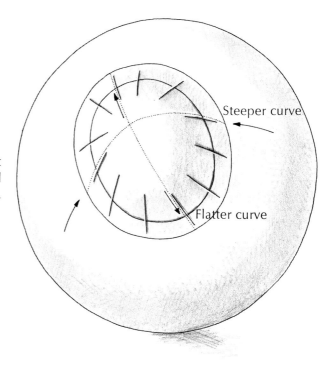

B. Oval button sutured into round recipient opening steepens the shorter meridian and flattens the longer meridian.

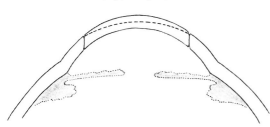

Flattened (hyperopic) meridian

Steepened (myopic) meridian

C. Flattened (longer) and steepened (shorter) meridians. Cross section.

EFFECT OF CORNEAL OPTICS ON CORNEAL AMETROPIA

As far as corneal optics is concerned, it is fortunate that about 95% of eyes are relatively standard from both anatomic and optical standpoints. Any pathologic alteration encountered must be considered a variation from the physiologic norm.

For the purposes of understanding the mechanism of a specific variation, we must first review the anatomy of the eye as it pertains to its optical function. The cornea is a segment of a sphere, 7.85 mm in radius, with a power of 43 diopters. A cornea of shorter radius has a correspondingly steeper curve and higher dioptric power; a larger corneal radius gives a flatter curvature and less power. For example, a 47-diopter cornea has a radius of 7.18 mm; a 39-diopter cornea has a radius of 8.65 mm (Plate 2-6, *A*). It can be seen from these figures that it requires a 0.67-mm decrease in the radius of one meridian (7.85 − 7.18 = 0.67) to induce an increase of 4 diopters of astigmatism (from 43 diopters to 47 diopters) in that meridian. On the other hand, it requires an 0.8-mm increase in radius (8.65 − 7.85 = 0.8) to induce a 4-diopter flattening of a 43-diopter meridian. It will be seen later that, in vivo, there exists a similar but more pronounced steepening-to-flattening ratio. In the Troutman corneal wedge-resection procedure, when a meridian is steepened deliberately to compensate excessive astigmatism, the steepening-to-flattening ratio is 2:1.

The corneal ring, defined as the junction of the cornea and the sclera, has a horizontal diameter of approximately 12 mm. The corneal ring is slightly foreshortened vertically. By reason of this smaller vertical radius, a steeper vertical meridian is induced, resulting in the physiologic, with-the-rule astigmatism (Plate 2-6, *B* and *C*).

Plate 2-6

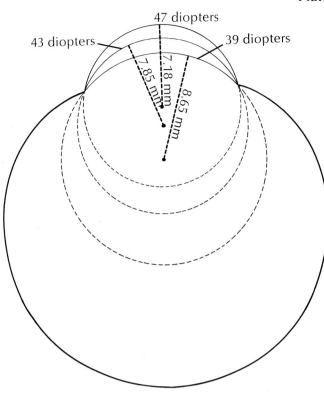

47 diopters

43 diopters

39 diopters

7.85 mm

7.18 mm

8.65 mm

A. Variation of corneal curvature expressed in radii and dioptric powers.

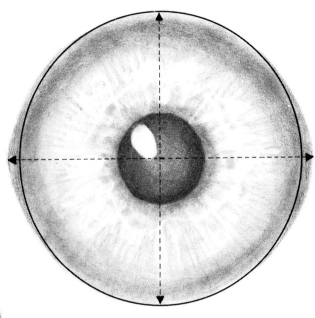

B. A corneal ring. A circle is drawn to illustrate better the vertical foreshortening of the cornea.

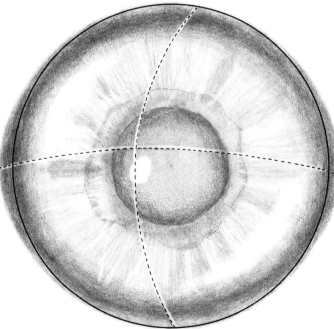

C. Steeper vertical meridian, resulting in physiologic with-the-rule astigmatism.

Peripherally, the cornea is slightly aplanatic, its curvature becoming increasingly flatter as the corneal ring is approached. Optically, it is the effective corneal radius (dioptric power), as measured at the optical center or visual axis of the cornea, that is important. In this optical zone, the normal cornea is approximately 0.5 mm thick. This thickness increases as the corneal ring is approached, stabilizing the critical central optical zone. For optical purposes, the cornea is homogeneous, and the miniscule differences in refraction of the five layers of the cornea and of the normal tear film are disregarded in any calculations. The power of the concave, internal surface of the cornea in contact with the aqueous is minimal and can be considered constant. An exception is an extreme internal distortion, such as is found in posterior keratoconus where the pathology creates a miniature concavo-convex lens, inducing greater myopia. In keratomileusis and keratophakia, which require very exact power calculations, this posterior curvature also is considered to be constant.

At the corneal ring, the softer, more flexible corneal tissue is overlapped by the leading edge of the tougher, more rigid scleral envelope, forming the scleral spur (Plate 2-7). Just distal to this junction, the radius of the posterior or scleral segment is significantly larger than that of the cornea. In explaining the mechanism and corrective manipulation of corneal optics, the sclera is considered only as a supporting structure as it contributes to the formation of the corneal ring. A very large variation in scleral radius is required to induce even a minimal alteration in corneal astigmatism. For example, extensive scleral buckling or scleral shortening procedures used in retinal detachment surgery rarely induce a change in corneal curvature. However, axial ametropia may be induced or compensated by scleral shortening operations at the equator or at the posterior pole. These procedures will not be considered in this volume.

OTHER OCULAR STRUCTURES OF SECONDARY OPTICAL IMPORTANCE

Other ocular structures that have secondary influence on the optical result of keratoplasty are the iris and the variation in size or in centration of the pupil in particular, as well as the lens and the vitreous (Plate 2-7, *B*). As will be seen, particular emphasis is placed on maintaining or reconstructing a stenopeic pupil centered at the optical axis of the grafted cornea. When possible, a traumatically disrupted or surgically iridectomized iris is repaired. An intact iris diaphragm and centered pupillary aperture reduce the glare and blur circles resulting from optical aberrations induced by the corneal graft-recipient scar.

Even minimal lens opacities, when coexisting with opacifying corneal pathology, reduce the vision more severely than anticipated from the clinical appearance of the individual pathologies. This is true also when an irregular or high astigmatism in the graft results from an otherwise successful keratoplasty. The surgeon may be tempted to remove the cataract

Plate 2-7

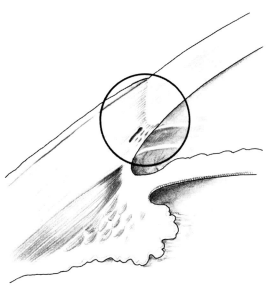

A. The circle indicates the anatomic position of the corneal ring. Cross section.

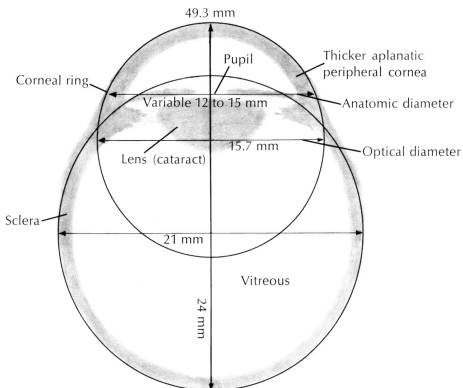

B. Relationship of the cornea to other ocular structures having secondary influence on the optical result of keratoplasty.

either simultaneously, in the first instance, or as a primary intervention, in the second. Often keratoplasty alone or, in the case of a high astigmatism, wedge resection or a contact lens will suffice to give the patient useful vision without having to remove the minimally cataractous lens.

Nevertheless, a cataractous lens that compromises significantly the vision must be removed. The patient is left then with an aphakic hyperopic defect, except in the rare instance of a highly myopic eye. In this case, the hyperopic aphakia can be compensated partially by deliberately inducing a steepening of the curvatures of the donor cornea. This is accomplished by using a graft larger in diameter than the recipient opening (see Plate 2-4, *B* and *C*). The residual hyperopic defect can be compensated by a spectacle lens, by a contact lens, or, in the older patient with no other significant anterior segment pathology, by an intraocular lens of appropriate power.

When an intraocular lens is placed during a combined keratoplasty and cataract extraction, it is difficult to predetermine exactly the required power of the intraocular lens. Though the lens power can be determined more accurately with an A-scan, the insertion of an intraocular lens at a second procedure (subsequent to a successful keratoplasty) is more likely to induce failure of the graft. In a combined procedure in the older patient, a 19.5-diopter, standard lens can be used. A preoperative A-scan or, at least, a B-scan ultrasound examination should be done. The lens power can then be adjusted, should the ultrasound indicate a significant posterior segment ametropia, as, for example, in a highly myopic eye. Also, when a graft larger than the recipient opening is used, the standard 19.5-diopter, intraocular lens will induce excessive residual myopia. To have better uncorrected distance acuity, the donor button should be the same size as or no more than 0.2 mm larger than the recipient opening. If a larger donor button is used, a weaker intraocular lens of approximately 16 diopters is indicated. Some residual myopia can be advantageous, particularly in the older patient, since it provides reading vision with no additional correction.

Vitreous opacities, which, if allowed to remain, would compromise the eventual vision result, are detected readily preoperatively by the use of B-scan ultrasound tomography. At surgery, obstructive opacities in the visual axis can be seen with the coaxial illumination of the microscope. In the aphakic eye, the optic nerve and macula are visualized easily through the recipient opening, with no need to use a contact fundus lens. Significant opacities are removed by using a vitreous sucking-cutting instrument (see Plate 10-7). In the phakic eye, the pars plana approach must be used to remove vitreous opacities.

In the rare case of a subluxated, tilted, or pathologically astigmatic lens, there is an induced astigmatic error only when the lens is on the visual axis. If this might compromise the result of keratoplasty, the offending lens must be removed either prior to or during the graft procedure.

Management of concomitant vision-obstructing iris, vitreous, or lens pathology is important to obtain the best final vision result. The potential effect of the pathology on the final optical result must be evaluated carefully and its correction included in the surgical plan.

EFFECT OF ANATOMIC AND OPTICAL DIAMETERS ON CORNEAL AMETROPIA

From the optical standpoint, the primary structure is the cornea, as limited by the corneal ring at the scleral spur. The anterior curvature of the standard cornea with a power of 43 diopters has a diameter of 15.7 mm (a radius of 7.85 mm) and a circumference of 49.3 mm. The optical diameter of the cornea must not be confused with its anatomic diameter measured at the corneal limbus. This limbal diameter can vary from 12 mm to 15 mm, averaging between 13.75 mm and 14.25 mm (Plate 2-7). Although the anatomic diameter of the cornea is not related directly to the dioptric power of the cornea, in general a larger cornea tends to be flatter, while the smaller cornea is steeper.

Physiologic, pathologic, or iatrogenic astigmatism is caused by the existing or induced distortion of the corneal ring and dome. The eventual surgical correction of the astigmatism is accomplished by altering the corneal curvatures and the shape of the delimiting corneal ring. The effect of a peripheral distorting force on a spherical surface is easily visualized (Plate 2-8).

An inflated balloon with a roughly spherical surface is compressed between the palms of the hands. Because of the constant air volume, the surface area remains constant. The previously spherical anterior surface is distorted meridionally as a result of compressing the diameter between the hands. This maneuver changes the surface curvatures but does not change the overall circumference. The meridian anterior to the hand-compressed surfaces of the balloon steepens, while the uncompressed meridian at right angles flattens as its diameter lengthens in proportion to the shortening of the compressed diameter. This demonstrates the effect of altering the shape of a corneal ring of fixed circumference on the curvatures of the corneal dome.

Plate 2-8

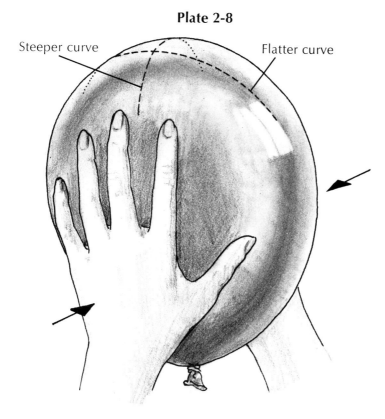

Steeper curve

Flatter curve

Demonstration of the effect of compression on the surface curvatures of a sphere of constant volume.

The surface area of the cornea also remains constant when an oval graft is placed in a round opening (see Plate 2-5). The corneal ring is induced into an oval shape to correspond to the shorter and the longer axes of the oval graft. The ring does not change in circumference, nor does the cornea change in area, just as the balloon does not change in these respects. As with the compressed balloon, steepening takes place in the meridian across the shorter diameter of the corneal ring.

A similar effect is obtained when a round graft is sutured to a recipient corneal margin from which a wedge-shaped quadrant of recipient corneal tissue was excised (Plate 2-9, A). This wedge resection of tissue induces two optical effects in the round donor button. One optical effect is that the radius is reduced in the wedged-out meridian. This meridian is steepened, while the meridian at right angles to it is correspondingly flattened (Plate 2-9, B and C). The second optical effect is that the total area of the surface of the cornea is reduced in amount by the area of the excised wedge. This flattens the entire cornea proportionately. The cornea becomes less powerful, causing spherical equivalent hyperopia (Plate 2-9, C). These optical effects are used to advantage in the Troutman wedge-resection procedure (see Chapter 11) to correct, postkeratoplasty, an excessive myopic astigmatic band in a clear graft. The combination of altering the shape of the corneal ring and the area of the corneal dome induces a combined astigmatic and axial correction. This technique may be used also at primary keratoplasty, when a preoperative astigmatic band can be approximately identified and quantified.

MEASUREMENT OF THE CORNEA—CLINICAL AND SURGICAL KERATOMETRY

In order to predict, to modify, and to assess postoperatively the optical result of penetrating keratoplasty, accurate consecutive corneal measurements must be made *before, during,* and *after* corneal surgery. Though it will not be possible always to measure the corneal curvatures accurately prior to surgery, the readings always should be attempted and at least a qualitative assessment made of the shape of the corneal ring. In the absence of accurate keratometric measurements, a qualitative distortion of the corneal ring, when detected prior to surgery, often can be corrected at least partially at surgery. A severe postoperative astigmatic band thus may be minimized or prevented.

Any clinical keratometer can be used to make quantitative measurements of the cornea. I use the Haag-Streit keratometer, which employs the Javal principle, and the Gambs keratometer, which incorporates two sets of targets, a Javal and a single and split-cross target. The latter instrument is

Plate 2-9

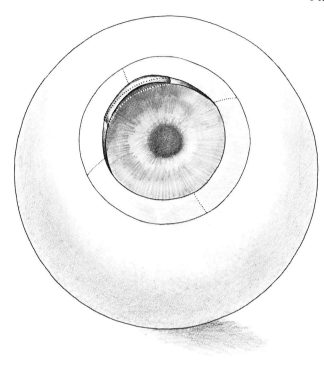

A. A wedge-resected recipient corneal margin (Troutman wedge-resection technique).

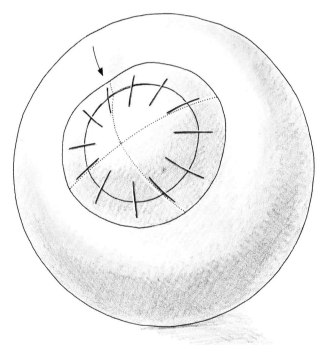

B. 8-mm circular button sewed in 8-mm wedge-resected recipient opening induces astigmatism and corneal hyperopia.

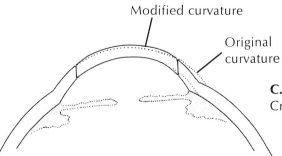

Modified curvature

Original curvature

C. Steepening in the wedge-resected meridian. Cross section.

useful, especially when an accurate measurement cannot be obtained easily using only the Javal mires. The crosses subtend a lesser angle to the corneal surface and, thus, may pick up more readily a readable central reflection.

I have used the Gambs instrument, as adapted by me and illustrated in Volume I, Plate 1-13, to measure curvatures from the vertical position .during surgery. However, the necessity of translating the keratometer to and from the operative field to take and then to correct for measurements proved to be too time-consuming. In addition, the surgeon was not able to monitor directly the effect of a surgical correction.

A similar adaptation of the Zeiss keratometer has been employed by J. I. Barraquer. His prototype instrument is illustrated in Volume 1, Plate 1-16. Though his instrument can be read directly through the microscope, it reads only a single meridian at a time, as does the adapted Gambs keratometer. The instrument head, the microscope, or both must be rotated for each meridian being read. In addition, zoom magnification is not available on the Barraquer surgical microscope, thus limiting significantly its surgical use. Reading the instrument is somewhat complex, since it requires monitoring on a specially adapted television unit operated by a technician.

Nevertheless, these two instruments demonstrate the feasibility of monitoring and modifying surgically induced corneal astigmatic bands not only during keratoplasty but also during other surgery on the cornea, such as cataract surgery.

My experiences have led me to develop a qualitative surgical keratometer, illustrated in prototype in Volume I, Plate 1-14. This prototype instrument has been modified to a production model, as illustrated here (Plate 2-10).

The individual incandescent light sources used in the original instrument proved not only to be insufficiently bright but also to vary individually in intensity and to blow out erratically, and they were difficult to replace. The six point-light sources of the original instrument were increased to 12. All 12 are now illuminated from a single light source projected into a master fiberoptic bundle. This bundle is split into 12 equal segments, which distribute the light to each of the 12 equidistant ports at the base of the circular keratometer housing. This provides not only the high intensity, cool light necessary for a continuous keratometer light ring projection on the cornea but also a shadow-free, ambient illumination of the surgical field, supplementing the illumination from the surgical microscope. In order to reduce the glare from multiple bright white light reflections and to differentiate between these and other reflections, a green filter is interposed in the fiberoptic system. A quantitative keratometer reticle is fitted to the eyepiece for the surgeon's nondominant eye. Its two concentric circles are used as a reference for the surgical keratometer projection, while its split cross hairs are used to space and to align sutures and to mark an astigmatic axis.

Plate 2-10

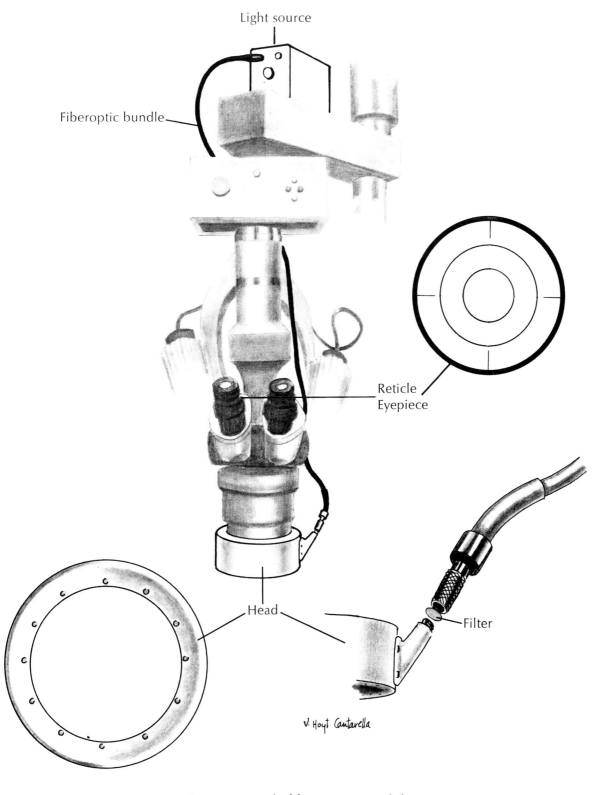

Light source

Fiberoptic bundle

Reticle
Eyepiece

Head

Filter

J. Hoyt Cantarella

**Troutman surgical keratometer as it is
attached to the Troutman surgical microscope**

The surgical keratometer is a qualitative measuring instrument with a function very different from that of a keratoscope, designed primarily to measure corneal topography. The surgical keratometer was designed specifically to aid the surgeon in the interpretation and correction of meridional corneal errors.

Quantitative measurement is possible with the use of a split-image prism device. The prism device splits, inverts, and superimposes the projected ring image. The eyepiece is rotated until the two half circles of dots match exactly, indicating the axis of the astigmatic band. The reticle images are then superimposed by adjusting the sutures to correct an indicated flatter or steeper band. In the prototype, when the splitting prism is in place in its ocular, the microscope can be used only monocularly. This limits the usefulness of this method of quantitative measurement.

Also, an electronically magnified surgical keratometer projection can be transmitted through the microscope beam splitter to a television screen on which a comparative projection is generated simultaneously. Differences between the projected images can be interpreted visually or by computer.

The interpretation of the surgical keratometer projection during the surgical procedure is discussed and illustrated in this and later chapters. However, a few words concerning the interpretation of the projection are in order here. A spherical cornea of approximately 43 diopters projects a corneal ring, at $20\times$ magnification, in an intermediate position between the two reticle circles (Plate 2-11, A). If the cornea is steeper than 43 diopters, the diameter and circumference of the projection decrease, displacing the light circle closer to or within the inner concentric ring (Plate 2-11, B). If the cornea is flatter than 43 diopters, the diameter and circumference of the ring increase, displacing the light circle toward or outside the outer concentric ring of the reticle (Plate 2-11, C). If the cornea is astigmatic, the circle of lights projected on the cornea assumes an oval shape (Plate 2-11, D). The flatter corneal meridian corresponds to the longer axis of the oval projection, and the steeper corneal meridian to the shorter axis. The approximate powers of the meridians of the astigmatic band can be interpreted by comparing the reticle circles to the oval reflection of the light ring. At $20\times$ magnification, the space between the two rings represents approximately 10 diopters.

Plate 2-11

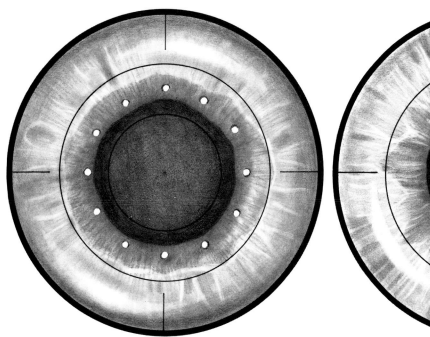

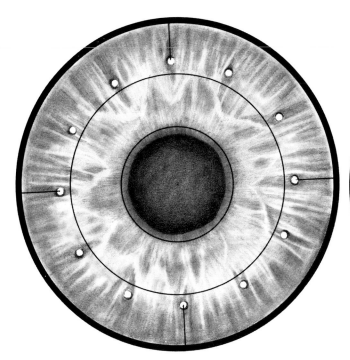

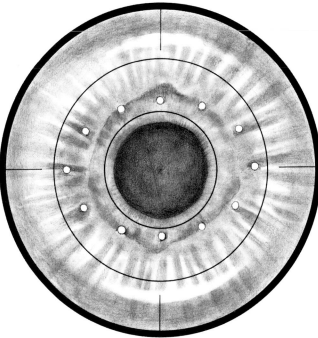

A. Projection of the Troutman surgical keratometer on a 43-diopter cornea. (20 X magnification.)

B. Projection of the Troutman surgical keratometer on reduced corneal diameter indicates steeper corneal curvatures. (20 X magnification.)

C. Projection of the Troutman surgical keratometer on increased corneal diameter indicates flatter corneal curvatures. (20 X magnification.)

D. Oval-shaped projection of the Troutman surgical keratometer indicates astigmatic cornea. Flatter meridian corresponds to the longer (horizontal) axis of the light ring. (20 X magnification.)

It is emphasized again, however, that the Troutman surgical keratometer is primarily a qualitative instrument. Interpretation of the projection depends on the experience of the surgeon, as well as on variations in technique, in the host or donor tissue, or in both. Only repeated and comparative measurements, in the context of the total procedure, will give an accurate referenced result for each case.

To determine the effect of intraoperative manipulation on preoperative measurements and to quantitate the final interpretation of the surgical keratometer, quantitative measurements must be taken postoperatively. Often, early in the postoperative course following keratoplasty—in penetrating keratoplasty in particular—regular mires cannot be observed or that portion of the corneal surface not distorted may be so small as to reflect only one mire. Though it is possible to obtain readings with the Troutman surgical keratometer during the early postoperative period, the information obtained has limited use for refraction. It is sufficient usually to wait until a more regular projection of the quantitative keratometer mire patterns is observed, so that accurate refractive measurements can be made. Interpretation of corneal curvatures can be obtained only by taking accurate preoperative, intraoperative, and postoperative measurements. It is the interpretation of the total data obtained, rather than any individual measurement, that enables the surgeon to use the surgical keratometer to its greatest advantage in the correction of meridional ametropia.

An immediate goal of corneal surgery, aside from obtaining a clear functional graft, should be to minimize suture-induced astigmatic aberrations. If reliable preoperative keratometric measurements are recorded and, if necessary, corrective tissue excision carefully performed, then with precise suturing under surgical keratometer control, the postoperative keratometry findings with the sutures in place should approach sphericity. Any deviation from this minimal "suture-in-place" postoperative astigmatism should be negligible when sutures are removed. The state of the art, however, is such that this usually is not the case. In spite of every precaution, sometimes distressingly large astigmatic errors occur. The Troutman wedge-resection procedure (see Chapter 11) was developed to correct these randomly occurring, excessive postoperative astigmatic errors. Here, too, preoperative measurement of the excessive astigmatic band, careful monitoring with the surgical keratometer during correction by wedge resection, and postoperative follow-up with periodic keratometric measurements are essential to a satisfactory anastigmatic final result.

SUMMARY

Success in keratoplasty is not just a clear graft. Success involves also the detection, interpretation, and surgical correction of optical aberrations that may precede or result from surgery for opacifying corneal pathology. This chapter has identified the causes of surgical ametropia and has indicated, briefly, some of the means for their correction. The succeeding chapters amplify these principles and apply them practically to individual operative situations.

CHAPTER 3

CORNEAL SURGERY– INDICATIONS AND OPERATIVE PLAN

General considerations
    Loss of clarity or optical irregularities
    Loss of continuity
    Active infection or inflammation
    Vision and condition of the fellow eye
    Keratometry and refraction
    Contact lenses
Chelation of corneal calcium deposits
Lamellar or penetrating graft
   Lamellar graft
   Combined penetrating and lamellar graft
    Suturing the lamellar graft

Penetrating graft
   Peripheral corneal defects
   Leukoma and staphyloma
   B-scan tomography
   Total corneal opacity
   Suturing the penetrating graft
    Simple penetrating keratoplasty
    Keratoconus
    Vascularized recipient cornea
Summary

GENERAL CONSIDERATIONS

From the operative standpoint, the indications for corneal surgery are relatively few. Since this textbook is limited to microsurgery of the cornea, this chapter classifies and describes the various corneal pathologies only insofar as each may dictate the operative plan or a portion thereof. It can be stated categorically, therefore, that *corneal surgery is indicated when the clarity or the regularity of the cornea is compromised to an extent such that vision is reduced below useful or acceptable levels. Corneal surgery is indicated also when the continuity of the cornea is threatened, so that irreparable damage or loss of an eye may result if its immediate repair is not effected.*

Loss of clarity or optical irregularities. When loss of clarity or an optical irregularity compromises vision, the surgeon must assess carefully to what extent concomitant physiologic or pathologic alterations affect the vision of the involved eye. It must be determined whether correction of a concomitant defect is indicated, either simultaneously or separately, or, indeed, whether correction of this defect might obviate the necessity for corneal surgery.

Loss of continuity. In the case of loss of continuity of the cornea by pathologic perforation or traumatic penetration, damage to ocular structures other than the cornea must be assessed and repair undertaken.

Active infection or inflammation. An active infection, present or suspected, an active, severe inflammatory process, or both must be controlled medically, insofar as possible, prior to any surgical intervention. The appropriate medical therapy alone or in conjunction with indicated surgical therapy should be instituted.

Vision and condition of the fellow eye. The vision and condition of the fellow eye must be assessed carefully. When the operable corneal pathology is bilateral, the first surgical intervention should be done on the eye for which the vision is compromised to the greater degree. This is done even in the presence of suspected functional amblyopia. Not uncommonly, useful vision results, and the patient more readily accepts surgery on the dominant eye. If the fellow eye has a normal cornea but is nonfunctional, an autograft may be considered should a homograft fail.

All clinical means of optical correction must be attempted before surgery is considered. A careful bilateral refraction is done on every case.

Keratometry and refraction. Keratometry is invaluable in identifying a corneal astigmatic band that cannot be detected by retinoscopic examination or that is difficult or impossible to elicit with subjective refraction. In some cases, it may be possible only to approximate the axis and power. If one keeps in mind a few simple principles, an accurate subjective refraction can be performed easily. In keratoconus, for example, invariably the cylinder is minus and greater than 5 diopters. In addition, the eye often has a moderate to high axial myopia. Placing a −6 cylinder with its axis corresponding to the flatter meridian and adding minus spheres can dramatically improve the patient's spectacle correction. Conversely, in a familial dystrophy, the cornea often is flatter than the physiologic mean and induces a moderate hyperopic astigmatism. If a +3 cylinder is placed with its axis corresponding to the steeper meridian and plus spheres are added, maximum acuity is obtained. The amount of the cylinder is smaller in familial dystrophy than in keratoconus and is measured accurately by the clinical keratometer.

Contact lenses. If a high or irregular corneal astigmatism cannot be neutralized with spectacle lenses, a hard or flexible contact lens is fitted and the vision reassessed. If a methylmethacrylate lens is not tolerated by the patient, an oxygen-permeable lens, such as one made from cyanoacrylate-butyrate or silicone, may be worn comfortably. The clear cornea, which does not tolerate well the hard or flexible contact lens and which is only minimally astigmatic, sometimes can be fitted successfully with a high-water-content, polymer lens. If the astigmatism is significant and not fully corrected by the soft contact lens, overrefraction may still give comfortable vision. The successful fit and comfortable wearing of a contact lens can obviate or significantly delay surgical intervention. When one eye requires surgery, contact lens correction of the *nonoperated* eye can give the patient more comfortable vision during the postoperative course.

CHELATION OF CORNEAL CALCIUM DEPOSITS

On occasion, opacifying corneal pathology can be removed by nonsurgical means and good to excellent vision restored. In band keratopathy and other corneal degenerations and irregularities, confluent deposits of calcium can obstruct the vision. These deposits usually lie beneath epithelium and extend no more deeply than superficial stroma. To remove them, the cornea over the affected area is denuded of its epithelium. The larger, discrete calcium plaques are then removed mechanically, using the edge of a razor knife, held at an angle to the corneal surface, or a curette. Residual calcium flecks are removed by using a solution of EDTA (disodium ethylenediaminetetraacetate dihydrate, 0.05 M). The EDTA combines with the calcium to soften and dissolve the calcium, facilitating its removal by debridement or subsequent irrigation.

This chelating solution is applied by means of a tube open at both ends and approximately the diameter of the corneal limbus. The application tube is easily made by cutting off about 1 inch from the top of a laboratory test tube and flaming the cut end. The finished, lipped top of the tube is placed on the globe to encompass the cornea. Sufficient pressure is applied to prevent escape of the EDTA solution introduced through the cut and flamed end (Plate 3-1). The solution in the tube is maintained in contact with the denuded cornea for a prolonged period, 8 to 10 minutes. Larger plaques of calcium are not dissolved readily by EDTA. Their attachment to the cornea, however, is loosened by the EDTA solution, and they are then easier to dislodge by debridement.

Though severely vision-obstructing opacities may be removed and apparent optical clarity restored, keratometry readings following chelation may demonstrate irregularities of the corneal surface. The optically clear but irregularly surfaced cornea often may be fitted advantageously with a hard or soft contact lens. Some of my patients have been improved from less than 20/200 vision to 20/40 or better, even to 20/20, as a result of simple debridement and chelation, though a spectacle or contact lens correction may be necessary for maximum acuity. When feasible, this technique avoids keratoplasty and can restore useful vision to the one-eyed patient or the patient who is a poor surgical risk.

Plate 3-1

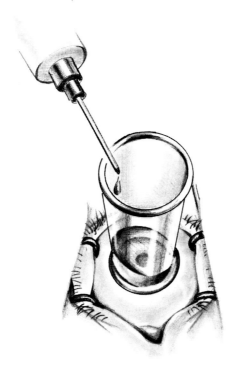

Application tube in place, maintaining chelating
solution in contact with cornea.

LAMELLAR OR PENETRATING GRAFT

When it is established that the vision-compromising corneal defect cannot be remedied by refractive or other nonsurgical means, the surgeon decides the type of keratoplasty—lamellar, penetrating, or a combination thereof—to be used and the size and shape of the graft.

Lamellar graft

When a lamellar graft is decided on for reconstructive or tectonic purposes, the donor button should be not only large enough but also of a shape to match the shape of the pathologic corneal tissue to be excised. While the shape of the graft should encompass the pathology, the resection should include the least amount of relatively normal cornea (Plate 3-2). Frequently, when a lamellar graft is required, the vision result is secondary to the reconstructive purpose of the graft.

One shape that can be used to repair a superficial pathology is a semicircular lamellar peripheral corneal ring (Plate 3-2, A) such as is used, for example, in the repair of an inferior peripheral corneal thinning.

Rather than the more commonly used circular, total corneal lamellar graft, a square lamellar graft may be used to repair a total anterior corneal opacification (Plate 3-2, B). The square shape provides a longer perimeter, hence a stronger peripheral scar, for the tectonic purpose of the graft. Also, the four peripheral sectors of recipient cornea along the four graft borders in the nonoptical peripheral zone minimize the possibility of peripheral vascular invasion.

In the case of a clear central cornea with severe circumferential peripheral pathology, such as in a marginal dystrophy, that threatens the continuity of the peripheral cornea or the regularity of the central cornea, a doughnut-shaped lamellar graft can be used (Plate 3-2, C).

To rectify the corneal lamellar defect, caused by resection of a pterygium or a symblepharon, in the corneal periphery, a segment of a circular graft may be used (Plate 3-2, D).

In less extensive pathology, a triangular graft can be used (Plate 3-2, E) for similar tectonic reasons that the large square-shaped graft is employed. This shape can effect repair of a central pathologic zone. It avoids the unnecessary excision of clear peripheral cornea and tends to prevent vascular invasion of the graft. A small, triangular lamellar graft may be used peripherally, rather than a segment of a lamellar circular button, to cover a peripheral corneal defect (Plate 3-2, F).

Combined penetrating and lamellar graft

A lamellar graft can be used also as a segment of a penetrating graft. This technique is used to repair circumferential or sector superficial periph-

Plate 3-2

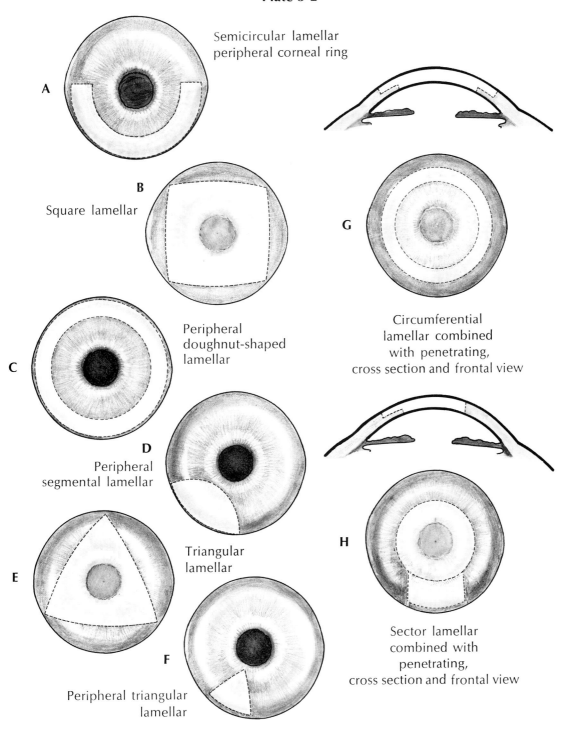

A Semicircular lamellar peripheral corneal ring

B Square lamellar

C Peripheral doughnut-shaped lamellar

D Peripheral segmental lamellar

E

F Peripheral triangular lamellar

Triangular lamellar

G Circumferential lamellar combined with penetrating, cross section and frontal view

H Sector lamellar combined with penetrating, cross section and frontal view

Various shapes of lamellar or combined lamellar and penetrating grafts that can be used to repair partial or full-thickness corneal pathology.

eral pathology and concomitant full-thickness central pathology (Plate 3-2, *G* and *H*). The combination of a penetrating and a circumferential lamellar graft is called a mushroom graft and is described in Chapter 7. If the superficial pathology involves only a sector of the periphery, a sector lamellar graft is used in combination with the central penetrating graft.

Suturing the lamellar graft. Various techniques are used to suture the different shapes of lamellar grafts described. In the case of a peripheral, doughnut-shaped graft, two continuous sutures are used (Plate 3-3, *A*).

In a semicircular lamellar graft, the squared-off ends must be fixed with interrupted or mattress sutures. A continuous suture is used to fix the remainder of the graft (Plate 3-3, *B*).

In a circular lamellar graft, a radially placed continuous suture causes torquing or an in-plane shifting effect, resulting in rotation and distortion of the lamellar graft in relation to its bed. Suture bites are placed diagonally to form a series of equal isosceles triangles. The suture thread is passed alternately through and then across the corneal incision in succeeding diagonal bites of equal length (Plate 3-3, *C*). The resulting pattern equalizes the individual loop tension and prevents the torquing that would result if the deep loops of the continuous suture were placed radially.

The torquing effect can be eliminated also by using interrupted sutures. However, interrupted sutures are more time-consuming to place, require a greater number of bites, and are more irritating to the tissue. Also, they do not lend themselves easily to adjustment to equalize suture-loop tension, especially when using the surgical keratometer.

Plate 3-3

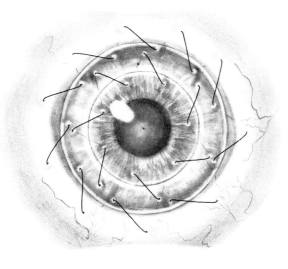

A. Two continuous sutures are used to fix a doughnut-shaped lamellar graft.

B. Suture pattern used for semicircular lamellar graft.

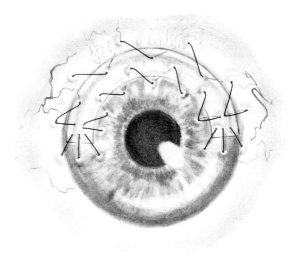

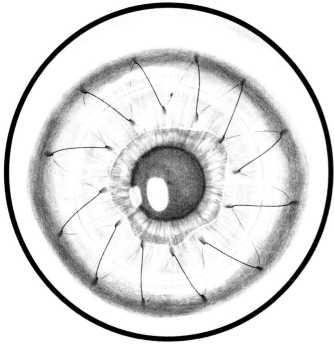

C. Antitorque continuous suture used for a circular lamellar graft.

A disadvantage of the square, the triangular, or the segmental graft is that the angular corners are difficult to suture accurately edge to edge. An overlying suture, a mattress suture, or an intracorneal suture bite can be used to draw or to compress a corner of the graft into the corresponding angle of the recipient cornea (Plate 3-4). Postoperatively, closure of a graft with angled corners is not as secure as is that of the curved edge graft.

Penetrating graft

Today the circular penetrating corneal graft is, by far, the most commonly performed keratoplasty procedure. Replacement of the full thickness of the cornea is usually selected, as it not only eliminates the primary corneal pathology but also offers the best opportunity for a good vision result. The type of pathology and the extent of the corneal opacification determine the size of the graft to be used, as well as the suture material and the suture pattern.

Closure of a corneal incision with other than elastic monofilament suture material will not be discussed. The choice of elastic monofilament material is now greater, since, in addition to monofilament nylon, a new suture material, polypropylene, is available. While polypropylene has the physical characteristics of nylon, its chemical composition renders it nonwettable and, therefore, unlike nylon thread, nonabsorbable over the long term. This property makes it more suitable for the management of certain corneal pathologies, especially in optical surgery requiring essentially permanent suture-loop tension.

No matter what the pathologic cause of the corneal opacity or optical defect, it is the location, the shape, and the degree of vascularization of the affected area that dictate the size of the penetrating graft and the closing suture pattern. For the purposes of this discussion, it is assumed that any opacity involves either the full thickness of the cornea or its posterior layers to a sufficient extent to require penetrating keratoplasty.

Plate 3-4

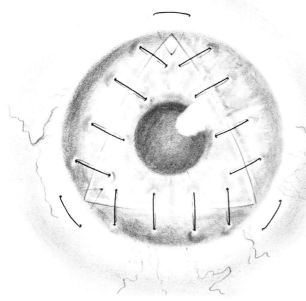

A. Mattress suture used to close corners of a triangular lamellar graft.

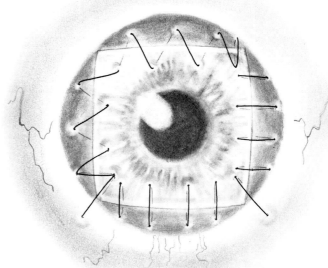

B. Alternate suture configurations to fix a square lamellar graft. Overlying interrupted sutures may be used to close angular corners.

C. Interrupted and continuous sutures used to close a semicircular lamellar graft.

Central, discrete opacities most commonly result from trauma, ulceration, or keratoconus. Sometimes the opacity may be more diffuse, approaching the corneal periphery, as in a familial dystrophy. Also, the opacity may originate in the endothelium, involving the posterior layers of the cornea, and result, eventually, in central corneal edema with the formation of corneal bullae. Such opacifications are predominantly avascular and usually do not involve other anterior segment structures. The exceptions include traumatic or iatrogenic corneal edema and bullous keratopathy, caused by endothelial damage at time of injury or cataract surgery. The more central, localized, and discrete the opacity, the more favorable is the cornea for penetrating keratoplasty. In most instances, the graft can be large enough to eliminate the pathology and, at the same time, to restore an optically clear and regular central area of cornea for a good vision result.

The graft is always centered in the optical zone of the cornea. In a cornea with curvatures within the normal range, that is, between 41 and 45 diopters, as measured preoperatively, the recipient opening should be 7 mm to 8.5 mm in diameter (Plate 3-5, A). To use a graft smaller than 7 mm may compromise the optical result, while a graft larger than 8.5 mm is more prone to graft reaction.

If the pathology is discrete, the trephine used should encompass the pathology and should be centered on the optical axis (Plate 3-5, B). If the pathology is more diffuse, such as in a corneal dystrophy or burn, and cannot be encompassed by an 8.5-mm diameter trephine, a smaller, 7-mm diameter, trephine is used, centered on the optical axis (Plate 3-5, C). Thus the periphery of the graft is farther from the vascular limbal zone.

When the donor button is cut from the endothelial surface of the cornea, the trephine blade used is 0.2 mm or 0.5 mm larger in diameter than that used for the recipient opening. As in lamellar keratoplasty, where a larger donor button is cut in order to reach the periphery of the lamellar excision, in penetrating keratoplasty, a larger donor button is used to provide a better fit of the donor button to the recipient cornea.

As will be explained further in Chapter 4 on the donor eye, when a corneal donor button is cut from the endothelial surface with the same diameter trephine used for cutting the recipient opening, a donor button 0.2 mm smaller in diameter than the recipient opening results. Thus, as it heals, the donor cornea flattens within the recipient ring and may induce hyperopia and, occasionally, a high astigmatic band.

Plate 3-5

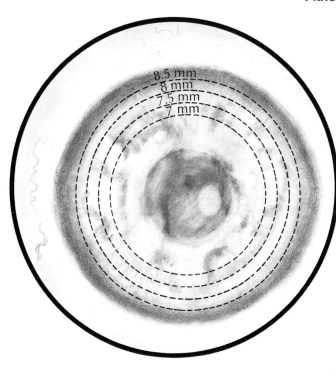

A. A comparison of commonly used trephine diameters.

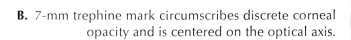

B. 7-mm trephine mark circumscribes discrete corneal opacity and is centered on the optical axis.

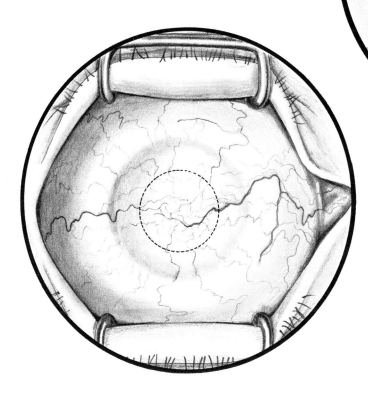

C. 7-mm trephine mark in a cornea with diffuse involvement.

In aphakic keratoplasty, as described in Chapter 2, the hyperopia of the postoperative aphakic eye can be reduced by deliberately using a corneal button 0.5 mm, or even 1 mm, larger in diameter, for example, an 8-mm donor button in a 7.5-mm recipient opening. This combination reduces, by as much as 5 diopters, the hyperopia that would result if the same trephine diameter were used for both the graft and the recipient.

An exception is in keratoconus or a myopic eye where a flatter than average postoperative corneal K may be desirable to compensate postoperative myopia. In keratoconus, in particular, the thinner peripheral cornea is somewhat more elastic than is the normal cornea. With a graft smaller than 8 mm, the button tends to protrude, inducing axial myopia that can be compensated by a flatter corneal curvature. I use the same trephine diameter (8 mm) to cut the donor button and the recipient opening in keratoconus. When keratoplasty is performed on the fellow eye, the donor-button size and the technique should be the same as were used for the first eye; otherwise a severe anisometropia may result.

Peripheral corneal defects. Occasionally, a peripheral corneal defect, such as a descemetocele or peripheral corneal perforation secondary to ulceration, may require penetrating keratoplasty. This type of defect is repaired by a circular penetrating graft of a diameter large enough to encompass the margins of the ulcerated area (Plate 3-6, A). If the cornea is perforated before surgery and the eye is soft, only an outline is made with the trephine and the excision is completed with scissors. The lower blade of the scissors is inserted through the perforation. A curvilinear cut is made radially, toward the trephine outline. The incision is extended along the marked circumference outline to complete the excision.

If the descemetocele is not perforated preoperatively, a lamellar dissection of the recipient is performed using the Troutman No. 1 corneal splitter (Plate 3-6, B). A thick lamellar graft is prepared and is used as a tamponade to cover the defect.

When the type of donor button to be used, lamellar or full-thickness, is in doubt, the recipient eye is dissected prior to preparing the donor button. Usually, in penetrating keratoplasty, the donor button is prepared prior to excising the recipient area. If an error is made in cutting the donor material, the surgeon is not faced with an open globe that must be closed with the only tissue usually at hand, the pathologic corneal button. In the case of a small peripheral perforation, however, the donor tissue available is usually sufficient to prepare a second, or even a third, button should the first one prepared not be suitable.

Plate 3-6

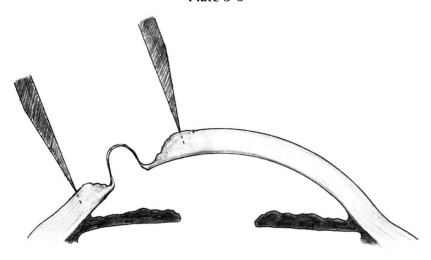

A. 4-mm trephine outlines peripheral corneal
defect. Cross section.

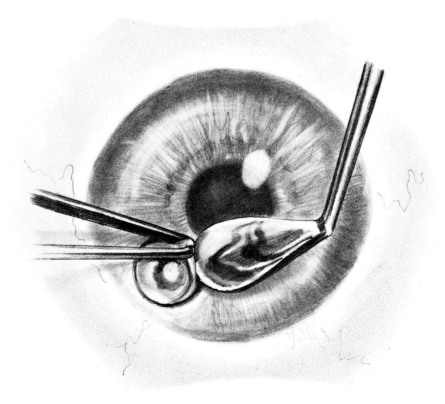

B. Dissection of outlined area using the Troutman
No. 1 corneal splitter in preparation for
thick lamellar graft.

Leukoma and staphyloma. Leukoma is a more extensive, often vascularized, corneal opacity, involving only the cornea. If the opacity involves internal ocular structures such as the iris, the lens, or both, it is a staphyloma. Each requires a somewhat different surgical plan.

In the event of a densely vascularized, central staphyloma or leukoma, the graft size often can be planned to encompass the pathology (Plate 3-7, *A* and *B*). Invariably, the invading vessels are a response to the pathologic tissue. When the pathologic tissue is removed, the blood vessel trunks atrophy and recede from the cornea; they recanalize only in the presence of a new irritant, such as uncovered suture material or knots. For this reason, 16-micron nylon or polypropylene suture material should be used in these cases. The knot is always buried and, when possible, in the donor button, not in the recipient cornea. Care is taken not to pass a suture needle into the recipient stroma in proximity to the cut end of a blood vessel.

Should the vascularized area extend to the periphery, it is not possible for the graft to encompass the pathology. In this instance, a flanged, composite graft, illustrated earlier in this chapter (Plate 3-2, *H*) and described in Chapter 7, can be used to advantage, especially if the peripheral corneal tissue is thin or soft. If the vascularization is superficial, as in herpetic keratitis, and the peripheral cornea is of normal thickness, a smaller, 7-mm or 7.5-mm, graft is placed centrally (Plate 3-7, *C*).

B-scan tomography. If the opacification in the staphylomatous cornea is partial, with some clear cornea peripherally, the extent of the involvement of the corneal scar to anterior segment structures often can be determined preoperatively. When corneal opacification is complete (Plate 3-5, *C*), a waterbath B-scan is necessary to determine the extent of lens and iris involvement.

I routinely use the Bronson B-scan tomograph (see Plates 10-1 and 10-2) without waterbath in the preoperative diagnosis and in the postoperative management of keratoplasty cases where posterior segment structures cannot be visualized directly. When the waterbath technique is not used, the information gleaned pertains only to the condition of the eye posterior to the iris-lens diaphragm. Prior to B-scan tomography, posterior segment pathologic conditions, such as vitreous opacification, retinal detachment, severe optic nerve cupping, and elongated myopic posterior segment, were all but impossible to detect in an eye with obstructive corneal opacities. Since the pathology can now be identified more readily, the surgical plan can be more effective not only in its execution but also in its eventual result. In the case

48

Plate 3-7

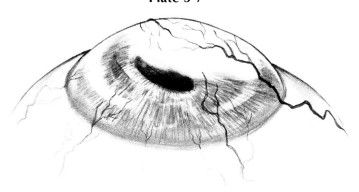

A. A dense, vascularized, central staphyloma
involving the iris.

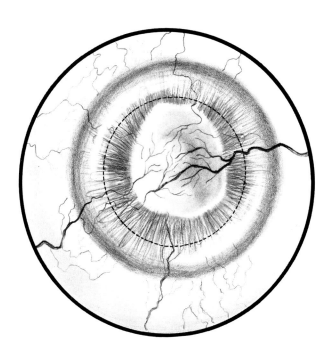

B. Trephined outline encompasses
the staphyloma.

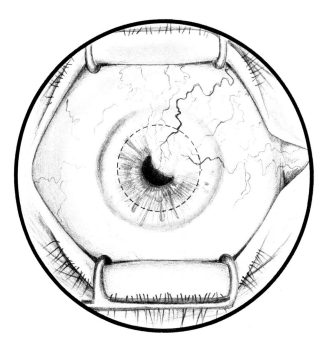

C. 7.5-mm trephined outline in a case of superficial
peripheral sector vascularization.

of extensive and irreparable posterior segment pathology, an unnecessary or futile surgical procedure can be avoided. On the other hand, should a retinal detachment or increasing vitreous pathology develop in a pathologic eye during preoperative observation, keratoplasty can be done immediately to allow simultaneous or subsequent repair of the posterior segment pathology under direct visualization. The B-scan provides more information in advance of the operation, and thus enables the surgeon to give the patient a more realistic diagnosis and prognosis.

Total corneal opacity. When a cornea is totally opaque and vascularized but B-scan tomography indicates that the posterior structures are relatively normal, it is better usually to use a smaller, 7-mm, penetrating graft (see Plate 3-5, *C*). For closure, 16-micron suture should be used. The smaller graft remains clear for a longer period of time than the larger graft. It permits direct observation of the anterior and posterior segment structures. Also, if the graft becomes opaque, the prognosis for a repeat homograft, for an autograft, or, as a last resort, for a keratoprosthesis can be better determined. In my experience, keratoprosthesis is indicated only in severe chemical burns where repeated homografts have failed; for even though a few spectacular results are obtained, few eyes survive functionally for more than 1 to 2 years postoperatively.

Suturing the penetrating graft

Simple penetrating keratoplasty. In keratoplasty for other types of pathology besides keratoconus, a single continuous, running, elastic monofilament suture is used for closure. Customarily, I use 20 to 22 equally spaced, through-and-through bites with a 22-micron suture (Plate 3-8, *A*). In the vascular cornea and in repeat operations, 16-micron suture may be used when the corneal diameter is small or when the graft margin approaches the vascular corneal periphery. The 16-micron suture, approximately one-fourth the cross-sectional area of the 22-micron suture, is more elastic. The suture bites must be spaced more closely; 28 to 30 equally spaced, through-and-through suture bites are needed to effect good closure (Plate 3-8, *B*). With 16-micron suture, secondary interrupted sutures are required more frequently to control temporary leaking just after suture placement. Because of its smaller diameter, the knot is less bulky. Not only is it easily buried, but also it tends to induce less tissue reaction than does the suture material of larger diameter, thus inhibiting the development of peripheral vascular invasion.

Keratoconus. In the case of keratoconus, a double continuous suture is used (Plate 3-8, *C*). This opposing continuous, radially placed pattern of closure provides firm, nontorquing apposition of the donor button and the peripheral keratoconic cornea. Twelve to 14 equally spaced, through-and-through suture bites are used in each opposing continuous suture.

Plate 3-8

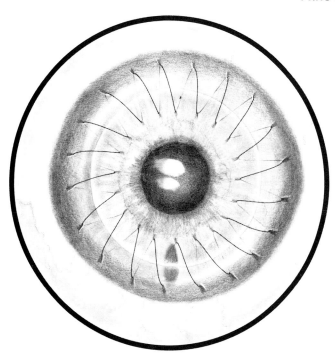

A. 22-micron single continuous suture.

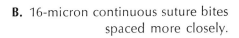

B. 16-micron continuous suture bites spaced more closely.

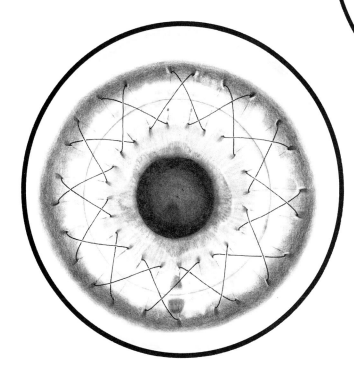

C. Double continuous suture pattern used primarily for keratoconus.

51

In a controlled study, I showed that the use of the double continuous suture, in combination with an 8-mm donor button cut from the anterior surface of an intact donor globe and an 8-mm recipient opening, resulted in a minimal (less than 0.5 diopter) spherical equivalent myopia. It was determined also that neither the type of suture closure nor the size of the graft significantly affected the amount of astigmatism postoperatively.

This important finding has made it necessary to seek other means of reducing or eliminating astigmatism from the graft. This is being accomplished at the primary procedure by deliberately varying the shape of the graft. The Troutman corneal wedge resection is used postkeratoplasty to correct a stabilized postoperative astigmatic defect.

Vascularized recipient cornea. Special care must be taken when suturing a graft to a vascularized recipient sector, since the donor button heals more rapidly to the vascularized tissue than to the clear peripheral cornea. This is one of the few instances where multiple interrupted sutures or a combination of interrupted sutures and a continuous suture may be preferred to a single or double continuous suture (Plate 3-9, *A*). The interrupted suture bites must be longer so that the thread crosses the vascular, usually somewhat softer, sector to reach the scleral spur. Suture bites of the usual length tend to loosen and to cut out of the softer vascular tissue soon after the operation, resulting in wound dehiscence or slippage. Postoperatively, it is often possible to remove interrupted sutures from the vascularized sector 2 to 3 months earlier than from the clear cornea. One should be very cautious about removing interrupted sutures from the clear cornea in less than 6 months, since healing is less rapid and late wound dehiscence more likely to occur than in the vascularized sector.

When a combination of continuous and interrupted sutures is used, the continuous thread should be 16 microns in size (Plate 3-9, *B*). After the 22-micron interrupted sutures have been placed radially, a 16-micron thread is placed with deep, diagonal, rather than radial, bites, so as not to torque the graft in its bed. When this combination is used, the interrupted sutures can be removed in the vascular sector first and later in the clear sector, about 2 months and 3 months postoperatively, respectively. The continuous suture is left in place for 6 months or longer, until circumferential healing is ensured.

Plate 3-9

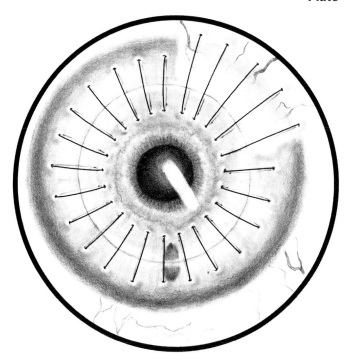

A. Use of multiple interrupted sutures. Note longer suture bites in vascularized sector.

B. Use of combination of 16-micron antitorque continuous suture and 22-micron interrupted sutures.

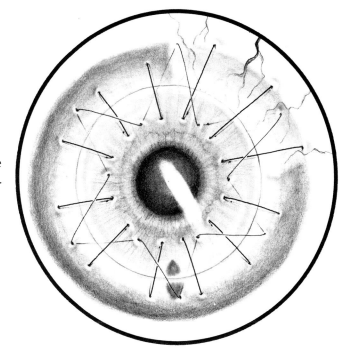

SUMMARY

The indications for corneal surgery have been outlined on the basis of the pathologically induced optical and topographic defects rather than on the basis of the specific pathology involved. The plan for operative intervention also is based on these criteria. Though it is recognized that the specific pathology involved may influence the prognosis of the graft, it does not follow that the surgical plan need be altered because of a different pathology.

In the case of lamellar keratoplasty, grafts of various shapes can be used to repair a defect without having to replace relatively normal tissue. Often the immediate objective is not the optical result, the purpose of lamellar keratoplasty being primarily tectonic or reconstructive.

On the other hand, in the penetrating graft, where the primary objective is optical, it may be necessary to sacrifice some normal corneal tissue in order to center optically the donor button. A circular, full-thickness donor button can be cut to match precisely the recipient opening. Accurate suturing and regular healing combine to give a more predictable optical result.

In penetrating keratoplasty, it is important always to excise as much as possible of the pathologic corneal tissue without approaching the corneal ring too closely. Trephining the recipient cornea should be central so that the apical portion of the centrally cut donor button is on the visual axis.

It is equally important to fixate the corneal button of selected size and shape to the recipient area in a fashion such that complete and adequate healing takes place without stimulating vascularization. Elastic monofilament suture material, either nylon or polypropylene, is best suited to this end. The fine, 22-micron or 16-micron, size is used according to the specific indications. The thread with the smaller diameter requires a greater number of suture bites for adequate closure. However, the reduced suture bulk lessens the potential for irritation and vascularization. Various continuous and interrupted suture patterns have been described. In general, the continuous suture pattern is preferred but may be reinforced or substituted by radial interrupted sutures when specific topographic or vascular situations obtain.

No operative plan is immutable, and conditions encountered at surgery determine the operative procedure to be performed.

CHAPTER 4

THE DONOR EYE

Eye-banking

Eye-bank operation

Enucleating the donor eye

Selection and preparation of the donor eye

    Slit-lamp examination and specular
      microscopy

    Preparation of the donor eye

Preparation of the corneoscleral segment

Cutting the donor button from the anterior
   surface

Cutting the donor button from the
   posterior surface

Selecting the size of the donor button

Summary

This chapter, in parts, may seem elementary to the ophthalmologist. However, it can be of value to eye-bank or technical personnel who work directly with or in an institution associated with ophthalmologists. In their early training, residents are asked also to assume eye-bank responsibilities. They, too, may find useful information on how to obtain, screen, and prepare the donor eye for keratoplasty. Therefore, some sections are written deliberately at a level more elementary than the rest of this volume.

EYE-BANKING

Ophthalmic surgeons, whether they do many, a few, or even no keratoplasties, should be familiar with the function of the source of supply of corneal donor material, the eye bank. I have had the good fortune, during most of my career in opthalmology, to be closely associated with The Eye Bank for Sight Restoration, Incorporated, in New York City. This organization, the first major eye bank in the United States, was conceived by Dr. R. Townley Paton and was incorporated as a nonprofit institution in February 1945. It was organized to supply ophthalmic surgeons with donor eye tissue for keratoplasty without cost to their patients. During 1976, the Eye Bank processed 2400 eyes, more than half of which were used for corneal transplantation procedures.

Over the years, individual ophthalmologists and lay organizations have started similar efforts in other localities. Most eye banks now in operation are members of a national organization, The Eye Bank Association of America. The national headquarters distributes organizational and operational literature, coordinates legislative efforts, and sponsors sectional and annual meetings of the membership. At these conferences, advances in eye-banking procedures and in medical and surgical management of corneal disease are discussed. Increased availability of donor tissue and improved techniques of preservation have led to an increasing number of ophthalmic surgeons performing keratoplasty successfully throughout the United States and Canada.

Dr. John Harry King, Jr., another pioneer in corneal surgery and eye-banking, established the International Eye Foundation, based in Washington, D.C. The Foundation distributes donor material to developing countries and sends teams of American surgeons to those countries to introduce modern techniques of keratoplasty and eye-banking. At the 1976 Second International Corneal Congress held by the International Eye Foundation, the accomplishments made in the last 12 years in the keratoplasty field were reviewed. More than 60 countries were represented on the list of speakers.

Without well-organized and well-financed eye-banking to ensure a steady supply of properly screened and selected fresh donor material, the success of keratoplasty, as we know it today, would not be possible. Every ophthalmologist should support eye-banking, both locally and nationally. Only in this way can we be assured that our surgical skill will ultimately benefit the patient.

EYE-BANK OPERATION

The means used to collect, to select, to preserve, and to distribute donor eyes are essentially the same, though they may vary slightly, according to the current practice of the local eye bank. The methods used by The Eye Bank for Sight Restoration, Incorporated, are described.

The Eye Bank, unlike many of its smaller counterparts, maintains a full-time staff, headed by a full-time director whose function it is to direct the Eye Bank in the collection of proffered donor material, to publicize its service and research activities, and to stimulate eye donations and the funds necessary to maintain the organization. Liaison is established between the Eye Bank and major hospitals whose incoming house staff is indoctrinated annually in the methods used to solicit and to collect donor eyes.

Individual donor cards are supplied on request. By this means, the next of kin of the potential donor will be aware of the donor's intentions. The Eye Bank should be notified as soon as possible after the death of the potential donor, since no more than 6 hours should elapse before the eyes are enucleated. In the New York area, on-call, trained personnel are available to remove the eyes within a few hours after notification of the death of a donor. When the call is received at the Eye Bank, the cause and time of death are ascertained, and an estimate is made as to the probable condition of the eyes. If a local ophthalmologist enucleates the eyes, local or state police often volunteer their services to deliver immediately the freshly enucleated eyes to the Eye Bank. Otherwise, a messenger service is dispatched to pick up the eyes and to deliver them to the Eye Bank. If no local ophthalmologist is available, on-call personnel or a resident is dispatched to perform the enucleation and to deliver the donor eyes to the Eye Bank.

ENUCLEATING THE DONOR EYE

A simple set of instruments (Plate 4-1, *A*), consisting of a solid-bladed lid speculum, blunt-pointed conjunctival scissors, muscle hook, dog-toothed forceps, and enucleation scissors is provided in a sterile pack. Sterile irrigation solution, rubber gloves, and eye caps to replace the enucleated eyes also are included. No surgical preparation or draping is done. The lid speculum is inserted (Plate 4-1, *B*), and the cul-de-sac is flushed with a sterile normal salt solution to moisten the cornea and to remove any loose material.

Plate 4-1

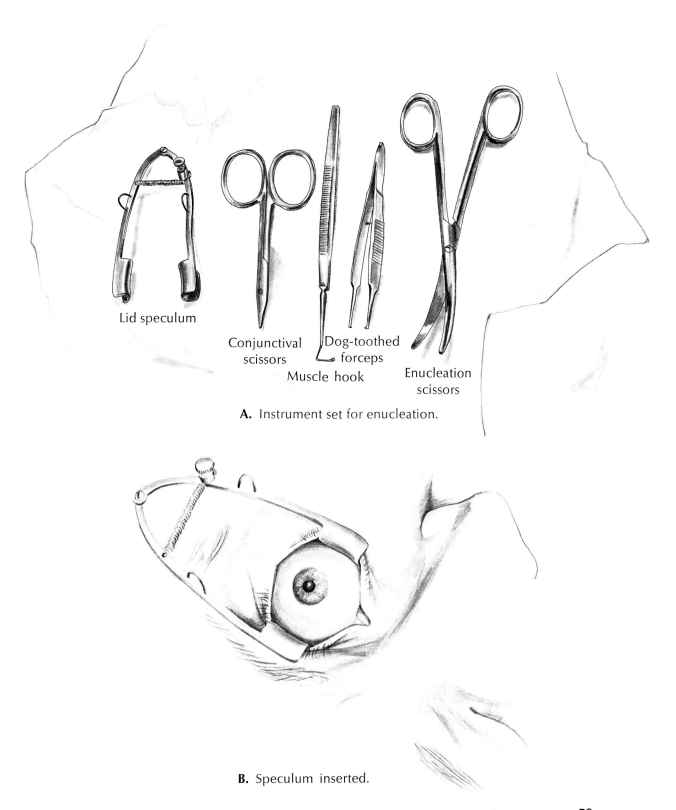

Lid speculum

Conjunctival
scissors

Dog-toothed
forceps

Muscle hook

Enucleation
scissors

A. Instrument set for enucleation.

B. Speculum inserted.

A peritomy is performed with the conjunctival scissors (Plate 4-2, *A* and *B*), leaving a minimal amount of conjunctiva at the corneal limbus. Blunt dissection of the subconjunctiva and Tenon's capsule isolates the rectus muscles.

Before the rectus muscles are cut free, the 12 o'clock meridian can be marked with indelible ink or a stitch in superficial sclera at the limbus (Plate 4-2, *C*). Later, this enables the surgeon to orient the cornea so that the vertical axis of the donor button coincides with the vertical axis of the recipient cornea. Each rectus muscle, in turn, is picked up with the muscle hook and cut adjacent to its insertion (Plate 4-2, *D*). The muscles should not be cut too close to the globe, since this may cause accidental perforation. Oblique muscles that can be identified are cut free. This often is a resident's first opportunity to locate and to cut an oblique muscle.

The enucleation scissors is introduced on the nasal side, since this is the shortest distance from the anterior aspect of the globe to the optic nerve (Plate 4-2, *E*). The optic nerve is cut as far posterior to the globe as possible. Remaining soft tissue is dissected to free the globe (Plate 4-2, *F*).

Plate 4-2

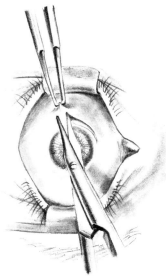

A. Peritomy performed.

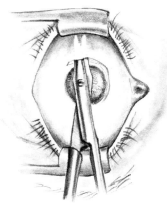

B. Dissection of subconjunctiva and Tenon's capsule.

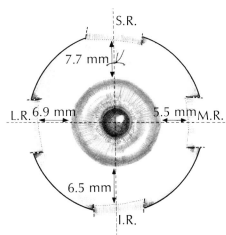

C. The 12 o'clock meridian is marked with a stitch. Anatomic relationship of rectus muscle insertions and surgical limbus of the right eye.

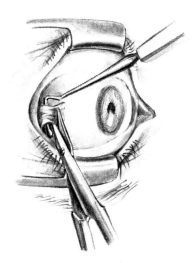

D. Isolating and cutting a rectus muscle.

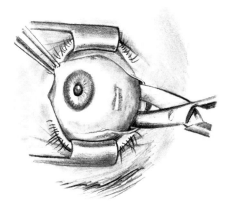

E. Enucleation scissors introduced on the nasal side to cut the optic nerve.

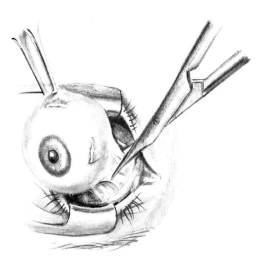

F. Cutting tissue to free the globe.

The eye is placed in a plastic, moist chamber containing a circle of wadded cotton wet with normal salt solution (Plate 4-3, *A*). The container, labeled with pertinent donor information, is closed tightly with a snap-on plastic lid and is placed in the Eye Bank outer shipping container, labeled with the name, address, and telephone number of the Eye Bank (Plate 4-3, *B*). The container may be kept in an ice-cooled thermos during transport, but it should never be frozen. Eye Bank containers are made available to all participating hospitals, as well as to participating ophthalmologists.

Plate 4-3

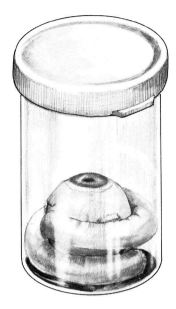

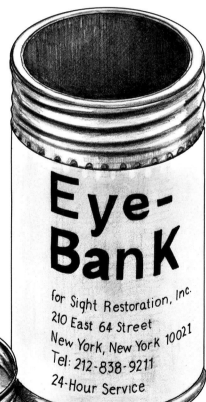

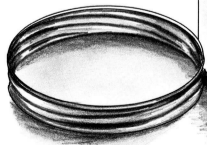

A. Eye in plastic, moist-chamber container.

B. Outer shipping container.

Eye-
BanK

for Sight Restoration, Inc.
210 East 64 Street
New York, New York 10021
Tel: 212-838-9211
24-Hour Service

SELECTION AND PREPARATION OF THE DONOR EYE
Slit-lamp examination and specular microscopy

When the eye is delivered to the Eye Bank, it is examined immediately under the slit lamp (Plate 4-4), and the Eye Bank technician decides whether or not the eye can be used for keratoplasty. If the donor material is suitable for keratoplasty, the surgeon on call is notified that donor tissue is available and will be delivered as soon as processed.

Plate 4-4

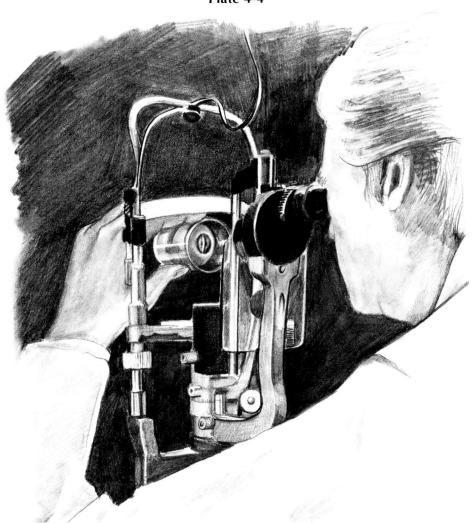

Slit-lamp examination of the donor eye.

The external and slit-lamp examination is important for gross screening of every eye received. The donor eye is usually hypotensive, with folding of endothelium and Descemet's membrane resembling striate keratopathy (Plate 4-5, *A* and *B*). As the eye is examined under the slit lamp, slight pressure is exerted on the sclera so that these folds disappear and the normal configuration and thickness of the cornea can be seen (Plate 4-5, *C* and *D*).

Plate 4-5

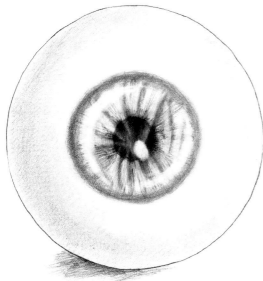

A. Frontal view.

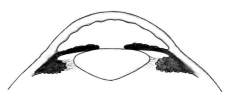

B. Cross section.

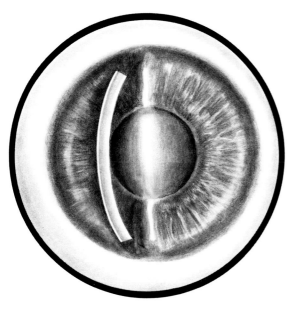

C. Folding disappears with increased intraocular pressure. Slit-lamp view.

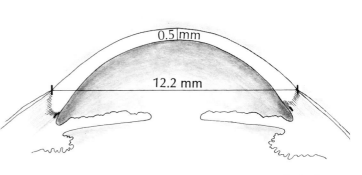

0.5 mm

12.2 mm

D. Normal configuration and thickness of ideal donor cornea. Cross section.

Folding of endothelium and Descemet's membrane in hypotensive donor eye.

If folding is severe and there is gross epithelial edema and dehiscences (Plate 4-6, *A* and *B*), pressure on the globe will fail to regularize the endothelial surface, and the cornea will remain thickened. A slit-lamp view of such a cornea shows the posterior folds to be sharp-edged and numerous (Plate 4-6, *C*).

Plate 4-6

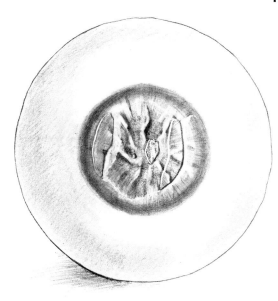

A. Frontal view.

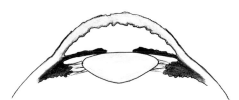

B. Cross section.

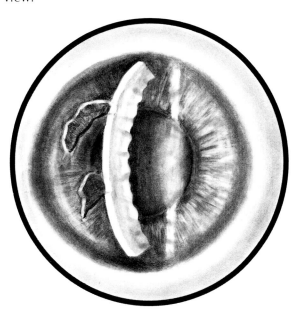

C. Increased pressure fails to regularize endothelial
folds or to reduce corneal thickness.
Slit-lamp view.

**Severe folding of cornea with epithelial
edema and dehiscences. Tissue
not suitable for keratoplasty.**

Surface irregularities can extend crater-like through Bowman's membrane into stroma (Plate 4-7, *A* and *B*). In some instances, a cornea that appears moderately clear may have extensive epithelial defects and dehiscences extending through Bowman's membrane. Such corneas should be rejected even when specular microscopy demonstrates normal endothelium. Conversely, in the absence of edema and sharp folds, epithelial dehiscences can be disregarded and the eye used (Plate 4-7, *C*).

In addition to external examination with the slit lamp, the donor cornea may be examined by specular microscopy. This additional evaluation may salvage a borderline eye, which might be rejected by slit-lamp examination. Conversely, an eye, particularly one from an older patient, may be acceptable biomicroscopically but under the specular microscope may show endothelial changes precluding its use for penetrating keratoplasty (Plate 4-7, *D*).

Plate 4-7

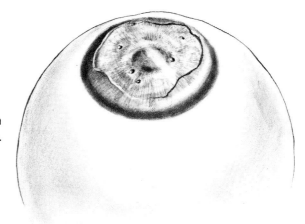

A. Crater-like dehiscences extending through Bowman's membrane.

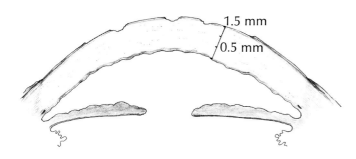

1.5 mm

0.5 mm

B. Crater-like dehiscences extending through Bowman's membrane. Cross section.

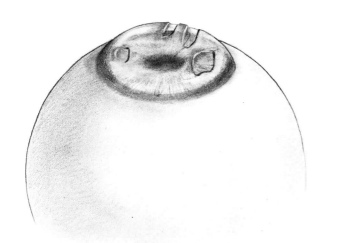

C. Epithelial dehiscences with normal corneal stroma and endothelium. Cornea suitable for graft.

D. Specular microscope photograph of endothelium with minimally enlarged cells but with numerous damaged cells. Tissue not suitable for keratoplasty.

Preparation of the donor eye

When the eye-bank technician determines that the cornea is acceptable for preservation, a culture is taken (Plate 4-8, *A*) and placed in brain-heart infusion broth (Plate 4-8, *B*) and incubated.

Since the eye is used as soon as possible after enucleation, the time elapsed may not have been sufficient to observe growth in the broth. For this reason, a donor eye from a patient with a history of septicemia or localized infection is rejected. Other diagnoses which preclude the use of donor eyes include leukemia or similar blood dyscrasias, large virus infections, such as Jacob-Creutzfeldt syndrome, and infectious hepatitis.

Following culture, the intact globe is flushed copiously with a normal salt solution containing penicillin and streptomycin. If the globe is to be delivered intact, it is placed in a fresh, sterile Eye Bank container and sent to the requesting surgeon.

Plate 4-8

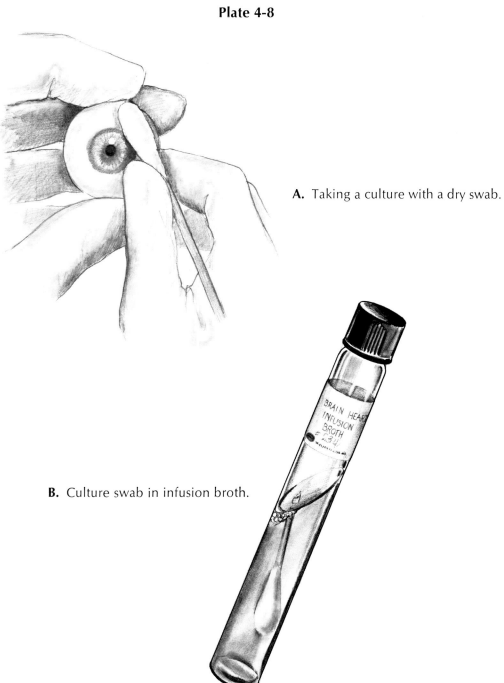

A. Taking a culture with a dry swab.

B. Culture swab in infusion broth.

Preparation of the corneoscleral segment

If the donor eye is to be prepared for tissue-culture medium preservation, it is placed in a laminar flow hood under ultraviolet light. Using sterile precautions, the laboratory technician removes the conjunctival remnants with a razor knife and scissors (Plate 4-9).

Plate 4-9

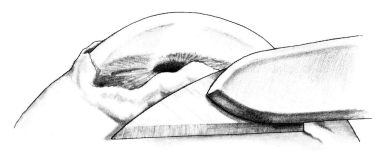

A. Dissecting the conjunctival remnants with razor knife.

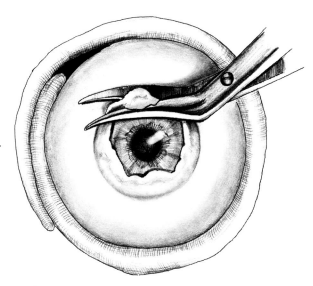

B. Removing the conjunctival remnants with scissors.

A partially penetrating circumferential scleral incision is made approximately 3 or 4 mm from the limbus (see Volume I, Plate 6-9). A razor knife is used to penetrate a section of the incision. The posterior blade of the cataract section scissors is inserted and the remaining thickness of the sclera is cut along the knife outline (Plate 4-10, A). Care is taken not to perforate the underlying uveal tissue. The edge of the sclera adjacent to the cornea is grasped with a toothed forceps. The corneoscleral segment is pulled up with as little distorting force as possible to break the attachment of the base of the iris to the scleral spur at the anterior chamber angle (Plate 4-10, B). The corneoscleral preparation is placed, endothelial side up, in a glass container filled partially with tissue-culture fluid (Plate 4-10, C).

Plate 4-10

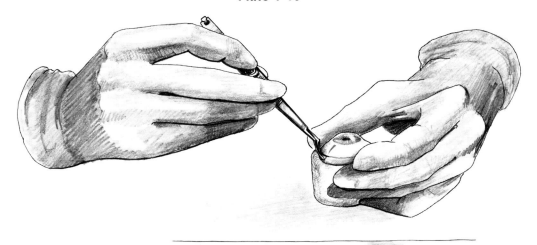

A. Cataract section scissors completing scleral incision along knife outline.

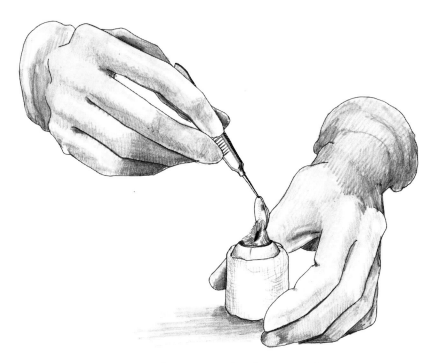

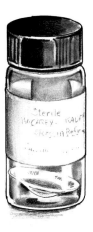

B. Removing the corneoscleral segment from its attachment to the scleral spur.

C. Corneal scleral segment in M-K tissue culture fluid.

Cutting the donor button from the anterior surface

When a fresh, intact globe is received, the surgeon may elect to cut the donor button from the corneoscleral segment in the manner previously described. Alternatively, the surgeon may elect to cut the corneal button from the anterior surface of the intact globe. In the latter case, the globe is removed from the eye-bank container (Plate 4-11, *A*) and wrapped in a gauze strip (see Volume I, Plate 6-9). A moistened cellulose sponge is used to remove loose epithelium (Plate 4-11, *B*).

Plate 4-11

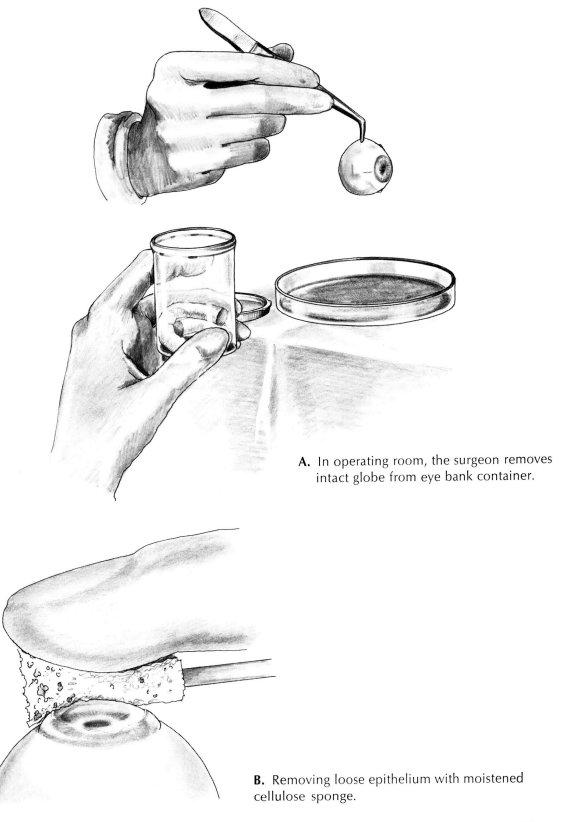

A. In operating room, the surgeon removes intact globe from eye bank container.

B. Removing loose epithelium with moistened cellulose sponge.

A trephine of the size selected is set for full penetration. It is placed vertically and centered on the cornea, steadied in position with the index finger, and rotated between the thumb and second finger by its knurled handle (Plate 4-12, *A*). As the globe is penetrated, it collapses. The trephine is withdrawn immediately or an irregular, sloping cut will result. A fine, curved corneal scissors (see Volume I, Plate 3-7) is inserted through the penetrated section, and the incision is completed (Plate 4-12, *B*). To prevent undercutting the donor button, the surgeon should hold the scissors in a position slightly overcorrected from the vertical and also should not exert excessive traction with the forceps. Before the donor button is cut free, the 12 o'clock meridian, corresponding to the scleral mark, can be identified by a superficially placed suture for orientation in the recipient opening (Plate 4-12, *C*).

It would be useful to know the keratometry readings of each donor cornea, but this is not practical. The K readings would make it possible to eliminate a cornea with high congenital astigmatism and to match selectively a flatter or steeper donor button to the recipient. Accurate keratometric measurements are not possible after the eye is enucleated, especially after it is dissected for preservation in a tissue-culture medium. However, when the corneal donor button is cut on the surface of a *spherical,* concave backing block, partial compensation of any preexisting distortion is effected. The donor button cut from the anterior surface of the intact globe will be spherical only if the donor cornea is anastigmatic. This is yet another reason why I believe a full-thickness donor button should be cut from the endothelial surface. When the intact globe is supplied, the anterior segment is excised by the surgeon in the operating room. The button is then cut from the endothelial side, in the same manner that a tissue-culture preserved preparation would be cut. The donor button is transferred to a Petri dish containing a balanced salt solution (Plate 4-12, *D*). The operation then proceeds to the recipient eye.

Plate 4-12

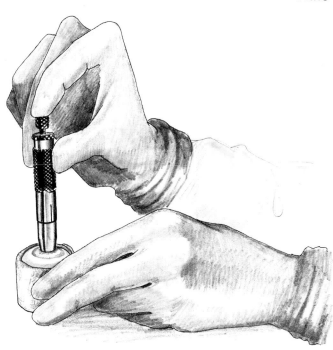

A. Trephining the donor eye.

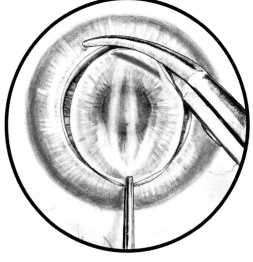

B. Excision of corneal button is completed with Troutman corneal scissors.

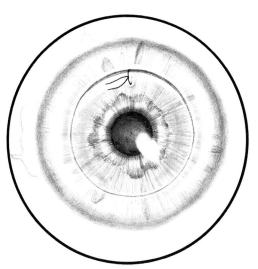

C. Orienting the donor button: suture placed at 12 o'clock.

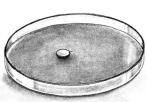

D. Excised donor button in Petri dish.

Cutting the donor button from the posterior surface

When the donor button is to be cut from the posterior surface, the corneoscleral preparation is placed in the concavity of a backing block. One of several Troutman instruments is used to cut the button. The simplest instrument is a Teflon block into which four cavities, two on each side, have been turned on a 7.5-mm radius, slightly steeper than the average corneal radius of 7.85 mm (Plate 4-13, *A*). The donor button edges cut on a 7.5-mm radius-of-curvature backing block are more vertical than those of a button cut on a less steeply curved block. This block is used with a disposable trephine blade, which first must be centered and balanced carefully on the posterior surface of the corneoscleral preparation. Then the trephine is pressed firmly with the thumb to penetrate through the cornea to the backing block (Plate 4-13, *B* and *C*). This technique can produce somewhat erratic results and often results in an irregularly shaped donor button when the thumb pressure is applied off the vertical axis. The trephine, and with it the underlying cornea, tend to slide up one side of the concavity as the cut is being made (see Plate 8-1). This slipping causes both shelving and ovaling of the button and can result in significant optical aberrations in the healed graft. Also, if the smooth concave surface of the block becomes marred from multiple use, it can cause the edge of the trephine to cut unevenly, resulting in an irregular graft edge.

Plate 4-13

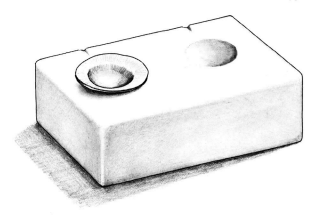

A. Four-concavity Teflon backing block. Corneoscleral segment in position for cutting.

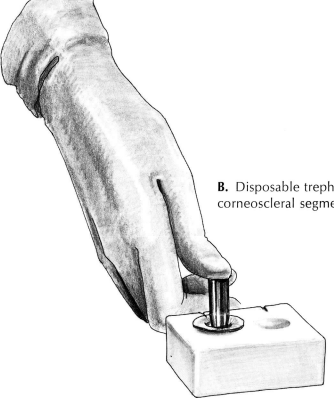

B. Disposable trephine used to penetrate the corneoscleral segment.

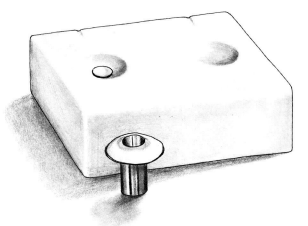

C. Excised donor button in backing block.

For these reasons, several cutting frames using a vertical piston guide for the cutter and a disposable backing block have been designed. In the Troutman model, the disposable backing block is cut with a double-curved concavity. The posterior aspect of the concavity is cut to a radius of 7.5 mm, slightly steeper than the average corneal curvature (Plate 4-14, *A*). A longer radius of 15 mm, corresponding to the scleral radius, is cut to the external rim of the first concavity to join it at the line of demarcation between the two concavities, with a diameter of 12 mm, corresponding to the limbal diameter. This double-curved concavity corresponds to the external double curvature of the corneoscleral button, which, therefore, sits firmly without distortion. A relief hole is drilled through and through centrally to allow fluid to escape from the concavity behind the button. The mild suction imparted by the escaping fluid helps to hold the button more securely in position. In addition, the centered hole serves as a point of reference for centering the corneoscleral button before cutting (Plate 4-14, *B*). The disposable block is mounted into a correspondingly sized, ring-shaped hole drilled partially into a flat, stainless steel plate. Since there is less tendency for the button to slide up the side of the double-concavity block during cutting, the donor button can be cut freehand more accurately than when using the four-concavity block (Plate 4-14, *C*).

Plate 4-14

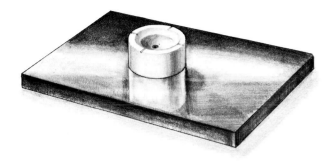

A. Disposable Teflon block with double-curved concavity set in stainless backing plate.

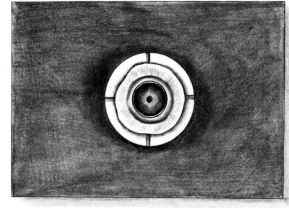

B. Corneoscleral segment centered on relief hole of Teflon block.

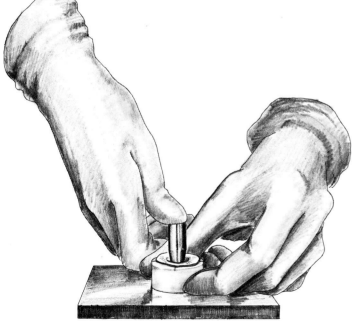

C. Cutting the donor button freehand on the disposable, double-concavity backing block.

85

However, the preferred method is to guide the trephine exactly vertically to the backing block by means of a piston passed through a guide frame fitted over the disposable block (Plate 4-15, *A* and *B*). The piston is designed to accept disposable blades sized from 7 mm to 11 mm (Plate 4-15, *C*). A screw adjustment expands or retracts the split ring, which centers and fixes the blade as it is held against the tapered shoulder of the piston (Plate 4-15, *D*).

Plate 4-15

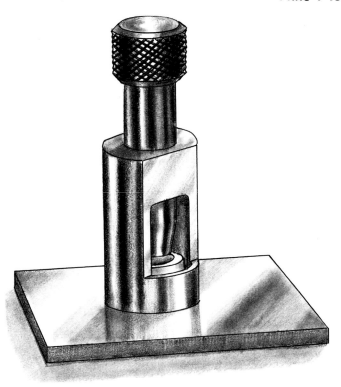

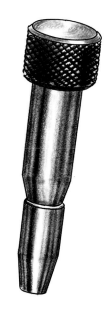

B. Piston fitted with
7-mm disposable blade.

A. Troutman frame-and-piston assembly
fitted over disposable block.

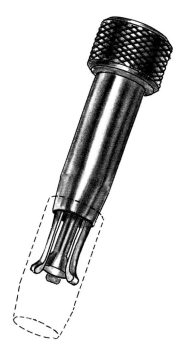

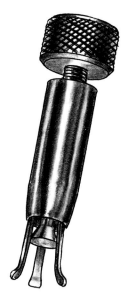

D. Detail of split ring, which expands to fix and
to center trephine blades of various sizes.

C. Troutman universal piston design accepts
disposable blades 7 to 11 mm in diameter.

Four fine anterior grooves on the block mark four meridians of the cornea so that the corneal button can be oriented (Plate 4-16, *A*). If a scleral marker has been used, one of the four marks will indicate the vertical meridian of the corneoscleral preparation. The block, with the button still in its concavity and covered with a few drops of tissue-culture fluid, is placed in a plastic Petri dish until used (Plate 4-16, *B*).

Plate 4-16

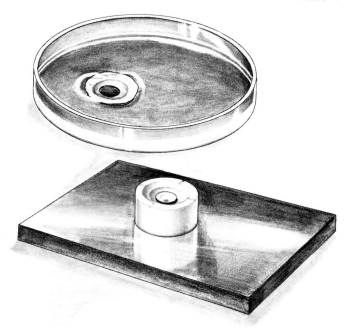

A. Donor button in backing block. Corneoscleral segment shows centered excision. Note meridian groove markings.

B. Donor button in M-K medium protected in covered Petri dish.

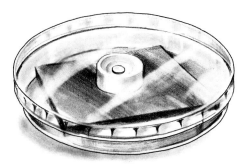

A similar, guided unit has been designed by Cardona and Roskothen. Each backing block is grooved individually to match the diameter of the trephine blade being used, in order to protect its edge. This obviates the necessity for a disposable block (Plate 4-17). Since the trephine blade passes into the groove as soon as it has cut through the cornea, the cutting edge of the blade is not dulled against the cutting block.

Plate 4-17

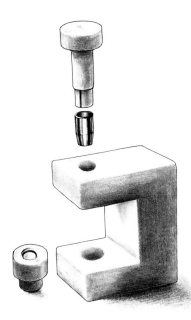

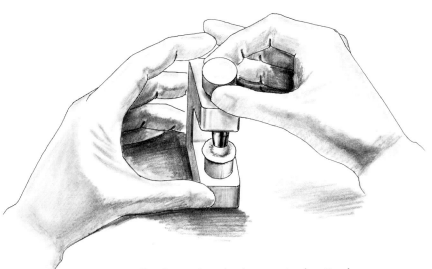

A. Cardona-Roskothen cutting-frame assembly with grooved backing block.

B. Centering the button in the Cardona-Roskothen cutting unit.

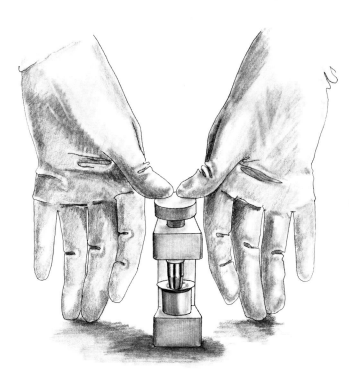

C. Cutting the donor button.

However, the pressure of the cutting edge of the trephine, pushing the cornea into the groove as it is being cut, distorts the soft corneal tissue (Plate 4-18, *A* and *B*). This causes cutting irregularities, the most serious of which is the narrowing of the anterior diameter of the cornea (Plate 4-18, *C*). Other irregularities include lipping, chipping, and ovaling or bias cutting of the donor button (Plate 4-18, *D*). A donor button cut with the Cardona-Roskothen unit and sutured into a recipient opening cut with the same-sized trephine blade flattens excessively when healed in place.

Plate 4-18

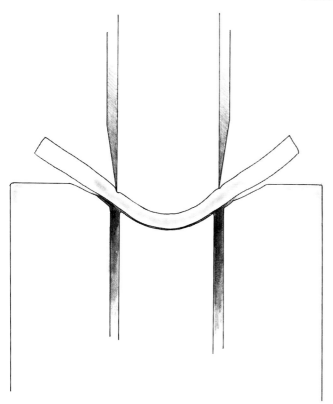

A. Beginning the cut in a grooved backing block. Cross section.

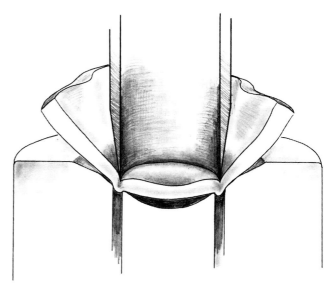

B. Corneal tissue distorted by trephine blade as it is being cut.

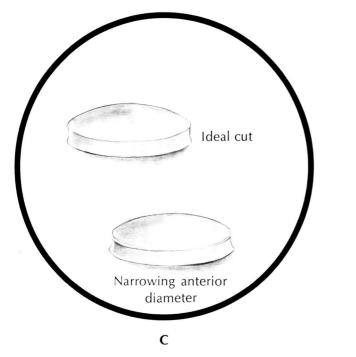

Ideal cut

Narrowing anterior diameter

C

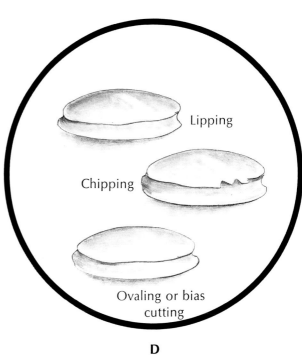

Lipping

Chipping

Ovaling or bias cutting

D

Ideal cut compared to cutting irregularities.

The Cardona-Roskothen unit requires a different piston for each diameter trephine blade. The Teflon piston guide, as with the Polack corneal graft punch (see Volume I, Plate 8-15), is not as accurate as is the stainless steel piston unit used in the Troutman donor cutting instrument. With the Troutman double-curved disposable backing block (Plate 4-19), such cutting irregularities are more easily avoided.

Plate 4-19

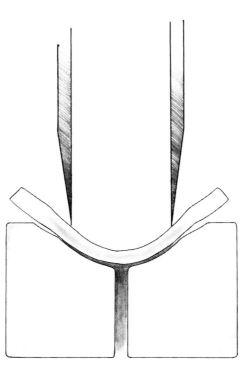

A. Troutman disposable solid backing block with double concavity and center relief hole: beginning cut. Cross section.

B. Trephine pressure does not cause distortion. Cutting irregularities are avoided.

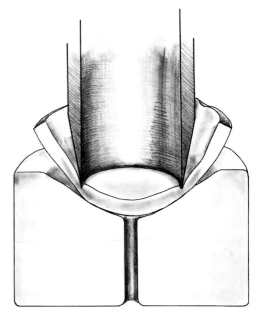

Selecting the size of the donor button

To avoid excessive suture tension on and flattening of the donor button, it is important that the donor button be approximately the same size and shape as the recipient opening into which it is to be sutured. Careful measurement of the trephine blades supplied by various manufacturers shows that the actual diameter of a trephine blade can vary by as much as 0.5 mm from the indicated diameter. The manufacturers have been apprised of this discrepancy, and most are currently producing standard-diameter trephine blades. Nevertheless, it is important for the surgeon to measure the diameters of the trephines to be used, especially when different-sized blades are to be used to cut the donor and the recipient.

I have determined that the donor button cut from the posterior surface with a 7-mm, 7.5-mm, or 8-mm trephine blade is smaller in diameter by approximately 0.2 mm than the recipient opening cut with the same blade. Therefore, to approximate the diameter of the recipient opening, the donor button should be cut with a trephine blade 0.2 mm larger in diameter than that used to cut the recipient opening. A cornea of normal curvature should result. Should a flatter corneal curvature be required for optical purposes, as in a keratoconic cornea, the same trephine blade or two blades of the same diameter should be used to cut both the donor and the recipient. When a steeper cornea is required to induce myopia or to reduce hyperopia, as in an aphakic eye, the trephine blade used to cut the donor button can be 0.5 mm, or even 1 mm, larger than that used to cut the recipient opening. In addition to producing a steeper cornea and a less hyperopic eye, a tighter apposition of the donor to the recipient is ensured—an important consideration in aphakic keratoplasty.

In lamellar keratoplasty, especially in a larger lamellar replacement, the donor button always should be cut larger than the recipient opening. The deep layer of a lamellarized cornea stretches slightly. Approximating the edges and suturing are more difficult if the donor replacement is the same size as the excised area.

SUMMARY

Today, the availability of good eye-bank material is taken for granted. This has not always been the case. We owe a great deal to the pioneers of eye-banking and to the local and national organizations that support eye-banking for giving us the opportunity to provide the patient with the benefits of microsurgical keratoplasty.

The procedure and techniques of The Eye Bank for Sight Restoration, Incorporated, have been outlined, as well as instrumentation used in the preparation of a donor button. Good donor tissue, well-prepared and precisely cut, is essential to obtain not only a clear graft but also an optically perfect graft by the various techniques outlined in the chapters to follow.

CHAPTER 5

INSTRUMENTATION

Introduction
Instrumentation for lamellar or penetrating
  keratoplasty
    Basic instrument set
    Basic donor cutting set
    Special or optional instruments

Description of instruments and their uses
  during keratoplasty
Special instrumentation
The surgical microscope
Summary

INTRODUCTION

The carpenter is no better than his tools. In Volume I, Chapter 1, the design principles of microsurgical instruments were discussed in considerable detail. Representative instruments, modified or developed especially for microsurgery of the anterior segment, were illustrated. Some aspects of their uses in microsurgery were discussed in Volume I, Chapter 3. Microsurgical instruments of prime importance, the fine suture needle and the monofilament elastic suture that the microsurgical needle arms, were presented in Volume I, Chapters 4 and 5. The design and function of the surgical microscope were detailed in Chapter 2.

In this chapter, microsurgical instruments and sutures and microscope requirements or modifications as used for keratoplasty techniques will be further detailed. New instruments or significant modifications of instruments are illustrated and their surgical applications described.

Ophthalmic microsurgical instruments are use-designed. For both penetrating and lamellar keratoplasty, specific instruments have been designed to grasp, to cut, or otherwise to penetrate, dissect, manipulate, and repair ocular tissue.

The basic microsurgical instrument set employed for lamellar or penetrating keratoplasty is described and illustrated in this chapter. A detailed description of some of these instruments, as used for one or another procedure exclusively or on special indication, is given. The needles and suture materials used during a keratoplasty procedure are described.

Finally, the surgical microscope is reviewed, and modifications introduced since the publication of Volume I, especially as they apply to keratoplasty technique, are described in detail.

INSTRUMENTS FOR LAMELLAR OR PENETRATING KERATOPLASTY

The instruments are separated into two categories, a basic set, boxed together and used for each case, and specialized instruments, individually sterile-packed to be available on demand. After each procedure, the basic set and any special instrument that has been used are checked functionally and visually under magnification. If an instrument is found to be dulled, damaged, or otherwise defective, it is repaired or replaced. Unless an instrument is prohibitively expensive or experimental, or the one-of-a-kind type, identical back-up instruments always should be available to replace damaged ones.

Instruments placed together on a tray or in a boxed set must be arranged so they do not touch each other during surgery or during sterilization. This is especially important when an ultrasound unit is used to clean instruments, as delicate metal tips of cutting edges may be fragmented on contact. When not in use and during cleaning, the tips or blades should be kept covered by protective plastic tubes or sleeves.

Basic instrument set (Plate 5-1)

The basic instrument set-up for keratoplasty, in the order of the probable use of instruments during surgery, is as follows:
3M aperture drape (individually sterile-packed)
Barraquer wire lid speculum
Troutman rectus fixation forceps
5-0 silk suture, on GS-3 Ethicon needle (individually sterile-packed)
7-0 silk suture, on GS-9 Ethicon needle (individually sterile-packed)
MICRA-Pierse needleholder
Troutman needleholder (curved tips)
Flieringa ring set, 12, 14, 16, 18, 20, 22, and 24 mm
MICRA-Pierse titanium rings, 12, 14, and 16 mm (or Girard expander)
MICRA-Pierse titanium tissue forceps, curved
Razor knife, MICRA-Pierse and Troutman angled
Trephine handle of size appropriate for procedure—6, 6.5, 7, 7.5, 8, 8.5, 9, or
    10 mm, individually sterile-packed
Disposable blade of size appropriate for procedure, corresponding to size of
    trephine handle, individually sterile-packed
Diamond knife with protective cover
Iris spatulas, 1 mm (2)
Troutman keratoplasty scissors, right and left (for penetrating kerato-
    plasty) (see Volume I, Plate 2-9)
Troutman keratoplasty scissors, right and left (for lamellar keratoplasty)
    (see Volume I, Plate 2-10)
Troutman corneal lamellar splitters, No. 1, No. 2, and No. 3 (for lamellar
    keratoplasty)
MICRA-Pierse tissue forceps, straight
Barraquer-de Wecker scissors, 5-mm blades (see Volume I, Plate 2-11)
MICRA-Pierse iris and suture scissors

Plate 5-1

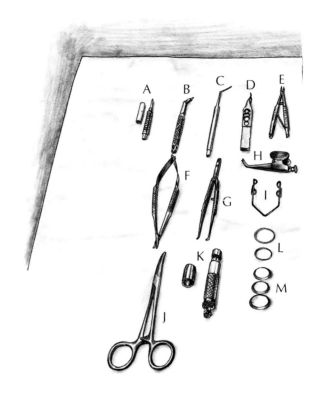

A. Diamond knife with protective cover
B. Troutman angled razor knife
C. Iris spatula, 1-mm diameter
D. MICRA-Pierse titanium tissue forceps, curved
E. MICRA-Pierse needleholder
F. Troutman needleholder, curved tips
G. Troutman rectus fixation forceps
H. Barraquer-de Wecker scissors, 5-mm blades
I. Barraquer wire lid speculum
J. Box-hinged hemostat
K. Trephine handle and disposable blade
L. Flieringa rings (2)
M. MICRA-Pierse titanium rings (3)

The basic instrument set for keratoplasty.

Vannas scissors
Harms tying forceps, straight (1 pair)
Troutman tying forceps, curved (1 pair)
MICRA-Pierse plain (P) forceps, straight
Troutman suture-handling forceps, pointed, on Barraquer-de Wecker handle (see Volume I, Plate 2-7)

Plate 5-1, cont'd

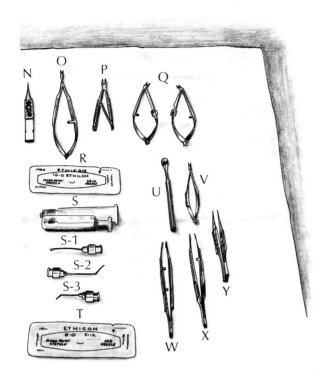

N. MICRA-Pierse titanium tissue forceps, straight
O. MICRA-Pierse iris and suture scissors, angulated
P. MICRA-Pierse razor knife
Q. Troutman keratoplasty scissors, right and left
R. 10-0, 22-micron monofilament nylon on GS-14 Ethicon needle
S. Syringe
S-1. Troutman olive-tipped irrigator needle
S-2, S-3. Irrigation-aspiration needle, 31-gauge, angled
T. 6-0 silk suture on GS-9 Ethicon needle
U. Paton graft transfer spatula
V. Vannas scissors
W. Troutman tying forceps, curved
X. Harms tying forceps, straight
Y. MICRA-Pierse plain tissue (P) forceps, straight

The basic instrument set for keratoplasty.

Box-hinged microhemostat (2)
Irrigation-aspiration needle, 31-gauge, angled
Troutman olive-tipped irrigator
10-0, 22-micron monofilament nylon or polypropylene armed with GS-14 Ethicon needle
6-0 or 7-0 braided silk armed with GS-9 Ethicon needle or equivalent

Basic donor cutting set (see Chapter 4)

Troutman-Amsler trephine piston punch set
  Universal piston punch (stainless)
  Backing plate (stainless)
  Backing block (Teflon)
  Piston guide (stainless)
Disposable trephine blade appropriate for procedure—6.5, 7, 7.2, 7.5, 8, 8.2, 8.5, 9, 9.5, 10, or 11 mm, individually sterile-packed
Petri dishes (2)
Paton transfer spatula

Special or optional instruments

Vitreous sucking-cutting instruments
  Rotoextractor, such as Douvas, Grieshaber, and Machemer
  Reciprocating, such as Kloti and Peyman
Cryoextractor set (Amoils type)
Retinal probe (for cyclocryothermy)
Motor-driven trephine, such as Barraquer-Mateus and Draeger
Lieberman single-point, cam-guided corneal knife
Barraquer lamellar microkeratome
Barraquer cryolathe
Lens disruption-aspiration device, such as Girard, Kelman (Plate 5-4, *B*), and Shoch types

Surgical microscope with surgical keratometer

DESCRIPTION OF INSTRUMENTS AND THEIR USES DURING KERATOPLASTY

Many of the instruments listed have been described in sufficient detail in Volume I. However, it is appropriate to describe others not so detailed or used for a specific technique during a keratoplasty procedure.

The *3M aperture drape* is a nonabsorbing, adhesive-backed drape placed so as to isolate the surgical field and to provide a run-off for fluid in order to maintain a dry surrounding field.

The Troutman *rectus fixation forceps* (Plates 5-1, *G* and 5-2, *A*, and see Volume I, Plates 2-8, 3-4, and 6-1) is used principally to grasp the superior rectus muscle (see Chapter 6). It may be used to grasp other rectus muscles should the surgeon elect to fix more than one muscle. It may be used also to grasp the Flieringa or titanium ring to manipulate the globe.

The *G-3 Ethicon curved ½-inch needle* for superior rectus suture, arming

Plate 5-2

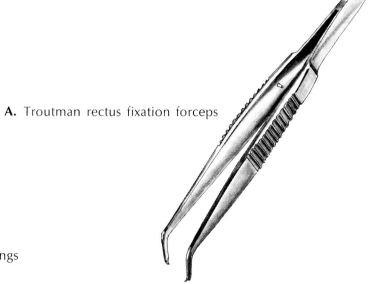

A. Troutman rectus fixation forceps

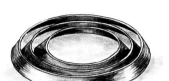

B. MICRA-Pierse titanium fixation rings

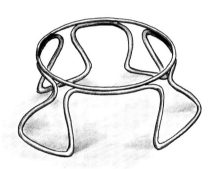

C. Girard scleral expander

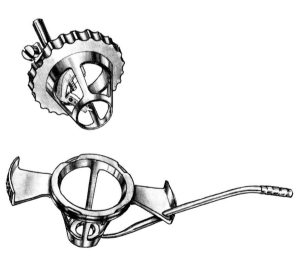

D. Lieberman single-point, cam-guided
corneal knife

101

5-0 silk suture, is a heavy-wire, relatively blunt needle used to position a rectus fixation suture. It is passed beneath the rectus muscle belly as it is elevated from the globe with the rectus fixation forceps.

GS-9 Ethicon 137° curved needle, arming a 7-0 silk suture (Plate 5-1, *T*), is a needle-suture combination that may be used alternately with the 5-0, G-3 armed suture to retract the globe. The fine spatula needle is inserted intrasclerally, just anterior to the rectus insertion (see Chapter 6). The same needle-suture combination is used with multiple intrascleral bites to fix either the wire Flieringa ring by interrupted sutures or the MICRA-Pierse titanium ring by a running suture.

A *box-hinged, small hemostat* (Plate 5-1, *J*) is used to drive the larger wire-diameter G-3 needle and to manipulate and position the globe by the rectus fixation suture or globe retraction suture. A microsurgical needleholder should never be used to drive a needle of a wire-diameter greater than that of the GS needle series, for the fine needleholder jaws will be sprung.

Hematoma, tearing the levator aponeurosis, or both can be caused by forcing a solid speculum blade, during separation or retraction fixation of the lids in preparation for or during a surgical procedure. Tearing of the levator aponeurosis or the levator muscle itself, by excessive or prolonged mechanical pressure from a lid speculum, is the most common cause of postoperative ptosis. The blades of the *Barraquer light-wire lid speculum* (Plate 5-1, *I,* and see Volume I, Plate 3-3) with flexible spring cannot be forced and do not hold lids forcibly in retraction. Consequently, speculum-related complications are avoided.

Flieringa rings (see Plates 5-1, *L,* 6-3, *A* and *B,* 6-6, 6-7 and Volume I, Plate 3-5) are circular wire rings available in sizes from 12 to 24 mm in 2-mm steps. The size usually used is 14 or 16 mm. The Flieringa rings are used primarily in aphakic keratoplasty. Using a GS-9 needle arming a 7-0 silk thread (see Volume I, Plates 2-15 and 3-5), the ring of selected size is sutured to the sclera with 4 or 8 interrupted intrascleral bites. The intermediate loops between selected bites (as illustrated in Volume I, Plate 3-5) are left intact to facilitate mobilization of the globe.

MICRA-Pierse titanium fixation rings (Plates 5-1, *M,* and 5-2 *B*), introduced since the publication of Volume I, are used for anterior segment stabilization and fixation in phakic keratoplasty. They are available in three sizes, with an inside diameter of 12, 14, or 16 mm. The outside diameters are 16, 18, and 20 mm, respectively. The ring is placed with its concave surface approximating a 2-mm ring segment of the sclera, toward the globe. It is fixed to the sclera by a running suture of 7-0 silk armed with a GS-9 needle. A running thread can be adjusted to equalize the tension between individual loops. This prevents the distortion of the cornea that can occur when interrupted fixation sutures are placed inaccurately or tied too tightly to the round-wire Flieringa ring.

102

The *surgical keratometer* (see Plate 2-10) is used to monitor the placement and suturing of both the Flieringa ring and the MICRA-Pierse *titanium ring*. Malplacement that might induce a corneal distortion can be detected by a distortion of the keratometer light ring, and the offending suture bite can be replaced.

Ring-fixation forceps (see Volume I, Plate 2-15) is made to grasp only the Flieringa ring and should not be used to grasp a MICRA-Pierse titanium ring. The latter ring can be fixed between the cupped tips of a straight or curved MICRA-Pierse corneal forceps. The thickness of the titanium ring edge corresponds to the opening of the cups. They must be engaged carefully, or the cupped tips may be bent or broken off.

The *straight MICRA-Pierse titanium cup-tipped forceps* (Plate 5-1, N, and see Volume I, Plate 2-16) is preferred to the *straight Bonn dog-toothed forceps* (see Volume I, Plates 2-8 and 2-16). The MICRA-Pierse forceps need not be turned during suturing, which is required when using the Bonn forceps so that its double-toothed tip engages better the vertical stromal edge of the cornea (see Volume I, Plates 5-9 and 5-11). Opposing cupped forceps tips, however, are not as forgiving of misapplication as are the dog-toothed forceps tips. If sufficient tissue is not engaged, the cupped tips can slip off readily or can become disengaged during the pressure of needle penetration, especially if the needle is not being driven radially. It is essential that needle passage be made directly from behind and continue beneath the anteriorly engaged forceps tip. Since the tips must grasp the wound margin radially to be most secure, the curved forceps should be substituted for the straight forceps when the patient's nose or forehead, the drape, or another obstruction prevents precise radial application of the straight forceps tips.

The *MICRA-Pierse curved tip forceps* (Plate 5-1, D, and see Volume I, Plate 2-17) is preferable to the Colibri-handled, 0.2-mm toothed corneal forceps. The latter cannot be turned to engage the double teeth, and a second pair of forceps with reversed teeth must be used. Since the MICRA-Pierse instrument has identical cupped tips on either side, no substitution need be made.

The *MICRA-Pierse titanium needleholder* (Plate 5-1, E, and see Volume I, Plate 2-20) is 8 cm long—short enough to be held within the palm of the hand as it is used. Even with straight tips it often can be manipulated through a greater range of positions and to better advantage in tight quarters than a longer curved-tip instrument. When required, needle angulation can be achieved by adjusting the lightly grasped needle with a closed tissue forceps and then more firmly closing the jaws to fix the needle at the angle selected for optimal penetration.

The *Troutman curved needleholder* (Plate 5-1, O, and see Volume I, Plates 2-18 and 2-19) has 12-cm long handles. Thus the spring rests across the edge of the index finger or on the anatomic snuff box, as does a pen or pencil, for lateral stabilization. I prefer the MICRA-Pierse needleholder for most microsurgical suturing because of its better balance and ease of manipulation.

The *MICRA-Pierse razor knife* (Plate 5-1, *P,* and see Volume I, Plate 2-20) is a blade breaker made for use with precracked blades only and should not be used otherwise, or it may be damaged.

The *Troutman short-angled blade breaker and razor knife* (Plate 5-1, *B,* and see Volume I, Plates 2-1 and 2-21) is a combination instrument, preferred because blades can be cracked to the desired shape and then used in the same instrument. The angle of the tips to the handle allows for better manipulation and use of the razor cutting edge.

Special *razor blades* for use with the razor knife are available from the several ophthalmic instrument manufacturers. These blades are formulated from a high carbon content steel to provide a consistently clean break and sharp tip. High chromium content or siliconized shaving razor blades are unsatisfactory for surgical use, for they are too soft, bending instead of breaking cleanly (see Volume I, Plate 6-5).

The *superblade* is a resharpened razor fragment set in a plastic handle. Since it is dulled quickly, it is used only to make precise incisions and then is discarded.

Corneal trephine blades (Plate 5-1, *K,* and see Volume I, Plate 2-23) are supplied by most manufacturers in a disposable model. Most manufacturers supply nondisposable handles in sizes to fit their varying sizes of disposable blades. These handles incorporate a depth-screw gauge to adjust the obturator within the trephine barrel in relation to the cutting edge. The surgeon is cautioned not to rely on the accuracy of such depth-setting devices. The length of successive disposable trephine blades can vary by 1 mm or more. Before an attempt is made to adjust the cutting depth of the blade, the trephine edge should be set level to the edge of the concave obturator tip. If the obturator is made accurately, a squarely ground blade edge will line up flush with the circumference of the obturator. The trephine depth gauge should be inspected and set under the microscope. High magnification is used also to check the blade edge before each use. The same handle is used to trephine a donor button from an intact globe as is used to trephine the recipient eye.

I have found a variation in diameter of as much as 0.3 mm in individual trephines marked as having the same diameter. This discrepancy can produce a serious distortion of the graft, especially if a disparate-sized donor button cut with a smaller-than-marked diameter blade is placed inadvertantly in a recipient opening made with a blade of larger-than-marked diameter. Known-diameter, disparate-sized graft and recipient opening can be used to advantage, however, as will be explained in subsequent chapters. Disposable trephine blades are used also with motorized trephines.

The *Lieberman single-point, cam-guided corneal knife* (Plate 5-2, *D*) is a manually operated, single-point, corneal cutting device that is fixed to the eye vertically by a low psi suction device applied over the sclera-conjunctiva peripheral to the cornea, just outside the corneal ring. A precut razor fragment, held at an accurate cutting angle by a clamp in a rotating bezel, is turned clockwise and cuts progressively into the cornea. The single point is guided by a cam incorporated in the cutter handle. The cam can be set to cut either a circular or an oval opening of a selected shape and diameter. The depth of the blade is advanced manually by a depth-setting screw turned counterclockwise as the progressive depth of the cut is monitored with the operating microscope.

Initially, the set screw is adjusted so that the tip of the razor blade just engages the corneal epithelium. A complete rotation of the cutting handle is then made. The mark made should correspond to a corneal mark made by the selected diameter trephine blade prior to placing the cam cutter on the eye. The blade is then advanced by a one-half turn of the depth-setting screw for each rotation. The handle is rotated and the blade advanced, in turn, until penetration is almost complete. The suction is released, and the cutting of the posterior lamella is completed with razor knife and corneal scissors. When properly employed, the razor knife cuts an accurate vertical edge and allows variation of the recipient shape to correct preexisting meridional errors.

Very accurate linear corneoscleral cutting is possible with the MUDO oscillating knife (O.K.) (Plate 5-3, *A*). MUDO is the Melbourne University Department of Ophthalmology under the direction of Professor Gerard Crock. The oscillating knife not only has been used routinely in anterior segment surgery performed by this group over the last 8 years but also has had an important role in experimental lamellar corneal grafting leading to the development of the contact lens corneal cutter (C.L.C.C.) (Fig. 5-3, *B*).

The C.L.C.C. allows extremely accurate and rapid microsurgical preparation of corneal buttons for penetrating graft. Further, because it makes exposure of Descemet's membrane possible over wide areas of recipient cornea, it promises to extend the indications for lamellar grafting.

Blades in both the O.K. and the C.L.C.C. do not cut the soft tissues of the conjunctiva, Tenon's capsule, or iris. Complete entry into the anterior chamber is thus safer than with traditional keratomes, trephines, or scissors.

The illustration shows the C.L.C.C. in use. The instrument can be flash autoclaved. It is controlled by hand, causes no distortion of tissues, requires no external fixation of the eye, and eliminates the need for separate puncture sites for anterior chamber injections of air or liquid while grafting is in progress. Unlike the Lieberman trephine, it does not require any suction apparatus. One of its more remarkable applications is in surgery of the conical cornea where, for the first time, it provides the surgeon with optically defined limits to the cone.

While both instruments have independent roles, they may be used together and in combination with donor holding devices (not illustrated here), which form a completely revolutionary system for corneal microsurgery. These instruments are being manufactured by Grieshaber.

The *Troutman keratoplasty (corneal) scissors* (Plate 5-1, *Q*, and see Volume I, Plates 2-9 and 2-10) have short, curved blades of equal length. The crossing of the blades is the reverse of that of cataract scissors. The lower blade closes inside the curve of the upper blade to make a vertical incision rather than a shelved incision (see Plates 6-10, 6-11, and 6-12, and Volume I, Plates 3-7 and 6-18). The scissors are never closed completely. When cutting a continuous incision, the scissors are not withdrawn until the incision is completed. The closing of the scissors tips is prevented by the interpositioning of a stop between the handles. The stop serves also as a catch to hold the scissors closed in order to protect the blades when not in use.

The *GS-14 Ethicon needle* (Plate 5-1, *R* and see Volume I, Plate 4-5) is a short, 5.5-mm, 160° curved needle with a steep curvature to penetrate more readily the cornea to the depth of Descemet's membrane or through and through. The wire size of the GS-9 and GS-10 needles is retained to provide a broad, sharp point and to provide better resistance to bending or straightening of the needle shaft. The tract cut by the needle is sufficiently large to

Plate 5-3

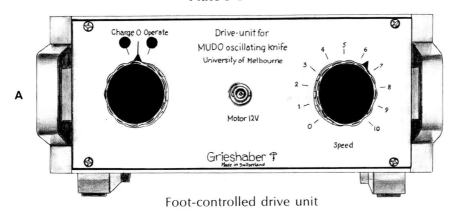

Charge O Operate   Drive-unit for
MUDO oscillating knife
University of Melbourne

Motor 12V

Grieshaber ₱
Made in Switzerland

Speed

A

Foot-controlled drive unit

Fitted with
oscillating knife

B

Drive motor in
autoclavable handle

C

MUDO oscillating knife and trephine.

permit the suture knot to be retracted or buried easily within it (see Volume I, Plates 4-7 and 5-15). Finer wire sizes are designated as GS-16 and GS-17 Ethicon needles. Similar needles are made by several other manufacturers to arm 10-0 monofilament nylon; especially sharp are the Alcon CU1, CU2, and CU3 needles.

Elastic monofilament suture thread (Plate 5-1, *R*) is essential to microsurgical technique and to the use of deep and, in particular, through-and-through suture placement. A new elastic monofilament suture thread made of *polypropylene* or *Prolene* (Ethicon) is available in fine microsurgical, *16- and 22-micron* diameters. This suture material has the desirable properties of being elastic and monofilament, but, unlike nylon, it is non-wettable and non-biodegradable. Nylon thread is absorbed eventually, though often not for several years in situ. However, when a portion of a loop dissolves, the remaining loosened thread can become irritating. For optical or anatomic purposes, it may be important to maintain tissue fixation or wound compression for a period longer than 1 or 2 years. The eventual dissolution of the nylon thread could be a functional disadvantage, for example, if used for intraocular lens fixation.

Polypropylene has been used for all the current ophthalmic microsurgical procedures in which monofilament nylon suture is being employed. My 2-year experience with polypropylene thread indicates that the surgical results using these two threads are essentially similar and, for all intents and purposes, the threads are interchangeable.

Because of its non-wettability, polypropylene tends initially to produce slightly more surface reaction than does monofilament nylon of the same diameter. As soon as epithelialization has taken place over the surface segment of the suture loop, the irritation resolves. The reaction around the suture is the same or less during the remainder of the postoperative period. In no instance has polypropylene suture been seen to biodegrade or the knot to untie during the period observed.

Polypropylene, because of its non-biodegradable feature, may eventually replace nylon as a more desirable elastic monofilament suture thread for ophthalmic microsurgery. Polypropylene promises also to be a better thread for use as iris suture, to fixate an intraocular lens implant to the iris (as in the Worst medallion lens), and to tie together the polypropylene loops through the iridectomy to suspend the Binkhorst four-loop lens.

The weight, action, feel, and angulation of the classic *iris (Barraquer-de Wecker) scissors* (Plate 5-1, *H,* and see Volume I, Plates 2-1, 2-2, and 2-11) are eminently satisfactory for several uses during keratoplasty. In particular, they are useful for microsurgery of the iris—sector, marginal, and peripheral iridectomies and iridotomies—and other incisions and excisions of the iris during anterior segment reconstruction. They are used also for Weck-cel sponge vitrectomy, since the angulation of these scissors provides an unimpeded view of the surgical area.

The *Vannas scissors* (Plate 5-1, *V,* and see Volume I, Plate 2-12) is a fine scissors, available either in stainless steel or in titanium, having many uses during keratoplasty. Their small size allows them to be used when the Barraquer-de Wecker scissors are too gross or cannot be held to cut at an optimal angle. The sharp tips of Vannas scissors enable the surgeon to make precise corneal cuts; for example, in the Troutman corneal wedge resection or in removing tags of corneal lamellar tissue remaining after faulty trephining or lipping of a recipient margin during corneal scissors excision. They are useful also for the precise cutting of the iris required to reconstruct the pupil.

The *iris-vitreous spatula* (Plate 5-1, *C,* and see Volume I, Plates 1-7 and 2-13) is an instrument used to probe, to sweep, and to disengage iris or vitreous. It is useful also in positioning an intraocular lens, since its fine diameter permits manipulation through the wound in an air-inflated or fluid-reformed anterior chamber, minimizing the possibility of corneal endothelial damage.

SPECIAL INSTRUMENTATION

During lamellar keratoplasty, *corneal splitting and dissecting spatula knives No. 1, No. 2, and No. 3* (see Volume I, Plate 2-13) enable the surgeon to dissect corneal lamellae manually either in sector or in toto. They are designed to remain within the selected lamellar plane of dissection (see Volume I, Plate 8-12).

Straight (Harms) and curved (Troutman) tying forceps (Plate 5-1, *W* and *X,* and see Volume I, Plates 2-7 and 5-2) are preferred for tying monofilament elastic suture material, both polypropylene and nylon of any microsurgical diameter. A needleholder or tissue forceps should never be used to tie monofilament suture material, especially not polypropylene. Polypropylene thread tends to shred and be weakened, without the surgeon being aware of it, by the roughened edges of grasping instruments other than tying forceps.

Other suture-handling forceps are pointed, sharp-tipped forceps; straight forceps, such as the MICRA-Pierse plain tip straight (P) forceps (Plate 5-1, *Y*); and angulated tip forceps such as the Troutman suture-handling forceps with the Barraquer-de Wecker–type handle (see Volume I, Plates 2-7 and 5-2). These forceps are used only rarely for tying and are useful primarily for removing suture loops or suture fragments that are adjacent to the needle tract and lying subepithelially (see Plate 14-2, *C* to *E*).

In optical surgery the *diamond knife* (Plate 5-1, *A,* and see Volume I, Plate 2-22) is ideal for making precise, regular incisions, such as in the Troutman corneal wedge resection procedure. It is used routinely for corneal cataract vertical incisions. Since it does not become progressively dull, as does a steel blade, and uniform cutting pressure can be maintained on the blade for the entire incision, the depth and angulation of an incision can be controlled precisely.

Recently, a resharpened and repointed razor blade fragment fixed to a disposable plastic handle, designated "superblade," has been marketed. Though this knife is not controlled as easily or as precisely as the diamond knife and does become dull quickly in use, it is much sharper and consistently more reliable than the cracked razor-blade knife. It is also much less expensive than a diamond blade, which is easily damaged if handled carelessly.

Presently, a number of *vitreous sucking-cutting instruments* (Plate 5-4, *A,* and see Volume I, Plate 9-16) have been developed following the original concepts of Machemer, Douvas, and Kloti. I have used primarily the Douvas and Peyman instruments, both of which have proved to be reliable and to maintain a predictable sharpness. They are quickly, if not inexpensively, repaired and are relatively easy to use from the anterior approach commonly employed in keratoplasty. Cellulose sponges also are useful in detecting vitreous remnants in the wound and on the iris and for fluid-imbibing (see Volume I, Plate 9-14).

The *Barraquer microkeratome* and *corneal optical lathe* have been developed especially for keratomileusis (the regrinding of a corneal lamella into a meniscus or hyperopic lens to correct myopia or hyperopia). It is used also in the keratophakia procedure, when a homograft ground into a convex lens is placed interlamellarly to correct aphakic hypermetropia. The microkeratome consists of a set of corneal suction rings that precisely guide the cutting of the corneal lamella by the microkeratome to a predetermined depth. The suction ring incorporates a grooved guide for the motorized microkeratome head containing a vibrating blade that smoothly excises an exact diameter and thickness of cornea.

A precise microlathe, incorporating a cryo headpiece, is constructed to fix the corneal lamella or homograft tissue and to freeze it with carbon dioxide. The corneal lamella or homograft is cut as a contact lens would be— to the optical power required to effect the desired optical correction of the cornea. In the case of keratomileusis, the anterior corneal lamella is shaped by the lathe. In keratophakia, it is the corneal stroma of a donor eye that is shaped by the lathe.

The results of this surgery have been described fully by José Barraquer.* The techniques have a broad application in the correction of high hyperopic and myopic errors. As a non-intraocular technique with minimal late complications, keratophakia or keratomileusis for aphakia should replace eventually the use of intraocular lenses, especially in the younger patient.

*From Barraquer, José, editor: Keratoplastia refractiva, vols. I and II, Bogota, Colombia, Instituto Barraquer de America.

Plate 5-4

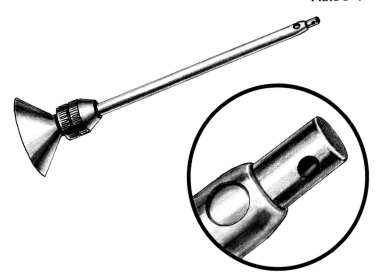

A. Douvas rotoextractor needle (vitreous sucking-cutting instrument).

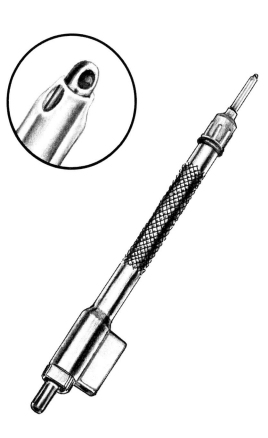

B. Infusion-aspiration tip for extracapsular cataract extraction (as used with Kelman phacoemul-sification unit).

THE SURGICAL MICROSCOPE

The surgical microscope currently in use is essentially the same as the prototype instrument (see Volume I, Plates 1-14 and 1-15). The current production model is known as the Weck IBSM or integral beam splitter microscope (Plate 5-5).

The *translation mechanism* has incorporated a "push-to-recenter" button and a rheostat speed control. The first enables the surgeon to return the microscope to the centered position between surgical procedures, and the latter adjusts the speed of in-plane travel of the microscope head, depending on the magnification used. Higher levels of magnification require a slower speed of translation.

The *coaxial illumination system* has been modified to include two fiberoptic light pipes ("twin beam"). Thus, coaxial illumination is directed in front of, as well as behind, the microscope objectives at an angle of 5° to the objectives. This coaxial illumination system is particularly useful for surgery at or posterior to the iris plane. The illumination that it provides anterior to the iris plane is too flat, destroying rather than enhancing detail. Only oblique illumination should be used for surgery anterior to the plane of the iris.

The *surgical keratometer* has light to the head ports provided by 12 fiberoptic bundles, illuminated, in turn, by a single, larger, fiberoptic bundle illuminated from the light box—but from a separate light source—used for the coaxial illuminators. The surgeon may use, interchangeably, one or the other system. The fiberoptic illumination of the keratometer is fitted with a green filter to reduce reflection and glare and to permit differentiation between the surgical keratometer reflexes and other light reflexes.

The *cine camera* unit now used is a specially manufactured Beaulieu, 16-mm unit with an automatic diaphragm. Procedures can now be filmed with perfect exposure at various magnifications or during zooming. The lens aperture opens automatically as magnification is increased. To ensure sufficiently bright illumination and to prevent fade-in and fade-out as the aperture adjusts at the beginning and end of photographic sequences, it is necessary to set the film speed indicator governing the automatic diaphragm aperture to 25, when 164 ASA film is used. This adjustment is necessitated by the light loss in the 50-50 IBSM prism system. This light loss from the IBSM system is noticeable also when the surgeon's field of illumination is compared to that of the assistant using a binocular zoom microscope, which views at an angle of 17° to the view of the surgeon. The illumination available to the assistant's microscope, which is not equipped with a beam splitter, is 50% brighter than that available to the surgeon's microscope. The assistant's biocular *coaxial* microscope attached to a part of the beam-splitter system of the surgeon's microscope has 50% less illumination than that available through the surgeon's microscope, since the light in this system enters through only one objective lens, as with a movie camera. An obvious,

Plate 5-5

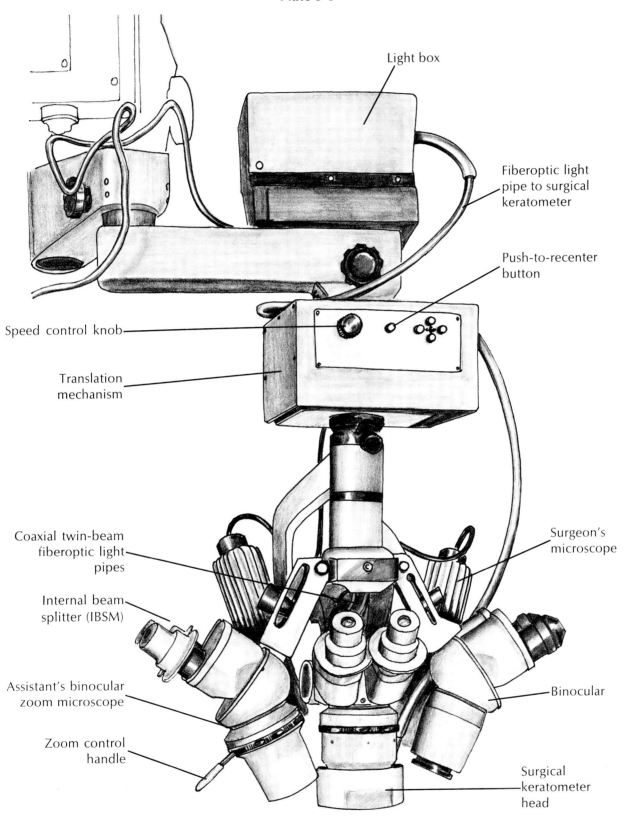

Light box

Fiberoptic light
pipe to surgical
keratometer

Push-to-recenter
button

Speed control knob

Translation
mechanism

Coaxial twin-beam
fiberoptic light
pipes

Internal beam
splitter (IBSM)

Assistant's binocular
zoom microscope

Zoom control
handle

Surgeon's
microscope

Binocular

Surgical
keratometer
head

Troutman IBSM surgical microscope.

but often overlooked, fact is that the image viewed through a beam-splitter system from a single port is monocular. Even when it is viewed through a biocular viewer, depth perception is absent. Surgical assistance through a beam-splitter system should be limited to surgery posterior to the plane of the iris.

When the oblique illumination system is used for anterior segment surgery, light may be increased by using the surgical keratometer as a light source. This unit provides a shadow-free light reminiscent of the multiple light source used for general surgical illumination systems.

A new microscope system under development will improve the depth of field and make possible the use of even higher magnifications. This system will partially offset the light loss of current systems and will allow the integral incorporation of the keratometer and true coaxial illumination.

In keratoplasty, the surgical microscope described may be used comfortably throughout its entire range of magnification, from approximately $5\times$ to $21\times$. Adequate illumination is available at all levels of magnification. The translation system facilitates centered continuous viewing at the highest available magnification levels, since the microscope head may be translated easily and quickly to any desired position without the necessity of reducing magnification. The translation system permits the surgeon to view directly the area of surgical manipulation in the center of the surgical field, where the microscope resolution and depth of field are highest.

The foot control has been redesigned with rocker-type switches that permit twice the number of functions as the older heel-toe pedal-type switches (Plate 5-6). With the present foot switch, rocking the left toe controls focusing, while rocking the left heel controls magnification. Rocking the right toe controls translation from right to left, and rocking the right heel controls translation from front to back. When both switches are depressed simultaneously on one side or the other, the microscope translates *diagonally.* Between the lateral foot switches is the tilt control, which is rarely used, since almost all corneal and cataract surgery should be done from the vertical position, where higher magnification ranges may be used and the surgical keratometer projection will not be distorted by angulation. In order to prevent accidental overriding and actuation of tilt control switches when actuating other controls, a combination handle and foot stop has been placed between the sets of pedals. Switches for additional functions, such as the switch to turn off the focal illuminator, the switch to control the camera, and a third, optional, accessory switch, are situated on a raised panel in front of the foot switches. These can be actuated by the left or right toe, as required. Manually operated switches have been discontinued except for special functions, since their use requires the surgeon to remove one hand from the operative field in order to actuate a given microscope function.

Plate 5-6

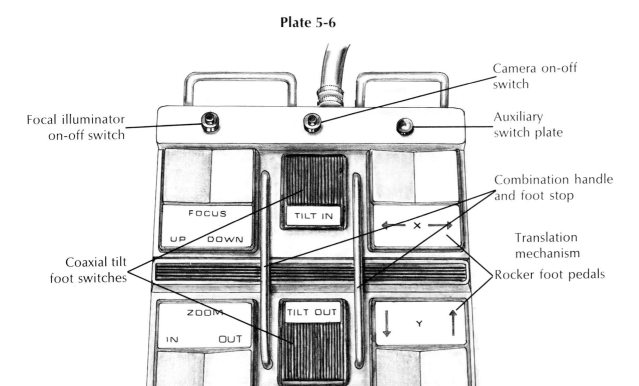

Camera on-off switch

Focal illuminator on-off switch

Auxiliary switch plate

FOCUS
UP DOWN

TILT IN

Combination handle and foot stop

← X →

Translation mechanism

Rocker foot pedals

Coaxial tilt foot switches

ZOOM
IN OUT

TILT OUT

↓ Y ↑

Foot-control panel for the Troutman surgical microscope

More sophisticated methods of control, such as voice actuation; light, color, or heat tracking; and computerized homing devices are being developed for use in future microscope designs. Ideally, these should allow the surgeon to center automatically the operative field with ideal light intensity for a given magnification. This will allow the surgeon better concentration of attention to the surgical procedure.

SUMMARY

Microsurgical instruments and suture materials used in the performance of keratoplasty have been listed, and some that were not covered in Volume I have been described. Most of the instruments are used in all types of keratoplasty. Other instruments of more specialized uses, not included routinely on the standard instrument tray, have been described also.

A thorough knowledge of the ophthalmic surgical microscope, ophthalmic microsurgical instrumentation, and needles and suture materials is essential for the execution of a minimally traumatic, precise, and effective keratoplasty procedure.

CHAPTER 6

COMMON TECHNIQUES

General considerations
Anesthesia, surgical preparation, and
    draping
Placing the lid speculum
Placing the rectus suture
Placing the fixation ring
    The Flieringa wire ring
    The MICRA-Pierse titanium ring
Cutting the recipient cornea with the
    trephine
Suction cutting frames, instrumentation,
    and technique
Cutting the internal corneal lamella
Iridectomy and iridotomy

Technique of midperipheral iridectomy
Iris surgery and suture—coreoplasty
    Technique of iris suturing
Transferring the donor button to the
    recipient
Suturing the graft
Placing the temporary interrupted sutures
Using the MICRA-Pierse titanium
    needleholder
Placing the continuous suture
Testing the integrity of the wound
Completing the operation
Summary

GENERAL CONSIDERATIONS

Some lamellar and penetrating keratoplasty techniques are common to almost every corneal surgical intervention. The particular techniques include those concerned with exposure and immobilization of the globe, preparation of the graft and the recipient bed, suture patterns and suture placement, and concomitant surgery of internal ocular structures, as well as surgery of the adnexa that may be done in preparation for or subsequent to definitive corneal surgery.

ANESTHESIA, SURGICAL PREPARATION, AND DRAPING

The general preparation of the patient for a microsurgical procedure has been outlined in some detail in Volume I, Chapter 7. The patient is quiet, adequately anesthetized, prepared, and draped. The surgeon is in position, with arms well supported. The microscope and the patient's head are stable in relation to each other. The microscope has been focused parfocally for optimal use of the highest magnification levels. The instrumentation has been selected and is appropriately and conveniently placed on the instrument table. Ancillary sterile instruments are immediately available, in case they are required. The operation may begin.

PLACING THE LID SPECULUM

The blades of the Barraquer light-wire lid speculum are held between the thumb and forefinger of one hand, and the spring is compressed lightly. The concavity of the upper blade retracts the upper lid margin while trapping the longer eyelashes under the anterior wire of the blade. With the thumb or forefinger of the other hand, the surgeon gently retracts the lower lid and slips the lower blade of the speculum around the lower lid margin. The tension on the spring is released, and the speculum is centered between the lids. The lids and globe are observed to ascertain that the speculum does not exert pressure. The speculum is used to elevate the lids, and the cul-de-sac is inspected for the presence of mucus or foreign bodies and is flushed again, if required (see Volume I, Plate 3-3). Once the surgeon is satisfied that the speculum adequately exposes the operative site, the operation proceeds to immobilization of the globe.

PLACING THE RECTUS SUTURE

Usually the superior rectus or an adjacent site is fixed by a suture to facilitate downward rotation of the globe. The superior rectus fixation forceps is positioned (see Volume I, Plate 3-4). As the muscle is held away from the globe, a 15-mm, ⅜ circle, reverse-cutting needle, arming a 5-0 silk suture, is passed beneath the belly of the muscle. This technique can cause hematoma of the muscle belly and can even result in partial paralysis of the superior rectus or levator muscle. Alternatively, a GS-9 spatula-type needle, arming a 6-0 or 7-0 silk suture, is passed intrasclerally, just anterior to the insertion of the superior rectus muscle (Plate 6-1). The muscle may still be held with the forceps to fix the globe during suture placement. A reverse-cutting needle should not be used for the scleral bite as it may penetrate the globe or cut out during placement. The suture is used to rotate the eye downward to ascertain that a good position and fixation have been obtained. Additional rectus sutures are placed, if required, using one of the techniques described.

Plate 6-1

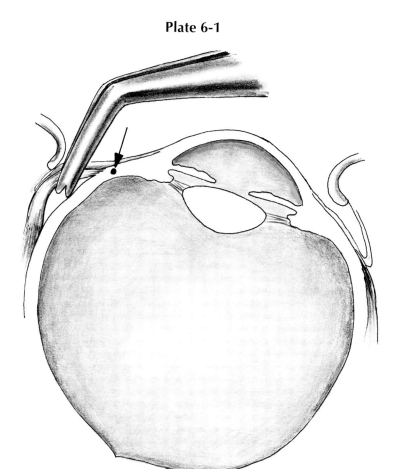

Position of intrascleral
retraction suture (arrow).

PLACING THE FIXATION RING

I routinely use a scleral fixation ring during phakic or aphakic kerato-plasty. Though the scleral ring was intended originally to reduce vitreous loss, it functions better to provide circumferential support for anterior segment surgery. In keratoplasty, during the removal of the pathologic corneal button and during subsequent suturing, the edge of the recipient cornea has less tendency to collapse inwardly or posteriorly, since the ring holds it in better position (Plate 6-2, *A*). Another advantage is that the ring, rather than the recipient corneal edge, can be grasped during needle passage. Grasping the ring to immobilize the recipient cornea avoids unnecessary trauma to the tissue (Plate 6-2, *B* and *C*). If vitreous loss occurs or if elective vitreous surgery is performed during the intervention, the ring is used to elevate the globe to prevent collapse of the posterior segment as vitreous is excised. The LeGrand ring (Plate 6-2, *D*) or the Girard scleral expander (see Plate 5-2, *C*) provides better support than a single ring. In some circumstances, elevating a single ring too forcibly can place excessive tension on the rectus muscles. The extraocular muscles compress the posterior segment of the opened globe from four quadrants, and vitreous is squeezed out of the eye. This must be borne in mind when vitreous loss threatens. Extreme care must be taken when manipulating the scleral ring, since the situation can be worsened rather than helped. Properly employed, a scleral ring or expander is of great value in routine surgery of the anterior segment, in surgery of the uvea and vitreous, and in management of iatrogenic vitreous loss.

Two types of rings are employed for routine keratoplasty, the wire-circle Flieringa ring (see Plate 5-1, *L*) used primarily in aphakic keratoplasty, and the flattened, hoop-type, MICRA-Pierse titanium ring (see Plates 5-1, *M*, and 5-2, *B*), used primarily in phakic keratoplasty.

Plate 6-2

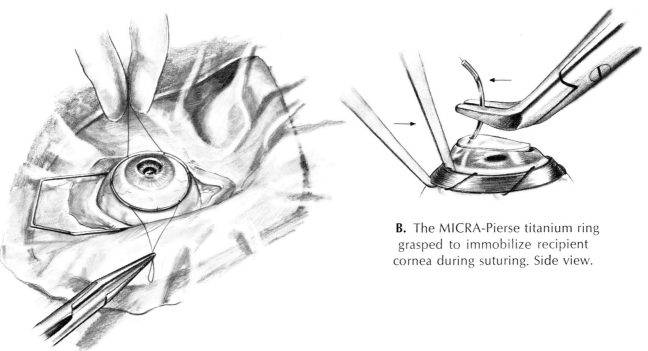

A. Flieringa ring used to prevent collapse of the globe.

B. The MICRA-Pierse titanium ring grasped to immobilize recipient cornea during suturing. Side view.

C. The MICRA-Pierse titanium ring grasped to immobilize recipient cornea during suturing. Frontal view.

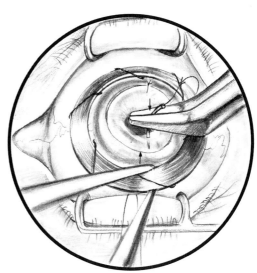

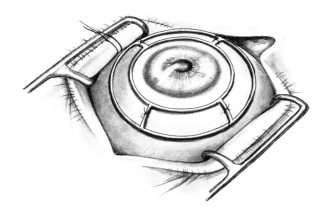

D. The LeGrand ring in place on the globe.

The Flieringa wire ring

A Flieringa circular-wire ring is placed to surround the limbus and is fixed to the sclera by four *interrupted sutures*. Though additional interrupted sutures require more time for placement, they also provide better anterior scleral support (Plate 6-3, *A* and *B*). To facilitate subsequent manipulation of the globe by the ring, a 4-inch loop of suture is left intact between the 10 and 12 o'clock bites and between the 4 and 8 o'clock bites. Additional interrupted sutures, when used, are placed between the loop-connected suture bites. A magnification of 8× to 10× is used to ensure exact insertion and positioning of each needle bite.

When tied to the rigid ring, a malpositioned suture distorts the opened globe. After trephining, the recipient opening will tent toward one or another of the poorly placed, ring-fixation sutures (Plate 6-3, *C*). To relieve the distortion of the recipient opening, the offending suture or sutures must be removed and replaced accurately. Failure to do so will result in malapposition as the graft is sutured in place, defective healing, and meridional optical distortion. An uncorrected recipient corneal distortion, resulting from a badly positioned ring-fixation suture, causes erroneous readings with the Troutman surgical keratometer. This prevents the surgeon from tensioning correctly the individual suture loops as they are placed and adjusted. For this reason, it is prudent, even if no distortion from the ring is evident prior to or during the placement and tensioning of the sutures, to recheck the surgical keratometer projection and to make a final suture adjustment after removing the ring.

Plate 6-3

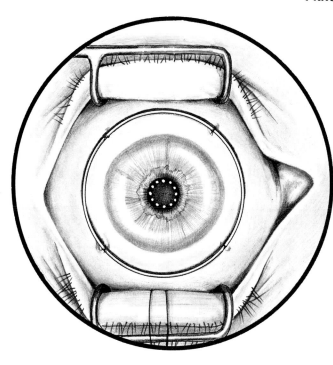

A. Four sutures fixing Flieringa ring (phakic keratoplasty).

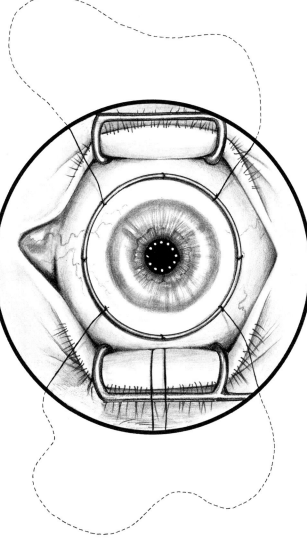

B. Flieringa ring fixed with eight sutures (aphakic keratoplasty).

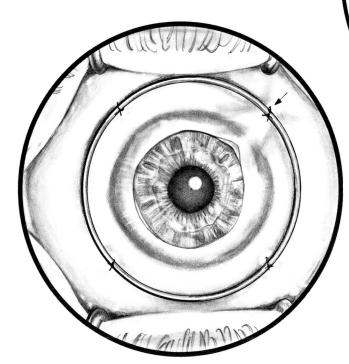

C. A too-tight, ring-fixation suture (arrow) distorts the recipient opening.

It is important to use a spatula needle to place the ring-fixation sutures. I prefer a fine-wire, spatula needle used for corneal suturing, the GS-9 Ethicon needle. The side-cutting point and edges of this needle pass easily intrasclerally. The 137° curvature and 7.2-mm length are ideal for the shallow, midstromal penetration required.

It is not necessary to incise the conjunctiva to expose the sclera for needle placement when fixing either the Flieringa ring or the MICRA-Pierse titanium ring. Neither is it necessary to fix the globe with another instrument. The needle alone should suffice when the following technique is employed.

To begin the needle passage when placing either a Flieringa ring or a MICRA-Pierse titanium ring, the needle is directed perpendicular to the sclera to engage and to fixate the sclera just posterior to the outer circumference of the ring as it is centered on the corneal limbus. As scleral resistance is met, the needle tip is turned gradually to the horizontal plane and passed radially and centripetally intrasclerally for a distance of 1 mm to 1½ mm. The needle is then turned abruptly toward the scleral surface, where it emerges from the sclera and the overlying conjunctiva (Plate 6-4, *A*) and is grasped with the needleholder and retrieved. If a radial or minimally angular, centripetal direction of pressure is maintained during needle passage, the globe, although tending to ride away from the needle, provides sufficient counterresistance for the needle to pass.

The 6-0 (or 7-0) silk suture is tied, using a 2-1-1 surgeon's knot (see Volume 1, Plate 3-5). Needle bites taken to fix a wire ring should not be longer than the width of the ring. If bites are too long, the sclera will buckle and distort the anterior segment when the suture loop is tied.

The MICRA-Pierse titanium ring

The MICRA-Pierse titanium ring is *always fixed with a continuous suture.* Since the ring is flat, the scleral bites can be longer than those used with a wire ring and sometimes are placed diagonally instead of radially. Six to eight equally spaced bites are usually required to fix the ring (Plate 6-4, *B*).

Regardless of the scleral ring used, the scleral bites must not be placed precisely at the 3 o'clock or the 9 o'clock meridian because of the likelihood of piercing a long ciliary vessel. A subconjunctival hematoma under the ring can cause the sclera to buckle. By using relatively high magnification (6× to 8×) to place the scleral suture bites, scleral vessels that could cause such bleeding can be visualized easily and thus can be avoided.

Continuous-suture fixation of a scleral ring is less likely to distort the globe. However, since the inner edge of the titanium ring is closer to the corneal limbus, great care must be taken to center the ring. Malpositioning of suture bites can decenter the ring to such an extent that it will interfere with later surgical manipulation of the cornea.

Plate 6-4

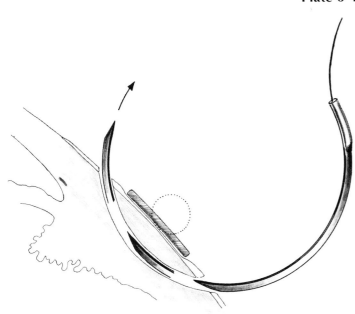

A. Intrascleral needle passage to fix scleral ring (bite may be longer when titanium ring is used). Cross section.

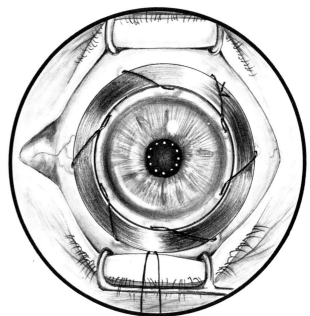

B. MICRA-Pierse titanium ring fixed with 6-0 silk continuous suture.

In order to ascertain whether the scleral ring has been placed and tensioned properly, the projection of the surgical keratometer is observed before and after fixing the ring (Plate 6-4, *B*). In this way, a distortion induced by the ring is detected readily and can be corrected easily prior to corneal trephining. When the titanium ring is used, the surgical keratometer reading is done before the continuous suture is tied. If a distortion is noted only after the knot is tied, the continuous thread often can be adjusted to correct the affected sector.

Once the ring is placed properly, so as not to cause any distortion, its first use is to help fixate the globe during trephining. The surgeon holds the ring with a MICRA-Pierse open-cupped–tipped titanium forceps. The superior rectus suture is held by the assistant to center and to immobilize the globe (Plate 6-5). During suturing also, the surgeon grasps the ring when driving the needle through the recipient cornea.

Plate 6-5

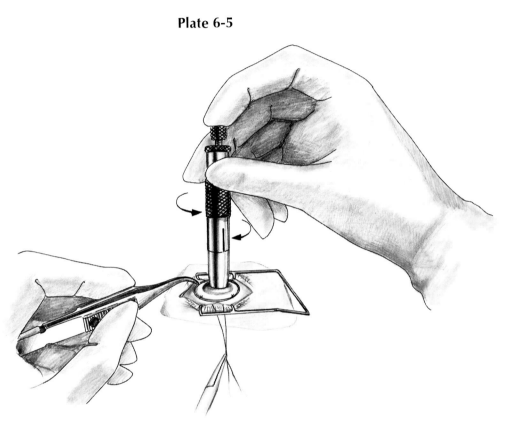

Holding the ring to steady the globe
during trephining.

CUTTING THE RECIPIENT CORNEA WITH THE TREPHINE

The eye is positioned and fixed so that the center or optical axis of the cornea is perpendicular to the objective of the microscope (Plate 6-6, *A*). The projection of the surgical keratometer aids the surgeon in centering the cornea. For keratoplasty, the microscope should always be in the vertical position, not tilted (see Volume I, Plates 1-6 and 1-7). For trephining, the microscope optics are zoomed to the lowest magnification, 4×. Under low power, the anterior globe and its relationship to the trephine can be visualized.

The cutting edge of the trephine blade is inspected under highest magnification and, if dulled or damaged, is replaced (Plate 6-6, *B*). The depth of the trephine cut is set by adjusting the obturator of the trephine handle for partial or full penetration, according to the requirements of the particular operative procedure to be performed (Plate 6-6, *C*).

Plate 6-6

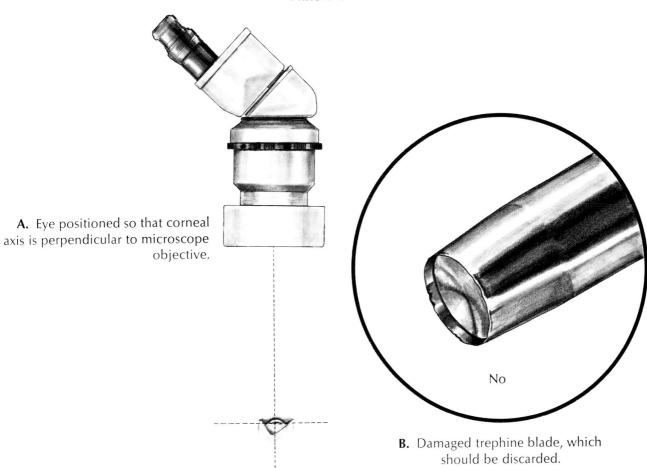

A. Eye positioned so that corneal axis is perpendicular to microscope objective.

No

B. Damaged trephine blade, which should be discarded.

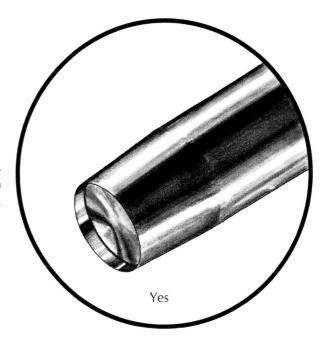

C. Blade suitable for trephining. Obturator retracted for 1-mm cutting depth.

Yes

The knurled trephine handle is held between the thumb and second finger, and the tip of the index finger is placed on the depth-setting screw on top of the handle. The trephine blade is placed on the cornea and centered, and the handle is rocked from side to side to verify its verticality by parallax. The thumb and second finger release the knurled handle while the position of the trephine on the cornea is maintained by pressure from the index finger alone on the top of the handle (Plate 6-7, A). The handle is again rocked gently from side to side to verify that the trephine blade is centered (Plate 6-7, B). If it appears not to be centered precisely, the handle is regrasped and the trephine lifted slightly off the corneal surface and repositioned. The surgeon should be satisfied not only that the trephine is in the proper position but also that the diameter selected is sufficient to include within its circumference the pathology to be excised.

The trephine blade is advanced into the cornea by slowly rotating the knurled handle between the thumb and second finger. The index finger exerts only the very lightest pressure as it steadies the trephine handle (Plate 6-7, A). The cut should be effected only by the weight of the trephine handle and the sharpness of the blade as it is rotated. Too much pressure on top of the trephine handle will distort a softened globe, and the blade will cut the cornea irregularly or obliquely. When penetration occurs because of excessive pressure, there is greater tendency for the uvea or lens to prolapse and be damaged by the trephine blade before the blade can be withdrawn.

During cutting, the trephine blade should be turned through a full 360° before reversing the direction of rotation. The blade edge is never equally sharp along its entire length. Rotating the cutting edge through 360° before reversing direction allows each point along the blade edge to cut around the full circumference of the incision, giving a more regular, even-depth cut.

As the trephine is rotated and the blade is advanced, slight side-to-side rocking motions are made to check verticality. The distortion or depression of the cornea, peripherally around the advancing blade, is observed carefully. An even depression of the recipient corneal edge adjacent to the blade indicates that the cut is continuing in a vertical plane. The trephine blade is not withdrawn from the incision until full penetration, as permitted by the trephine obturator, has been achieved or a gush of aqueous or softening of the globe is observed. Should the blade be removed accidentally, duplication of the cut, distortion of the incision, or both may result when the trephine blade is replaced. Therefore great care must be taken when reintroducing the blade in its groove. When the positioning is doubtful, it is better to continue the incision under direct observation with razor knife and scissors.

When a motor-driven trephine is used, it is more difficult to determine whether the trephine is being held perpendicular to the cornea. Since the cutting action of a motor-driven blade is in one direction only and is more rapid, there is less feedback than with a manual trephine. It becomes doubly

Plate 6-7

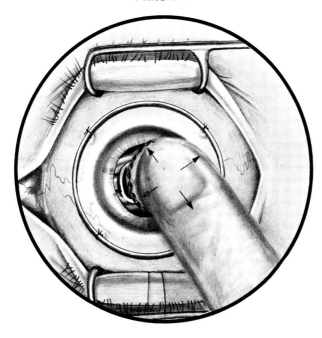

A. Index finger maintains position
of the centered trephine.

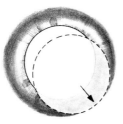 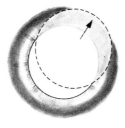

B. Trephine handle is rocked gently
to verify centration.

important, when using a motor-driven trephine, not to err in the initial placement or vertical positioning of the instrument, since a defective cut is almost ensured before the error can be observed and corrected. Nevertheless, an instrument such as the Barraquer-Mateus motor-driven trephine cuts precisely when used correctly.

SUCTION CUTTING FRAMES, INSTRUMENTATION, AND TECHNIQUE

Ideally, a cutting frame fixed to the globe, the orbital rim, or both and supporting a motor-driven or manual trephine in a position vertical to the cornea would allow the blade to cut precisely perpendicular to the center of the cornea and optical axis. Several types of frames that are fixed to the globe by suction have been used to support cornea-cutting instruments. As an example, the lamellar microkeratome of José Barraquer employs a suction ring to fix the microkeratome cutting-blade guide to the cornea during the precise lamellar corneal excision required for his keratomileusis and keratophakia procedures. Lieberman has designed a suction-fixed frame for his single-point, cam-guided corneal cutter. The disadvantage of suction fixation has been the increase in intraocular pressure induced by the negative pressure on the globe. As the guided knife or trephine blade penetrates the eye, the lens and iris diaphragm prolapse onto the knife blade or through the wound. This seems to be less of a problem with the Lieberman suction ring than with the Barraquer unit. Nevertheless, cutting irregularities and damage to intraocular structures are still possible.

To assemble the Lieberman cam cutter, a precisely cut razor-blade fragment is mounted in the jaws of the cam-cutter blade holder. The tip of the single-point blade is set so that it clears the cornea. The cam-cutter unit is placed to rotate within the suction-fixated frame. The knife blade is advanced by a depth-setting screw turned counterclockwise in quarter rotations.

To use the Lieberman device, the surgeon grasps the finger holds of the suction-ring-fixated cutting frame between the thumb and index finger of the nondominant hand (Plate 6-8). Under low magnification (4×), the suction ring is placed to encompass the limbus. It is centered by equalizing the rim of sclera between the suction rim and the corneal limbus or the pupil while observing through the microscope. Moderate (15 inches of water) suction is then applied and the suction ring fixes firmly to the perilimbal conjunctiva.

The depth-setting screw is turned counterclockwise until the tip of the razor-blade fragment just touches the corneal epithelial surface. A 360° clockwise rotation of the cutting frame is made by turning the knurled circular bezel between the thumb and forefinger of the dominant hand. This rotation must be clockwise, for the angle of the cutting edge of the razor fragment is slightly inverted so it will rip rather than cut down through the cornea as it rotates. Following each clockwise rotation of the cutting frame, the razor-blade tip is advanced *counterclockwise* in quarter turns of the depth adjustment screw, so that the blade point cuts progressively deeper until it reaches the level of Descemet's membrane. Since the single, cam-cutter knife blade is maintained perpendicular to the cornea by the suction frame, the thickness of the cornea is incised vertically in any regular shape, as determined by the shape of the cam used. When the knife is observed to

Plate 6-8

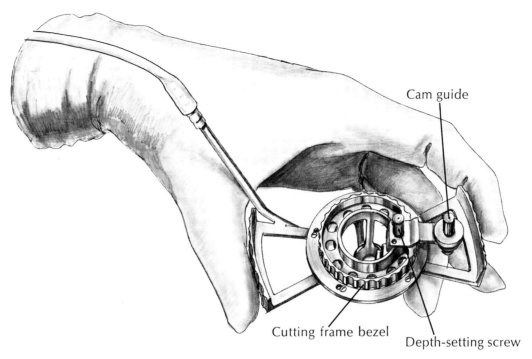

Cam guide

Cutting frame bezel

Depth-setting screw

Lieberman cam cutter grasped by finger
holds of suction-ring frame (cam cutter
and adjusting screws assembled to frame).

penetrate the anterior chamber slightly, the suction is stopped and the unit withdrawn. After initial penetration, usually only a very thin posterior lamella or Descemet's membrane remains to be cut. Incision of the remaining deep lamellar layer is completed with a diamond knife or scissors.

With the single-point cutter, it is possible to adjust the knife blade selectively to cut deeper in a sector where the cornea is thicker. A single-point cutter has the added advantage that by changing the cam on the cutting frame, the same unit can be used to make not only different-diameter circular cuts but also oval-shaped cuts. Thus, a round or oval graft of dimensions selected to compensate specific optical or pathologic defects can be cut precisely.

CUTTING THE INTERNAL CORNEAL LAMELLA

If the internal corneal lamella is left intact deliberately, the depth of the incision is verified by gently separating the wound margins, using the tip of a razor knife to depress the proximal wound lip (Plate 6-9, *A*). The incomplete incision is opened into the anterior chamber between 8 and 10 o'clock (for the right-handed surgeon) or between 2 and 4 o'clock (for the left-handed surgeon) using a diamond or razor knife (Plate 6-9, *B*). As soon as the chamber is entered, the blade is reversed to cut upward to extend the incision into the anterior chamber with greater safety (Plate 6-9, *C*).

Plate 6-9

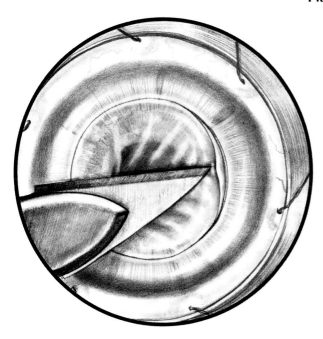

A. Verifying depth of trephine cut.

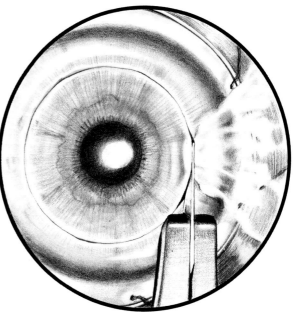

B. Initial penetration into the anterior chamber.

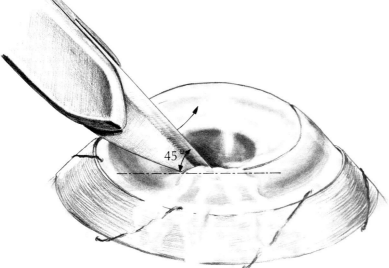

C. Position of blade reversed to extend incision along initial penetration.

45°

From the 9 or 3 o'clock position, the right or left corneal scissors is manipulated more easily to complete the cut. The blades of the Troutman corneal scissors are set uncrossed, the lower blade passing inside the curve of the upper blade to produce a more vertical cut. The inferior blade enters the incision, as would a spatula (Plate 6-10, A), with the flat of the blade held tangential to the surface of the iris. Once the blade is in the chamber, it is turned so that both blades coincide with the incision line and are vertical to the cornea. In fact, the blades are best held in a slightly overcorrected position to ensure that they engage the cornea perpendicularly (Plates 6-10, B, and 6-11, B).

To obtain the smoothest edge possible, the incision is cut continuously. The scissors blades are not quite closed as the tips are advanced. To facilitate this maneuver, the Troutman scissors are equipped with a stop between the handles to prevent the scissors tips from quite closing to their tips. The tip of the upper blade is kept in the trephined cut which serves to guide the scissors as it is advanced (Plate 6-10, B).

Plate 6-10

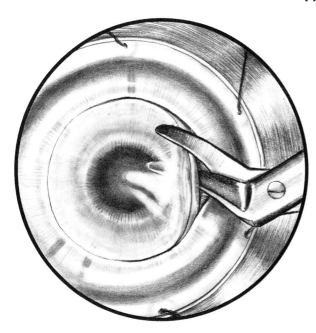

A. Lower blade of corneal scissors introduced as a spatula to avoid engaging iris.

B. Blades turned to engage cornea perpendicularly. Upper blade guides scissors cut in trephined groove.

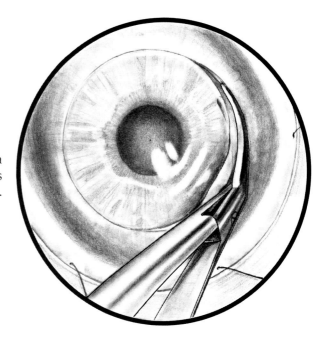

The lower blade is lifted up slightly to open the trephined cut and to keep the lower blade away from the iris (Plate 6-11, *A* and *B*). The thin posterior lamella is easily cut in small sections. If the scissors blades are opened only slightly and advanced in the groove for the next cut, it will be impossible to cut out of the trephined incision line. If the scissors blades are held at an angle, a posterior shelf or undercut will result (Plate 6-11, *C*).

Plate 6-11

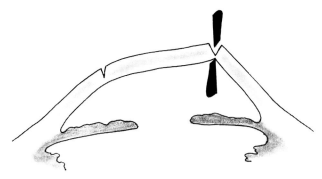

A. Lower blade elevates cornea away from iris. Upper blade guides incision plane in trephined cut. Cross section.

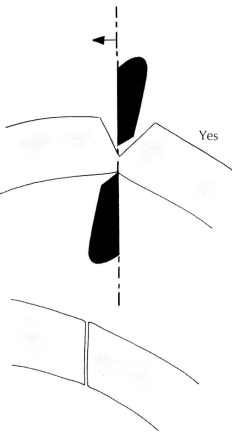

Yes

B. Scissors blades held in slightly overcorrected position to produce vertical cut below. Cross sections.

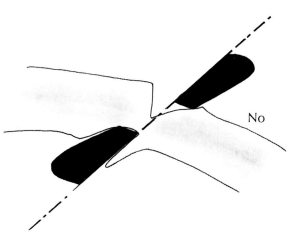

No

C. Scissors blades held incorrectly produce posterior shelving. Cross sections.

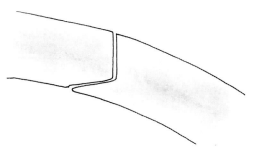

When approximately one-half the circumference has been cut, the MICRA-Pierse open-cupped titanium forceps are used to grasp the pathologic corneal button at its edge at a point 90° to the meridian of the advancing cut of the scissors. This prevents the scissors blades from buckling the cornea and producing an irregular cut as the blades are closed (Plate 6-12, A). Care is taken not to exert too much traction on the button with the forceps because the posterior corneal lamella and Descemet's membrane may be pulled inside the anterior trephined edge of the recipient opening. Then, as the posterior lamella is cut, the stroma and Descemet's membrane retract behind the vertical recipient edge to create an undercut edge. This may cause a posterior wound dehiscence or an astigmatic band (Plate 6-12, B).

When the scissors excision of the recipient corneal button is completed, fluid is sponged from the recipient opening and the iris. Residual tags or lips of deep lamellar tissue can then be visualized readily. To remove a fragment of deep lamellar tissue, the surgeon grasps it gently near one end with an open-cupped titanium forceps and excises it with the corneal scissors (Plate 6-12, C). Again care is taken not to exert excess traction on the lamellar fragment or the recipient wound edge will be undercut (Plate 6-12, B).

It is essential that the recipient cornea be resected accurately, since a defectively cut incision cannot be repaired. A defective incision invariably results in defective apposition of the graft and, should the graft survive, an optical distortion.

Plate 6-12

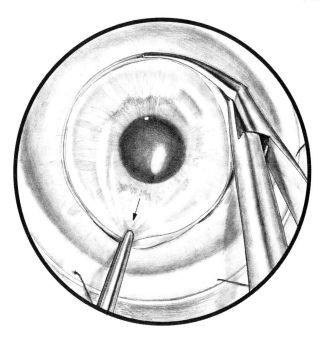

A. Countertraction with MICRA-Pierse forceps aids scissors excision of the button.

B. Excessive traction on pathologic button causes undercutting of recipient rim as button is cut. Cross sections.

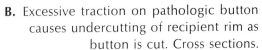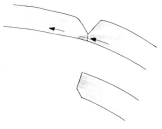

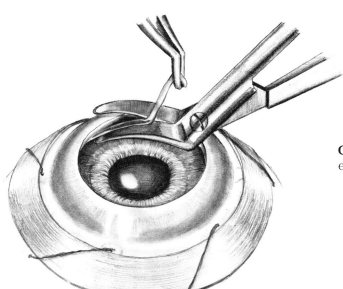

C. Posterior recipient lip being excised with corneal scissors.

IRIDECTOMY AND IRIDOTOMY

When the iris is intact and normal, I perform a *midperipheral iridectomy* in all cases of phakic or aphakic keratoplasty to prevent possible pupillary block. Iris sphincter atrophy and paralysis can occur from an unrelieved intraoperative pupillary block prior to or during suturing of the graft to the recipient or postoperatively. Observing this precaution, I have not encountered any cases of iris paralysis and atrophy, as Urrets-Zavalia and others have reported following keratoplasty for keratoconus. In the usually young keratoconic patient, increased posterior pressure often causes forward movement of the lens and iris diaphragm during suturing of the graft. Necrosis of the iris central to the recipient edge can result as the lens presses the iris against the cut edge of the recipient and prevents peripheral escape of aqueous, causing further increase in the pressure. A simple midperipheral iridectomy relieves the pupillary block and prevents pressure build-up to the level at which strangulation of the sphincter can occur.

In aphakic keratoplasty or in combined cataract and keratoplasty, one, or sometimes several, midperipheral iridectomies are used. These will prevent postoperative pupillary block caused by formed vitreous or postoperative inflammatory reaction, especially when extracapsular extraction of the cataract is performed. Prior to keratoplasty, the normal pupil is neither constricted nor dilated deliberately by medication. In any event, a pathologic iris usually cannot be constricted or dilated, but this should be determined preoperatively because coreoplasty may be required.

Technique of midperipheral iridectomy

With the open-cupped titanium forceps, which is held in the nondominant hand, the iris midperiphery is grasped just under the superior edge of the recipient opening.

Under magnification of 8× to 10×, the sphincter muscle can be seen readily and must be avoided. It is important that the forceps tips do not grasp the sphincter muscle. When the iris is held at the correct level, there should be little distortion of the sphincter. Care is taken also not to disinsert the iris root by pulling up the tissue too forcibly.

As the dilator tissue muscle is brought forward by the forceps tips, a small piece of the iris is cut off just under the forceps tips, using the Barraquer-de Wecker scissors (Plate 6-13, *A*). As the iris retracts, a small lozenge-shaped opening, rather than the triangular-shaped opening typical of peripheral iridectomy, appears. When correctly placed, this oval opening straddles the edge of the posterior aspect of the recipient opening (Plate 6-13, *B*). By coaxial microscope illumination, the red reflex should be visualized through the iridectomy opening. If the iridectomy is incomplete, the retained posterior pigment layer is dislodged with a 1-mm spatula. This remnant is seen more often in brown eyes than in blue eyes. Rarely is there indication for peripheral or sector iridectomy in penetrating keratoplasty.

Plate 6-13

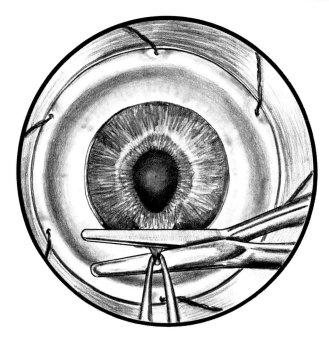

A. Midperipheral iridectomy being cut with Barraquer-de Wecker scissors.

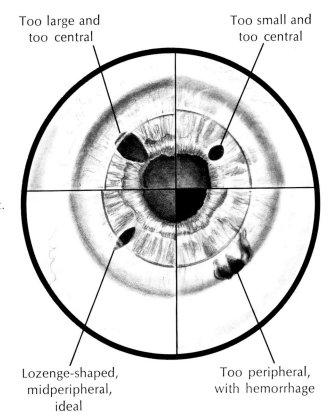

Too large and too central

Too small and too central

B. Iridectomy: ideal and incorrect.

Lozenge-shaped, midperipheral, ideal

Too peripheral, with hemorrhage

IRIS SURGERY AND SUTURE—COREOPLASTY

To interrupt the iris sphincter, or otherwise to excise or incise a portion of the iris diaphragm, increases the likelihood of anterior synechia, closure of the angle, an eccentric pupil, or glare that reduces the function or the final visual acuity or both. In keratoplasty, there often is need for coreoplasty to repair a disrupted iris or to recenter or repair a pupil distorted by inflammation, surgery, or trauma.

Radial sphincterotomy or sphincterectomy may be done, using the Vannas scissors, to enlarge a small pupil or to reposition an eccentric pupil. In the latter case, a sphincterectomy or sphincterotomies often are done in combination with suture of an iris coloboma. In enlarging a small, fixed pupil, such as can result from prolonged administration of miotics, an improved cosmetic result can be obtained with four or more small radial sphincterotomies rather than with a single, deep, radial iridosphincterotomy (Plate 6-14, *A* and *B*). Small tags of tissue, which may remain between the short sphincter incisions, can be trimmed away with Vannas scissors to make a rounded-out, more normal-appearing margin.

When an iris coloboma is present, made at previous surgery, by trauma, or, unavoidably, during an extensive iris dissection at the same intervention, one or two edge-to-edge iris sutures are used to close the dehiscence.

Coreoplasty can be used to restore the continuity of the iris diaphragm and simultaneously to recenter the pupil. If, for example, there is a superior iridectomy and the pupil is displaced upward, a series of small radial sphincterotomies are made in the inferior iris border. Then a marginal sphincterectomy is done to create a new inferior pupillary border (Plate 6-14, *C*). Finally, the enlarged superior coloboma is closed with two sutures to produce a round, central pupil (Plate 6-14, *D*).

Plate 6-14

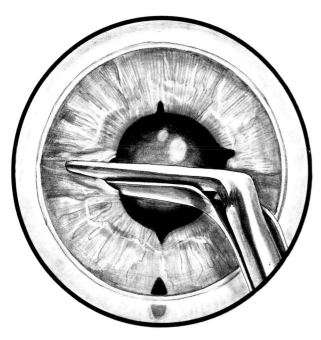

A. Multiple sphincterotomies used to enlarge a small, fixed pupil.

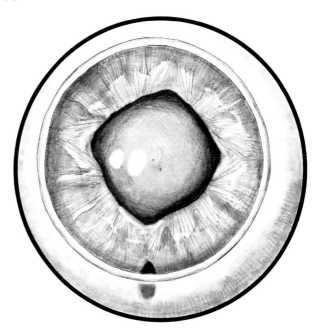

B. Final result. Note midperipheral iridectomy.

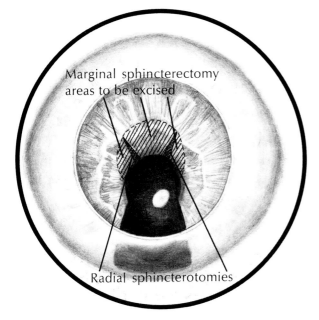

C. Recentering of pupil by radial sphincterotomies and marginal sphincterectomy prior to suturing iris coloboma.

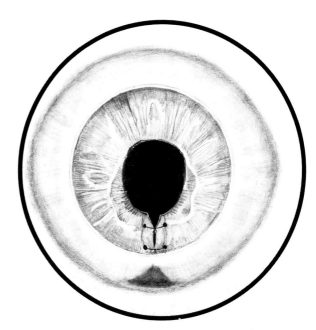

D. Centered pupil with sutured iris coloboma.

Technique of iris suturing

The GS-14 needle, armed with a 22-micron monofilament polypropylene thread, is used to suture the iris. Though 16- or 22-micron monofilament nylon suture material may be used, it is not recommended; for it biodegrades in time, and the repaired iris tissue may pull apart spontaneously. If nylon suture material must be utilized, the larger-diameter size will take longer to absorb.

At 12× to 15× magnification, the smooth-tipped or open-cupped titanium forceps is used to pick up the iris at the free edge radial to the point where needle penetration is planned. The GS-14 needle or the BV-5 special coreoplasty needle, a 160° curved, taper-point, round no. 4 wire needle held firmly with the MICRA-Pierse titanium needleholder, is passed through and through the iris just behind the tips of the forceps (Plate 6-15). It is very important not to pass the needle at a distance from the tips of the forceps. The iris is so elastic it will be pushed away by even the sharpest needle point, causing tearing or disinsertion. As the iris is impaled, it is held on the needle shaft. The tissue forceps can then be released to grasp the opposing iris border. Without releasing the needle from the needleholder, the point of the needle is brought under the fixated opposing iris border and up through and through the iris stroma to emerge just distal to the tips of the forceps. The needle is released, carefully regrasped close to its tip, and pulled through to the thread with the needleholder.

A GS-14 needle must be grasped precisely on its flat surface or it may be twisted suddenly by the needleholder. The round-shaped needle is preferred for coreoplasty. If the iris tissue to be sutured is quite separated, it may be necessary to pass the needle one pillar at a time, or the iris can be torn.

Only a short length of thread, about 10 cm, should be used to provide for tying. If a coloboma suture is preplaced, for example, before a lens extraction or an intraocular lens insertion, a longer thread is used in order to be able to loop the central portion of the thread out of the way. In addition to the thread looped between, an equal amount of thread, about 5 cm, should be left to each side of the coloboma for tying. Though a 3-1-1 tie can be made with the Harms tying forceps, a simple square knot will suffice, since there is usually no tension on the tissue. Care is taken not to close the first loop too tightly, but just tightly enough to hold the tissue in apposition. When the square knot is locked firmly with a third tie, the Vannas scissors are used to cut the thread ends as close as possible to the knot. The razor knife should not be used to cut off the suture threads, since it is not possible to hold the threads sufficiently taut against the soft iris tissue.

In 10 years of experience with iris sutures, 90% for which monofilament nylon was used, I have seen no untoward reactions nor any case of disruption of the sutured iris. It has been shown in the interim that, contrary to popular belief, the iris does heal when sutured. Since the dissolving nylon may have some chemical effect on the angle or on the endothelium, now that nonbiodegradable polypropylene is available, it is preferred.

146

Plate 6-15

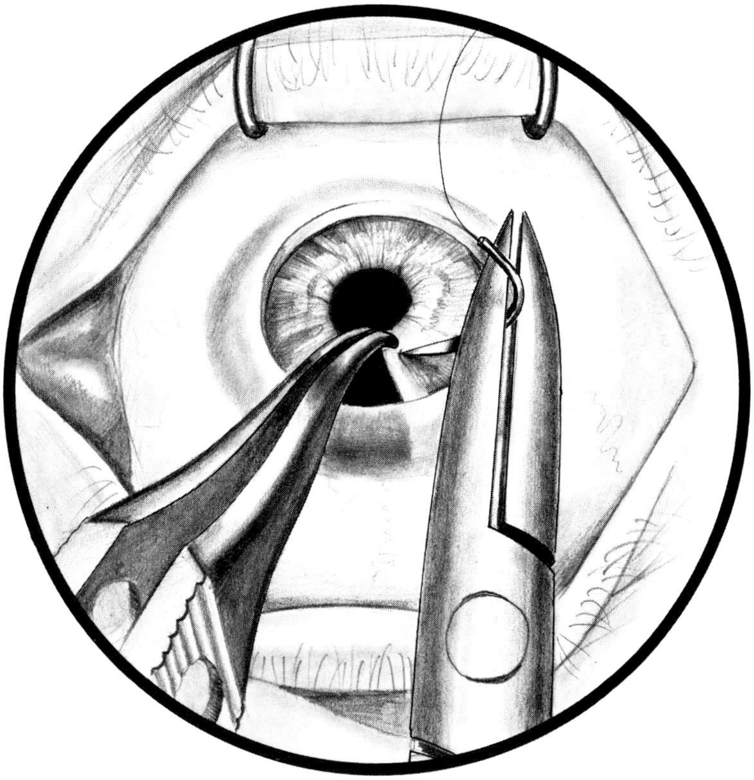

Iris suture used to close a
superior coloboma.

TRANSFERRING THE DONOR BUTTON TO THE RECIPIENT

Using the fenestrated Paton spatula, the donor button is transferred from the Teflon backing block to the recipient eye, care being taken not to touch the endothelial surface with any instrument. The spatula is turned to place the graft in the recipient opening (Plate 6-16). If the button is of disparate size or shape from the recipient opening or its vertical meridian is marked, it is fitted to or aligned with the corresponding meridian or marking of the recipient cornea.

Plate 6-16

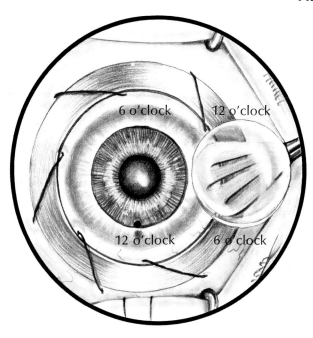

A. Donor button on fenestrated Paton transfer spatula.

B. Spatula inverted to place the button in the recipient opening.

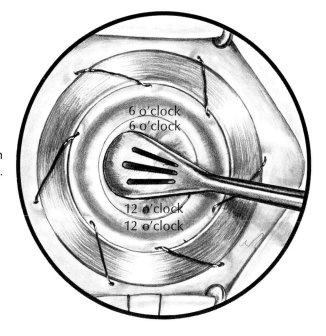

149

SUTURING THE GRAFT

The various suture patterns used to fix lamellar and penetrating grafts to a recipient cornea were discussed in Volume I, Chapter 6. In Chapter 5 of Volume I, the handling of needles and sutures was discussed in some detail. Deep-to-Descemet's-level and through-and-through suturing, as used at the corneoscleral limbus with a shelved cataract incision, were described briefly and were illustrated. Suture placement following lamellar keratoplasty and for repair of trauma was presented in Volume I, Chapters 8 and 9.

In penetrating keratoplasty, the appositional surfaces, though usually vertical, are often disparate in thickness. No matter which suture configuration is used—continuous, double continuous, interrupted, or a combination—accurate placement of the individual suture bites for full-thickness, radial apposition is essential for accurate anterior-posterior corneal alignment and optimal wound healing (Plate 6-17, A).

The techniques for suturing the donor button to the recipient edge differ somewhat from those described for suturing more peripherally at the corneoscleral limbus. They are essentially the same, however, for all types of penetrating keratoplasty. I employ both deep-to-Descemet's-level and through-and-through suturing to close a keratoplasty wound. When surgical conditions permit, through-and-through sutures are used preferentially, since they provide better full-thickness apposition (Plate 6-17, A), especially of the posterior aspect of the incision, and more rapid, secure healing of the full thickness of the wound. In addition to a better anatomic result, there is an improved optical result.

In the following discussion, a through-and-through passage of the needle is described. The deep-to-Descemet's-level suture placement is illustrated but not described in the text, since the needle passage is identical to that in through-and-through passage except for the depth of placement. I use deep-to-Descemet's needle insertion only when the needle tends to catch the iris readily or when corneal tissue is so fragile that a number of through-and-through punctures might cause a severe aqueous leak. In the latter instance, deep-to-Descemet's bites may be alternated with through-and-through bites, for example, in a continuous suture.

PLACING THE TEMPORARY INTERRUPTED SUTURES

A donor button must always be fixed by temporary interrupted sutures. No fewer than six sutures are placed prior to the insertion of the running suture (Plate 6-17, B). If less than six sutures are used, particularly in a larger-sized graft, an operculum flap of corneal tissue is formed between each pair of suture bites. Maintaining a formed anterior chamber, accurate placement of the continuous suture is more difficult. It is important, especially during through-and-through continuous suturing, to reform

Plate 6-17

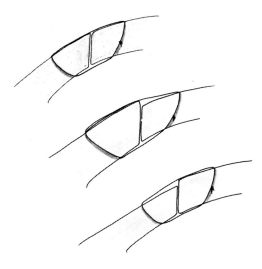

A. Disparate thickness of appositional surfaces requires full-thickness suture bites for optimal closing alignment. Cross sections.

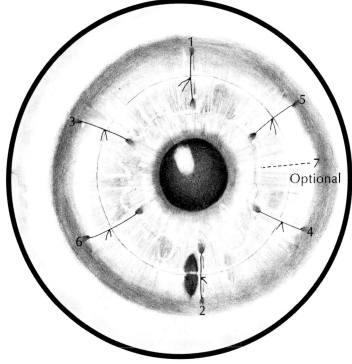

B. Six temporary interrupted sutures in place, in the order of insertion.

the chamber from time to time to be sure that a shred of iris tissue is not caught in a suture loop. One or several additional preplaced sutures may be necessary; for example, during a combined keratoplasty and wedge-resection procedure.

The first interrupted fixating suture is placed at the 6 o'clock position. The suture bites are always taken from donor to recipient. The donor cornea is grasped across its anterior edge with the open-cupped MICRA-Pierse titanium forceps. The forceps tips grasp about two-thirds of the vertical thickness of the corneal edge and a corresponding amount of the adjacent anterior corneal surface. It is essential to grasp an amount of corneal tissue sufficient to ensure good stabilization of the button before attempting to pass the needle. A microbite of tissue will not hold against needle pressure. The teeth of the forceps will punch or tear out a piece of cornea (Plate 6-18, A). *The surgeon must learn not only to grasp the cornea correctly, but also to grasp the cornea only once for each needle passage, to keep trauma to the donor tissue edge to an absolute minimum.* For accurate manipulation, the tissue forceps is always held in the surgeon's nondominant hand, the needleholder in the dominant hand. Microscope magnification during needle passage should be from 10× to 15× or higher.

With the donor tissue grasped firmly between the teeth of the forceps, the GS-15 needle, held at the center of its shaft by the needleholder, is placed perpendicular to the cornea, the point entering just proximal to the anterior forceps tip (Plate 6-18, B and C). *The point of the needle should not be to the right or to the left or even 0.5 mm behind, but precisely centered just proximal to the forceps tip.* The needle shaft should almost touch the end of the forceps tip as the needle is passed under it (Plate 6-18, D). The needle is directed vertically until it penetrates Bowman's membrane.

Plate 6-18

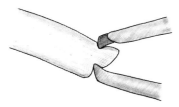

A. Microbite of tissue: danger of tearing or losing grasp of cornea (Bonn forceps). Cross section.

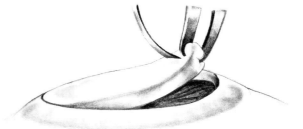

B. Correct tissue grasp with needle in insertion position (open-cupped forceps).

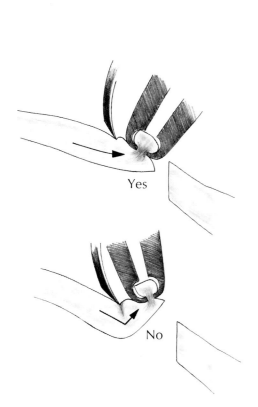

Yes

No

C. Detail of correct and incorrect tissue fixation for needle passage. Cross sections.

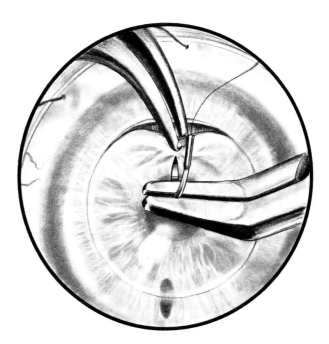

D. Needle precisely centered for insertion.

153

The needle is then directed slightly toward the edge as it passes through the corneal stroma to penetrate Descemet's membrane and the endothelium just proximal to the vertical cut edge of the donor button. Once the needle has been passed through the donor button, the needle point is tipped upward about 30°. This everts the edge of the cornea so that the needle point can be visualized as it exits (Plate 6-19).

Plate 6-19

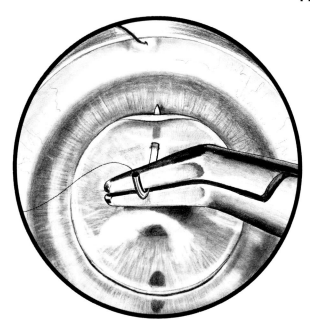

A. Needle passage through and through donor button.

B. Needle passage through and through donor button. Cross section.

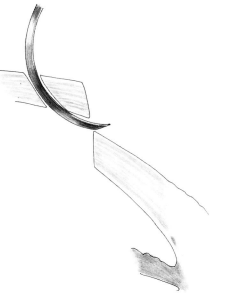

155

When the needle point appears, the edge of the donor button is aligned horizontally and vertically to the edge of the recipient cornea (Plate 6-20, *A* and *B*). The tip of the needle is inserted just posterior to Descemet's membrane and the endothelial surface of the recipient cornea. Then, using the recipient cornea as a backstop, the needle is pushed under and then parallel to the posterior surface of the recipient cornea for about 0.75 mm and is then turned upward abruptly at an angle of 90° to penetrate the endothelium, Descemet's membrane, the stroma, and Bowman's membrane to exit (Plate 6-20, *C* and *D*).

Plate 6-20

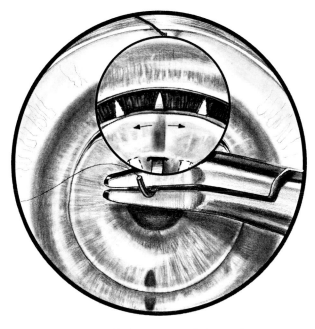

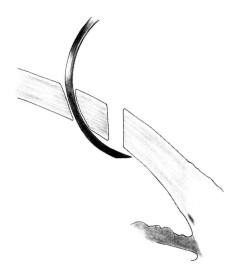

A. Horizontal alignment of donor button and recipient cornea.

B. Vertical alignment achieved by dropping the needle point under recipient corneal edge. Cross section.

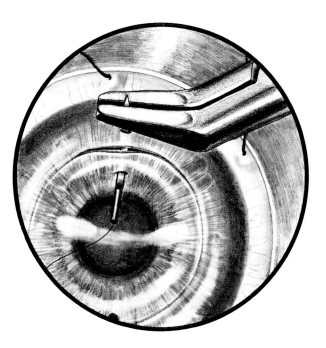

C. The needle exiting from recipient cornea.

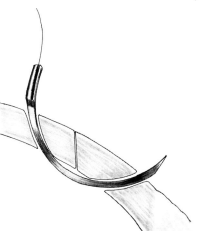

D. Through-and-through needle passage exiting from recipient cornea. Cross section.

As the needle is passed between the cornea and the iris, the tip always must remain bright and in view. A sudden disappearance of the shiny tip or a dulled look may indicate that the iris is caught (Plate 6-21, *A*). The surgeon should then draw back the needle point to disengage the iris. The shaft of the needle can be used as a spatula to keep the needle point from catching the iris (Plate 6-21, *B*).

Plate 6-21

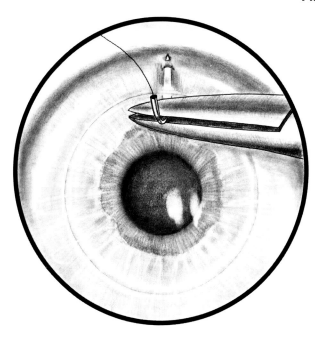

A. Needle catches iris.

B. Back of needle pushes iris away.
Cross section.

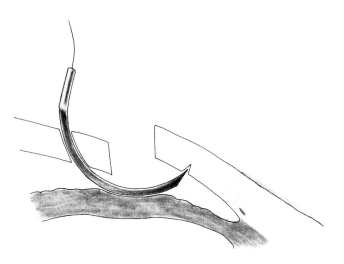

If catching the iris is a continuing problem, through-and-through suturing should be abandoned in favor of deep-to-Descemet's-level suture placement. The needle is introduced into deep stroma on the recipient side, just anterior to Descemet's membrane to avoid accidentally catching the iris. Without grasping the recipient cornea, but steadying the globe by grasping the fixation ring, the surgeon turns the needle to pass vertically through the stroma to exit through Bowman's membrane and the epithelium (Plate 6-22, *A* to *D*). The length of each recipient bite, whether through and through or deep to the level of Descemet's membrane, should correspond roughly to that of the bite through the donor button, 0.75 mm to 1 mm in length. When Descemet's membrane–level bites are passed through the recipient edge, care must be taken not to depress the donor button with the needleholder as the needle is turned to exit. Severe damage to the endothelium can result (Plate 6-22, *E*).

Plate 6-22

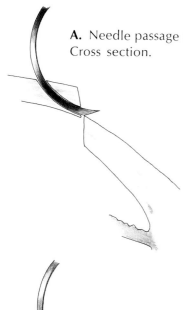

A. Needle passage at Descemet's level. Cross section.

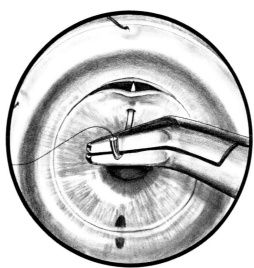

B. Vertical alignment achieved by dropping the needle point to engage the recipient corneal edge at Descemet's membrane.

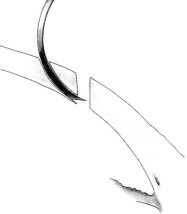

C. Cross section of **B.**

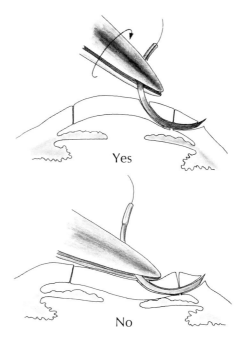

Yes

No

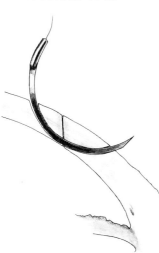

D. Needle passage at Descemet's membrane exiting from recipient cornea. Cross section.

E. Needleholder must not depress donor button. Cross sections.

The needle is not released from the needleholder until the needle exits sufficiently for the shaft to be grasped far enough behind the cutting edge to minimize the possibility of damage to the needle tip. The needle is placed on the cornea and the thread is pulled through with tying forceps, leaving about 2 cm protruding from the needle entrance point. A 3-1-1 tie is made with the tying forceps. The surgeon holds the thread ends taut as the assistant cuts them off about 5 mm from the knot with Barraquer-de Wecker scissors. The thread ends are left long in order to be identified more easily for removal after the continuous suture is placed (Plate 6-23, A).

A second interrupted suture is placed at 12 o'clock, slightly to one side of the midperipheral iridectomy, to avoid possible damage to the lens during needle insertion (Plate 6-23, B). When tying the second or succeeding interrupted sutures, the first triple throw may tend to loosen before the second throw locks the knot. The triple throw can be fixed at the recipient needle opening by twisting the threads 180° and pulling the collapsed knot just to the orifice. The second throw can then be placed without the knot loosening. Since this sometimes forms a slipknot, only the third throw should be pulled up tightly, or too tight a suture loop may be formed (Plate 6-23, C).

Four or more additional suture bites are taken in sequence (see Plate 6-17). The identical technique is used for through-and-through or deep-to-Descemet's-membrane–level radial suture placement for each interrupted or continuous suture bite.

Plate 6-23

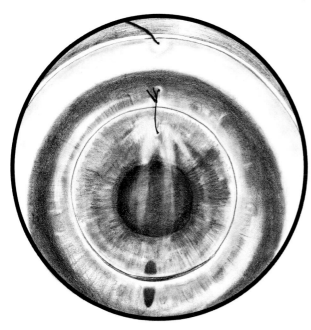

A. First interrupted suture in place.

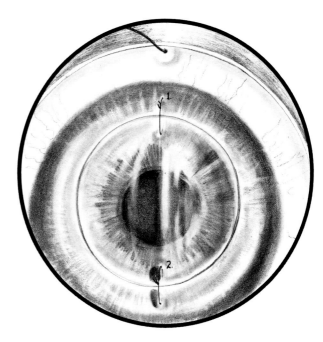

B. Second interrupted suture in place.

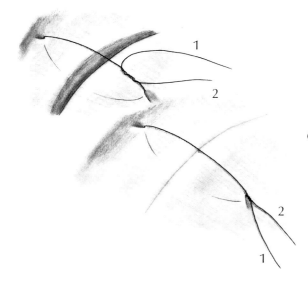

C. Locking triple loop under tension.
Reverse threads and pull collapsed
loop into needle orifice.

USING THE MICRA-PIERSE TITANIUM NEEDLEHOLDER

The MICRA-Pierse titanium needleholder, illustrated inserting the needle to Descemet's level (Plate 6-24), is used somewhat differently from the Troutman 45° needleholder, shown in the illustrations of through-and-through needle passage (see Plates 6-18 to 6-20). The MICRA-Pierse needleholder is preferred, since it can be held within the palm and can be manipulated more easily in tight quarters, where it can be rotated smoothly as it is held with the thumb and first two fingers (Plate 6-24).

Plate 6-24

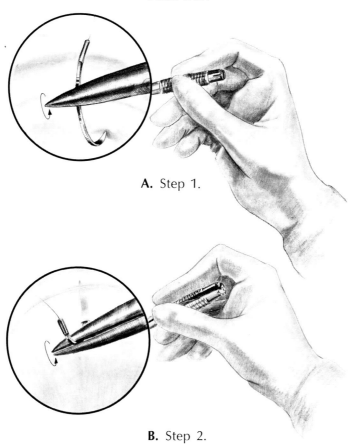

A. Step 1.

B. Step 2.

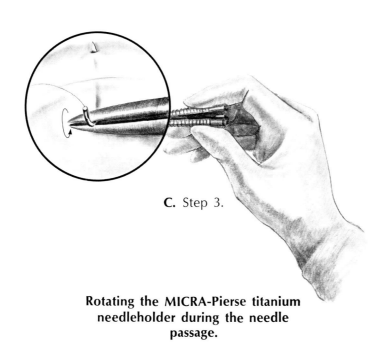

C. Step 3.

**Rotating the MICRA-Pierse titanium
needleholder during the needle
passage.**

However, since the tip of the MICRA-Pierse needleholder is straight and comes to a fine point, the needle must be held correctly (Plate 6-25, *A*). If it is held too close to the needleholder tip ends, it will pop out of the needleholder tips during passage (Plate 6-25, *B*). When the needle is being used next to the nose or in a deep orbit, the needle shaft often must be tilted or twisted slightly in the needleholder tips to be in a position to enter the cornea at the correct angle (Plate 6-25, *C*). In placing a continuous suture, a slight change in the position of the needle shaft between the tips of the needleholder is required for each insertion of the needle (Plate 6-25, *D*).

Plate 6-25

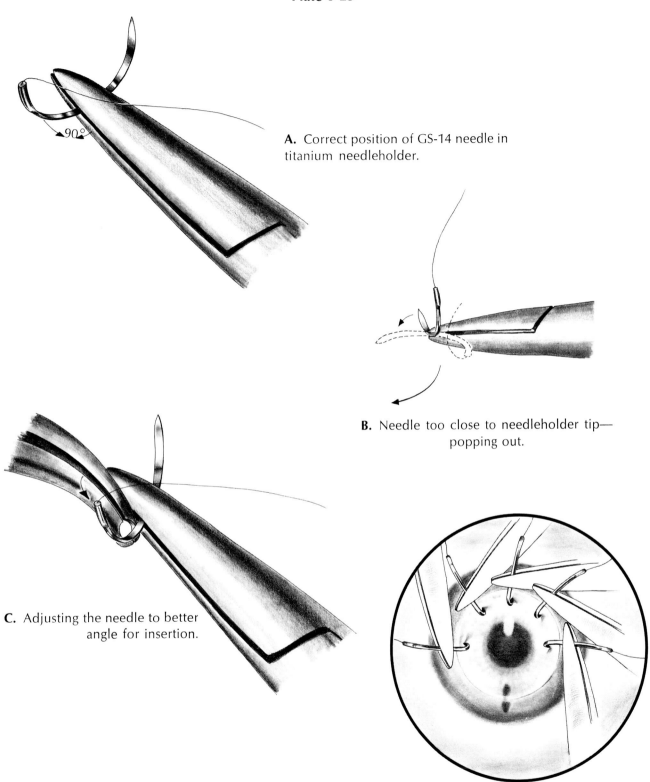

A. Correct position of GS-14 needle in titanium needleholder.

B. Needle too close to needleholder tip—popping out.

C. Adjusting the needle to better angle for insertion.

D. Positioning the shaft to ensure radial passage of GS-14 needle during continuous suture placement.

PLACING THE CONTINUOUS SUTURE

Continuous suture bites are placed radially, through and through, just as are the interrupted bites. As each succeeding bite of continuous suture is placed, the following thread loop can become locked or entangled by the needle or the thread as it is drawn up from the recipient. This can be avoided by using tissue forceps in the nondominant hand to hold the intermediate loop out of the way to the side opposite the direction of passage. Since most of the following loop will be out of the microscope field and not visible to the surgeon, it should be handled gently (Plate 6-26). The assistant, usually working with lower magnification, should observe the loop and warn the surgeon if it is in danger of being tangled or broken.

Plate 6-26

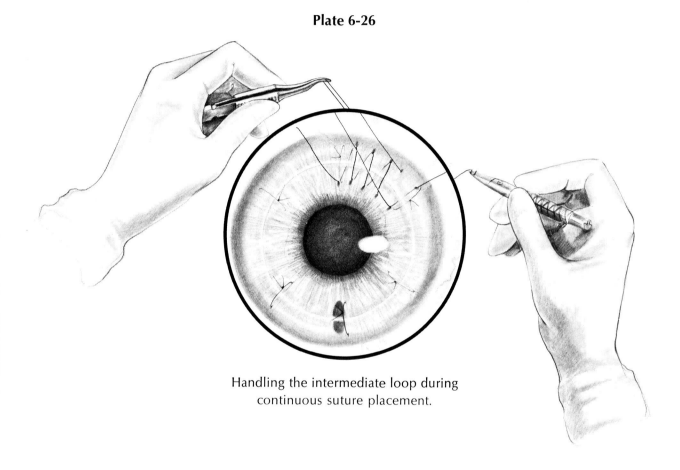

Handling the intermediate loop during
continuous suture placement.

In placing a continuous suture, it is not always possible to place every bite through and through. If desired, alternate bites may be placed to Descemet's membrane level. The needle tract of a through-and-through bite may leak aqueous temporarily. The 20 or 25 through-and-through suture bites make 40 or 50 tiny holes through the thickness of the cornea. Usually, however, only a few leak, and never for more than a few hours following surgery. I have not experienced delayed reformation or loss of the anterior chamber from leaking through-and-through needle tracts.

Since continuous suture bites are equally spaced, it may happen that a bite will coincide with an interrupted suture loop. The interrupted suture will interfere with proper placement of the tissue forceps. To ensure proper placement, a forceps tip is introduced in the incision, a short distance from the interrupted suture, where it can be inserted easily. The forceps tip is then slid along the incision to just in front of where the needle will engage the tissue at the correct level (Plate 6-27, A).

When the continuous suture bites are completed, before tying the knot, each loop successively is pulled centripetally with the curved tip of the closed tying forceps (Plate 6-27, B). This maneuver takes up the slack in the thread. The loose ends of the suture threads are locked by a single triple throw going in the opposite direction. The suture loops are individually tensioned by pulling up each loop gently with a tying forceps and, while holding it with a second tying forceps, pulling up the succeeding loop hand over hand until all loops have been tensioned (Plate 6-27, C). At this time the tying of the knot is completed using three single throws.

Interrupted fixation sutures should be removed with a razor knife and tying forceps immediately after the continuous suture or sutures are placed and tied and the knots buried (Plate 6-27, D). Invariably, the interrupted fixation sutures loosen and torque out of radiality when a single continuous suture is tightened and tied. Only in the rare instance in which only interrupted sutures are used to close a wound can some interrupted *fixation* sutures be left in place.

It is necessary sometimes to place secondary interrupted sutures to control a persistent leak between too-widely placed continuous suture bites. Secondary interrupted sutures may be used also to compensate an astigmatic band, detected by the surgical keratometer, that cannot be compensated by adjusting the continuous suture loops. Such secondary interrupted sutures are left in place, usually for 6 weeks to 3 months postkeratoplasty. They are placed, in depth, to the middle third of the stroma; shorter bites are used than for the fixation or the continuous sutures.

Plate 6-27

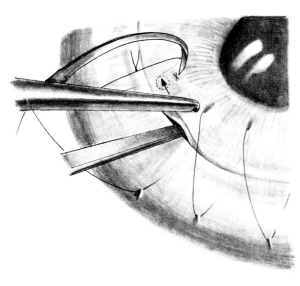

A. Forceps are introduced between wound lips, then slid into position for needle bite near interrupted suture loop.

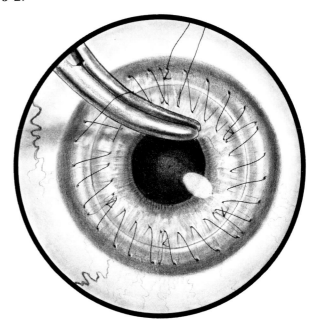

B. Closed curved Harms forceps to pull up slack in continuous suture (clockwise).

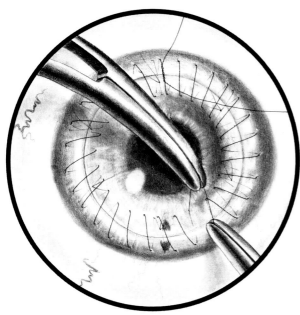

C. Hand-over-hand technique to distribute tension on continuous suture (counterclockwise).

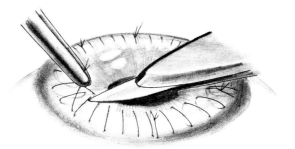

D. Removing the interrupted fixation sutures.

An antitorque suture pattern, such as is described for lamellar keratoplasty, may be used also in penetrating keratoplasty when a single continuous suture is used. While it is more difficult to place the suture bites diagonally, the resultant force is radial and appositional. This is in contradistinction to radially placed bites in a single continuous suture that tend to turn or torque the donor button in the recipient bed. Because of the wider spacing required to place the continuous suture, secondary radial interrupted sutures are needed between the continuous bites. I prefer to use radially placed, double opposing, continuous sutures for a penetrating graft when torquing must be prevented, since they provide firmer radial apposition without the necessity for interrupted sutures.

TESTING THE INTEGRITY OF THE WOUND

An absolutely watertight closure of the wound must be obtained in order to prevent early loss of the anterior chamber, to prevent anterior synechia formation, and to ensure firm, even, long-term healing. When the chamber cannot be well maintained at the close of the procedure, it may be difficult to identify exactly the source or sources of a leak.

When suturing is completed, all air bubbles are evacuated and the anterior chamber is refilled with basic salt solution. An anterior chamber formed with air may not be water tight. Also, retained air bubbles prevent accurate reading of the surgical keratometer.

The chamber usually is readily filled by forcing a stream of basic salt solution through the incision, circumferentially around the recipient to the graft margin, using the Troutman olive-tipped needle (Plate 6-28, A). This technique fills the anterior chamber without the need to introduce the needle between the lips of the incision, which sometimes loosens the sutures or induces prolapse of iris or vitreous.

If the anterior chamber fails to reform completely because a sector of the iris is incarcerated in the wound, a 1-mm spatula is introduced through an opposite sector of the incision to free the prolapsing tissue (Plate 6-28, B). It may be necessary to introduce basic salt solution directly, inserting the tip of a 30-gauge angled needle between suture loops in a tight sector of the incision. The needle should be introduced carefully, obliquely over the iris, not over an iridectomy or the pupil, for the iris may be forced anteriorly to incarcerate.

Plate 6-28

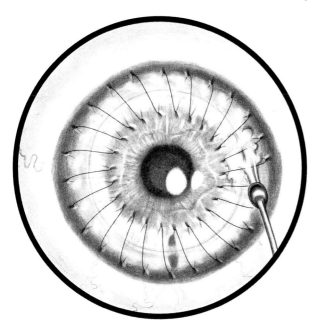

A. Forcing a stream of basic salt solution to reform the chamber, using Troutman olive-tipped needle.

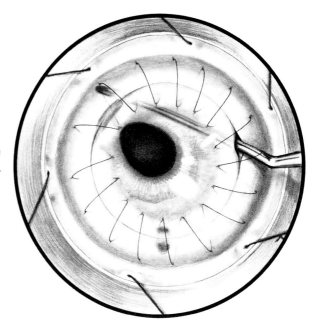

B. 1-mm spatula used to free a section of incarcerated iris.

When the anterior chamber has been filled, the eye is normotensive, and there are no apparent leaks or synechiae. A 1% fluorescein solution is dropped on the globe to cover the cornea completely from limbus to limbus. A persistent aqueous leak produces a telltale bright green flush (see frontispiece). Continuous suture loops are adjusted, tightening the sutures in the area of the leak, loosening those in an apparently too-tight area. This adjustment is refined by observing the surgical keratometer projection, which will identify for the surgeon the loose (usually the flatter meridian) and the tight (usually the steeper meridian) sectors that require adjustment (Plate 6-29). If adjusting the sutures fails to control the leak, a secondary interrupted suture or sutures are placed in the appropriate sector. The leak-controlling sutures are placed with short superficial bites in the anterior one-half to two-thirds of the stroma. The anterior chamber depth and iris position are examined carefully with the slit lamp of the surgical microscope as a final check against incarceration or synechiae. Spatulation of the iris is performed again, as required.

The elasticity of the continuous suture thread recovers soon after surgery. The recovered suture elasticity, combined with swelling of the graft edge, will effectively close a leaking area, and the secondarily placed interrupted sutures usually can be removed within 6 weeks after surgery. Nevertheless, the thread ends should be cut to the knot and the knot buried in tissue, as are the knots of sutures to be left in place for longer periods.

Plate 6-29

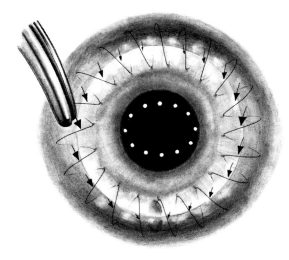

A. Adjusting the sutures to compensate for a meridional distortion.

B. Meridional distortion compensated (use slight overcorrection).

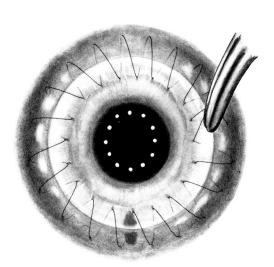

COMPLETING THE OPERATION

The scleral fixation ring is removed by cutting the fixating suture loops with a razor knife, individually in the interrupted sutures or every other loop of a continuous suture. Following the removal of the fixation ring, the corneal curvatures are again monitored by the surgical keratometer, with the eye normotensive and the speculum lifting away the lids (Plate 6-30). Necessary adjustments are made, and a final test with fluorescein is done to be sure that no new leaks have been caused by the suture adjustment. One limb of the superior rectus suture is cut with the razor knife, and the suture is removed from beneath the muscle or from its intrascleral tract anterior to the muscle. The slit lamp is used again for a final check on the position of the iris and the depth of the chamber before the lid speculum is removed.

Plate 6-30

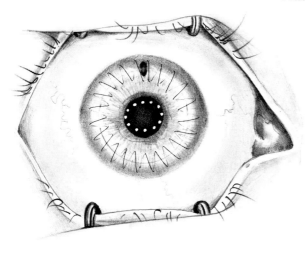

A. Pressure from lid speculum induces meridional error in soft eye.

B. Final appearance after refilling anterior chamber and elevating speculum away from the eye.

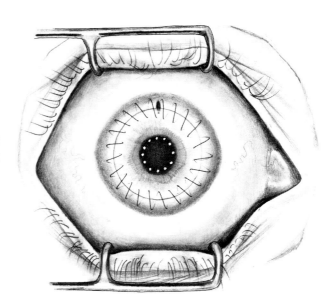

The lid speculum is removed by grasping the spring end of the speculum as it rests over the external canthal area and rotating the blades 90° (Plate 6-31, *A*). The speculum upper and lower lid retractors will be released as they turn into the canthi without it being necessary to hold or retract the lids.

A unilateral dressing is applied (Plate 6-31, *B*) with a protective shield (Plate 6-31, *C*). After the first postoperative dressing, the shield is used without a patch to protect the eye during sleep. The shield is adjusted so that it presses on the bony orbit and not on the globe (Plate 6-31, *D*).

SUMMARY

Techniques common to most keratoplasty procedures have been introduced and described in this chapter in the hope of eliminating some redundancy in the chapters to follow. As specific operative interventions are described in subsequent chapters, some of the techniques discussed here are repeated or amplified in the context of the particular procedure. The techniques described constitute the major technical functions of the surgeon during any given keratoplasty procedure and should be practiced until they become so familiar as to be performed almost automatically. Their execution should be so precise and uniform as to minimize or eliminate those anatomic or optical aberrations that might result from less-than-adequate performance of them. The surgeon who wishes to perform accurately other simple or complex microsurgical procedures should practice the common techniques described in this chapter on animal or eye-bank eyes until they become second nature. Only then will the surgeon be able to attempt the more technically demanding keratoplastic procedures with a reasonable chance of optical, as well as technical, success.

Plate 6-31

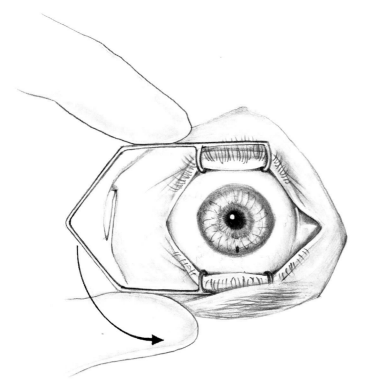

A. Removing the lid speculum
by rotation.

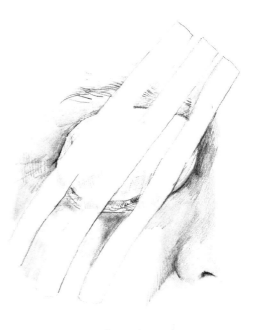

B. Unilateral patch.

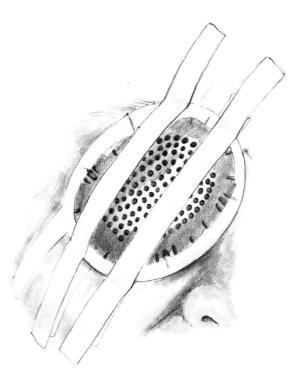

C. Protective shield (used without
patch after 24 hours).

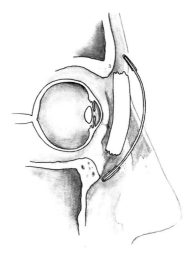

D. Shield supported on bony orbit.
Cross section.

CHAPTER 7

LAMELLAR KERATOPLASTY TECHNIQUE

General considerations
Preparation of the lamellar recipient bed
Technique for successive lamellar
  dissections
Suturing the lamellar graft
  Placing the interrupted fixation sutures
  Placing the antitorque continuous suture
  Final adjustment of the antitorque
    continuous suture

Lamellar keratoplasty combined with
  penetrating keratoplasty
  Preparation of the recipient eye
  Preparation of the donor mushroom
  Suturing the mushroom to the recipient
Lamellar flanged penetrating keratoplasty
Lamellar keratoplasty in keratomileusis and
  keratophakia
Keratoprosthesis
Summary

GENERAL CONSIDERATIONS

Simple lamellar keratoplasty technique has been described in some detail in Volume I, Chapter 8. Lamellar keratoplasty is reserved primarily for tectonic or reconstructive purposes. However, in keratomileusis or keratophakia, its primary function is optical. The various shapes and sizes of lamellar grafts used for tectonic repair were described and illustrated in Chapter 3. Almost any conceivable pattern of lamellar replacement can be formed by a combination of linear and curvilinear incisions to fit the lamellarized recipient bed. The French, and in particular Paufique, are responsible for the concept of and continuing interest in lamellar keratoplasty. Lamellar techniques are still practiced much more extensively in France, where they are often used effectively for vision as well as for tectonic grafts.

PREPARATION OF THE LAMELLAR RECIPIENT BED

Preparation of the lamellar recipient bed in relation to pterygium was described in Volume I, Chapter 8. A description of partial or total corneal lamellar dissection was not given. The nature and extent of the pathology determine the surgical plan for dissection of the corneal lamellae. Three major factors must be taken into consideration—the size, the shape, and the depth of the lamellar excision to be performed. Since any one, or all, of these factors may vary during the course of a given dissection—in contradistinction to penetrating keratoplasty—*the preparation of the donor graft lamellar dissection should be delayed until the recipient dissection is completed.* It is possible also that unsuspected posterior corneal pathology may necessitate a combined lamellar and penetrating keratoplasty. In this instance, if a lamellar graft already has been prepared and if a second donor eye is not available, it would be necessary to close the penetrating incision with the lamellar donor tissue or even to replace the pathologic button to preserve the globe.

The *size* of a lamellar excision depends on the extent of the pathology. However, since lamellar grafts usually are tectonic in function, they tend to be large, often extending to the periphery of the cornea. If a sector of the recipient cornea is relatively normal and is not removed in the dissection, the *shape* of the lamellar excision will be varied to conform to that of the pathology.

The *depth* of the dissection is determined by the vertical extent of the pathology. If the diseased cornea is of irregular thickness or curvature, a dissection to the full depth of the pathology must be avoided at the first lamellar excision. A second or even a third lamellar dissection to relatively normal stroma may be required. The lamellar peeling or tearing technique, advocated by E. Malbran, may be used to advantage in case of extreme variations of thickness and curvature (Plate 7-1, *A*). This is done after peripheral lamellar dissection. The lamellarized cornea is grasped with one or two forceps and forcibly separated in plane over a thin or irregular area centrally, as in a severe keratoconus.

TECHNIQUE FOR SUCCESSIVE LAMELLAR DISSECTIONS

After the usual preparation and draping, a Barraquer light-wire speculum is inserted and a MICRA-Pierse titanium ring of appropriate diameter is fixed with a 6-0 silk running suture. Under low magnification, 6× to 8×, a trephine blade of appropriate size is used to outline the pathology. A partially penetrating incision is made with the trephine (Plate 7-1, *B*) and deepened or extended with a diamond knife or a razor knife.

If, for example, an 11-mm circular incision is used and successive lamellar dissections to three-fourths the corneal depth are performed in a superficially and irregularly scarred cornea, the following procedure is employed. Under slit-lamp illumination of 15× to 20×, a section of the outlined incision is selected where corneal tissue appears to be relatively normal in lamellar arrangement and thickness. Using a diamond knife, the surgeon deepens vertically to one-half corneal thickness a 45° section of the trephine-outlined incision in the selected wound sector (Plate 7-1, *C*). The No. 1 spatula is passed between the corneal lamellae at the depth of the incision. The dissection is extended in the tissue plane by forward pressure combined with lateral sweeping movements of the serrated knife edge (Plate 7-1, *D*), care being taken to remain in the established lamellar plane. The dissection is extended to the limit of the No. 1 spatula blade length. The No. 2 spatula extends the dissection to the corneal apex. To complete the dissection to the periphery on the other side of the corneal apex, the No. 3 spatula is used. The curvature of the No. 3 spatula blade is the reverse of that of the No. 1 and the No. 2 blades to correspond to the reversed curvature of the cornea beyond the corneal apex (see Volume I, Plate 8-12). The reversed curvature minimizes the possibility of the edge of the blade moving out of the plane of dissection (see Volume I, Plate 2-13). The lamellar dissection is completed from a single entrance sector. If, during the dissection, the plane is lost or an area of severe scarring is encountered, the outline circumference is deepened and the dissection is continued in a deeper plane to encompass the troublesome area. The lamellar flap can then be grasped and torn in plane across the thin scarred section (Plate 7-1, *A*). This dissection is facilitated by cutting carefully with the razor knife the separating tissue at the lamellar plane junction.

If slit-lamp examination reveals the remaining posterior lamellae to be clear, the excision is complete, and the donor lamellar graft may be prepared. If the opacity extends more deeply or additional unsuspected pathology is seen, one or several more posterior lamellae are removed, using the same technique (Plate 7-1, *E*). Each lamella must be completely dissected and excised before dissection of another lamella is started.

Plate 7-1

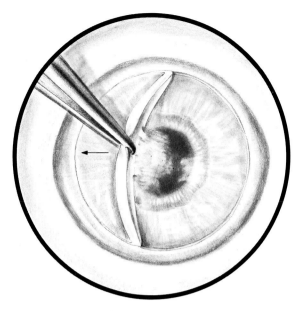

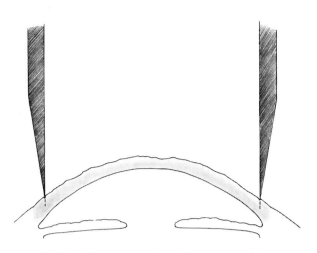

B. Partially penetrating 11-mm trephine incision. Cross section.

A. Lamellar peeling technique: alternative to sharp dissection at corneal apex.

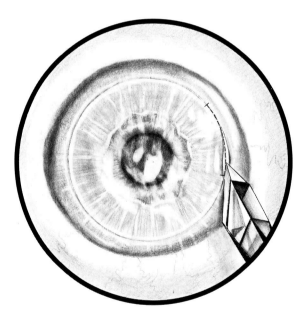

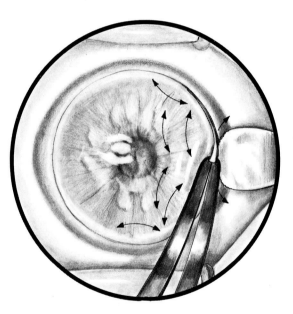

C. A 45° sector deepened vertically.

D. Lamellar dissection with Troutman No. 1 serrated corneal splitter.

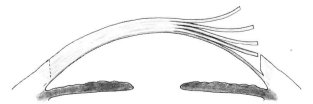

E. Successive dissections of corneal lamellae. Cross section.

183

SUTURING THE LAMELLAR GRAFT

The most widely employed, accurately cut, and easily fitted and sutured lamellar graft is the circular one. It is cut with a trephine 1 mm larger in diameter than that used to outline the lamellar recipient bed, 12 mm in the case illustrated. When a lamellar graft cut with the same-sized trephine is used for tectonic repair, especially when the preliminary trephining and dissection are deep, stretching the thin, elastic, posterior corneal lamella of the recipient makes closure difficult. Closure is facilitated if paracentesis is performed and some aqueous removed before the lamellar graft is sutured into position (Plate 7-2).

Placing the interrupted fixation sutures

Prior to the paracentesis, one edge of the graft may be sutured in place and several preplaced sutures inserted on the opposite side and left untied (Plate 7-2, A). Following the paracentesis, the preplaced sutures are tied to fix the graft (Plate 7-2, D). Additional interrupted sutures or an antitorque continuous suture is placed, as required.

Plate 7-2

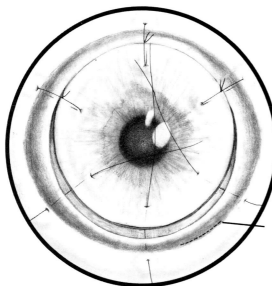

Paracentesis position

A. Preplaced sutures prior to paracentesis.

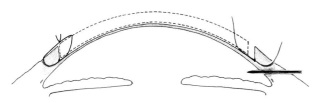

B. Position of paracentesis. Cross section.

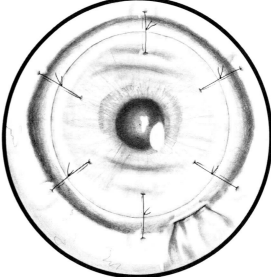

D. Interrupted sutures in place.

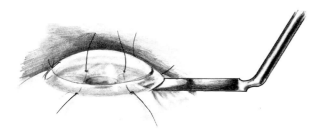

C. Graft falling into position following paracentesis.

Placing the antitorque continuous suture

The deeper bites of the antitorque continuous suture are placed diagonally, rather than radially, preventing rotation of the lamellar graft in its bed. The diagonal deep bites are spaced so that the intermediate overlying thread of each suture loop is equal in length but opposite in its direction of pull to that of the deep diagonal bite.

It is not necessary to place the suture at an angle in the thinner, more pliable, lamellar graft tissue. A 1-mm bite of the *full thickness* of the corneal lamella is grasped firmly between the cupped tips of the MICRA-Pierse tissue forceps (Plate 7-3, *A*). The GS-14 needle is introduced just proximal to the anterior forceps tip and is passed vertically through the thickness of the graft. The needle is engaged at the junction of the posterior lamella and the vertical cut edge of the recipient cornea. The needle then is passed *diagonally,* at the required angle, in the posterior lamellar plane for approximately 1 mm. The needle point is turned up abruptly to exit approximately 1 mm distal to the edge of the recipient cornea (Plate 7-3, *B*). The needle is retrieved. The next pass is made at the same angle, beginning at a point on the donor lamella so that the overlying thread from the preceding bite equals the deep bite in length, but opposes it in direction of pull, forming the two equal vertical sides of an isosceles triangle. To reference each point of junction, the overlying thread from the preceding bite is drawn down across the wound to establish the direction of the overlying loop. The length of the suture loop is marked with the needle tip at the point of entrance of the succeeding deep bite (Plate 7-3, *C*). When the needle is inserted, it should be left in situ until referenced for length and direction to the preceding deep and overlying bite (Plate 7-3, *B*).

Final adjustment of the antitorque continuous suture

When the antitorque continuous suture is placed, adjusted, tightened, and tied, the interrupted fixation sutures, the ring suture, and the superior rectus suture are removed. The projection of the surgical keratometer is viewed to monitor the final adjustment of the individual continuous suture loops. This ensures the firm, even apposition of the graft-recipient edges and the lamellar base. In lamellar refractive keratoplasty, use of the antitorque continuous suture and the surgical keratometer to monitor the adjustment of the suture tension is essential to an optimum optical result.

After the speculum and drapes are removed, a monocular modified pressure dressing is applied. No ointment is used because it might seep between the lamellae. Every effort is made during the surgery to keep the interlamellar face free of foreign bodies.

186

Plate 7-3

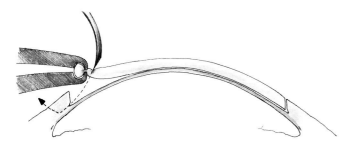

A. GS-14 needle track from donor lamella through recipient edge. Cross section.

B. Diagonal position of the needle for antitorque continuous suture as it passes through recipient lamellar plane.

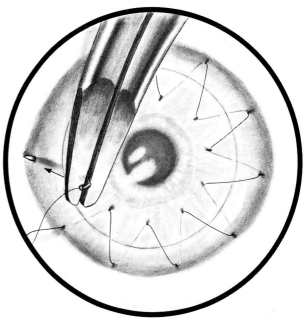

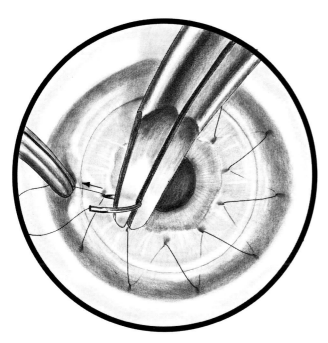

C. Referencing the position and angle for succeeding needle passage in antitorque suture placement.

LAMELLAR KERATOPLASTY COMBINED WITH PENETRATING KERATOPLASTY

When there is extensive peripheral corneal pathology and thinning and full-thickness central opacification, it is useful, occasionally, to combine lamellar keratoplasty with penetrating keratoplasty.

Preparation of the recipient eye

The periphery of the recipient corneal pathology is outlined with a trephine (Plate 7-1, *B*). Using a razor knife or, preferably, a diamond knife, a 45° section of the partially penetrating trephined incision is deepened to about one-half the thickness of the cornea (Plate 7-1, *C*). A lamellar dissection of the cornea is carried out as described, but only to the depth necessary to establish a plane of dissection under the *peripheral* pathology. The lamellar dissection is completed circumferentially and centrally using the No. 1 corneal splitting knife, followed by the No. 2 and No. 3 knives, as required (Plate 7-1, *D*). Though one dissection in depth may suffice, successive thin lamellar dissections may minimize the danger of perforation (Plate 7-1, *E*). The corneal lamella is resected to sufficient depth to ensure a uniform lamellar bed. When the peripheral pathologic area is completely dissected, the central penetrating incision is outlined with a 6.5-mm trephine (Plate 7-4, *A*).

Preparation of the donor mushroom

The operation then proceeds to the donor eye, from which a donor "mushroom" is dissected. For the donor, a 12-mm trephine is used for the peripheral, partial penetration, and a 7-mm trephine is used for the central penetration to ensure a better fit and better optics. A fresh globe should be used for this dissection. A tissue-culture preserved cornea can be used only if the mushroom is prepared from the intact globe in advance. Since circumferential peripheral lamellar replacement is to be prepared, the boundary of the peripheral lamellar flap is outlined with the larger-diameter, 12-mm trephine to ensure an accurate fit.

When only a sector lamellar replacement is required, as in a flanged graft, the lamellar section is outlined freehand with a razor knife or with a template corresponding in size and shape to the recipient dissection.

The lamellar dissection is carried out circumferentially with only the No. 1 spatula and centrally to approximately the diameter of the planned central trephined penetration (Plate 7-4, *B* and *C*).

Plate 7-4

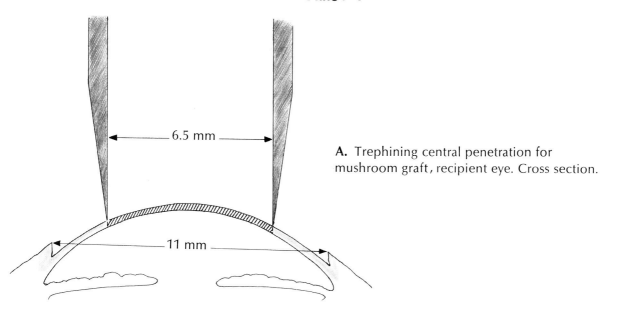

A. Trephining central penetration for mushroom graft, recipient eye. Cross section.

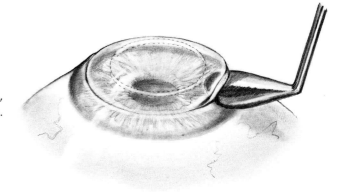

B. Peripheral lamellar dissection, donor eye.

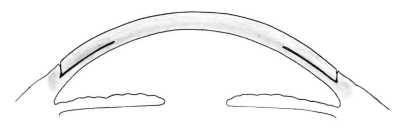

C. Peripheral lamellar dissection, donor eye. Cross section.

189

The lamellar flange is purse-stringed with 8-0 virgin silk armed with a GS-9 needle (Plate 7-5, *A*). The purse-string of over-and-over bites is drawn up tightly to bunch the lamellar tissue so that it will fit inside the trephine barrel as the blade cuts the penetrating portion of the graft (Plate 7-5, *B*). An open, disposable 7-mm trephine blade, placed over the bunched-up tissue, is rotated between the thumb and forefinger to penetrate the deep lamella into the anterior chamber. The excision is completed, as necessary, with corneal scissors. The purse-string suture is cut and removed to free the peripheral lamellar flap.

The penetration in the recipient is completed with trephine and scissors, and a midperipheral iridectomy is performed.

Plate 7-5

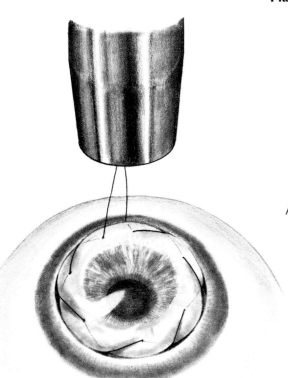

A. Purse-string of peripheral lamella.

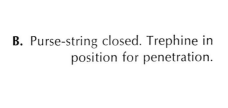

B. Purse-string closed. Trephine in position for penetration.

Suturing the mushroom to the recipient

The graft is sutured in place using four or six through-and-through, interrupted sutures to fix the edge of the penetrating portion of the mushroom to the edge of the penetrated lamellar dissection. The first of these through-and-through interrupted sutures is placed and tied. All the remainder are placed and then successively tied.

To place a suture, the junction of the lamellar portion and the penetrating portion of the mushroom is grasped with the MICRA-Pierse tissue forceps. The anterior tip of the forceps is angled to overlay the proximal edge of the penetrating portion of the mushroom. A GS-14 needle is introduced vertically from just behind the anterior tip of the forceps to penetrate the full corneal thickness (Plate 7-6, *A*). The point of the needle is brought under the nonfixated recipient lamella for 1 mm and is then turned straight up to exit. The donor lamella is again grasped just radial to and 1.5 to 2 mm from the first entrance point of the needle in the graft. The needle is passed vertically up through the donor lamella just proximal to the forceps tip to exit (Plate 7-6, *B*).

Plate 7-6

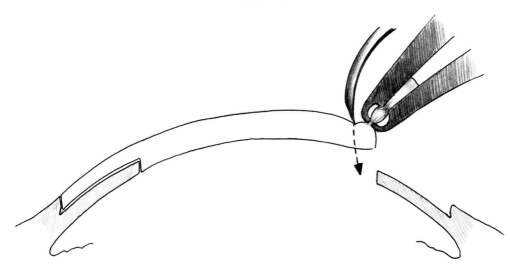

A. Placing the through-and-through suture
in the penetrating portion of the
mushroom graft. Cross section.

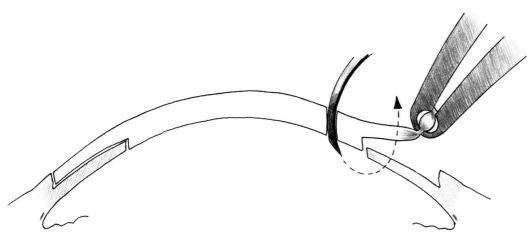

B. Completing the through-and-through
suture bite. Cross section.

193

The first suture is tied to fix one point of the button. The remaining interrupted suture bites are then all placed and finally tied, fixing the penetrating portion of the mushroom graft securely through and through to the edge of the penetrated recipient flange. As these interrupted sutures are tied, the surgical keratometer is used to prevent excessive tightening of individual loops. The peripheral lamellar edge of the donor button is sutured to the edge of the lamellarized periphery of the recipient with an antitorque continuous suture (Plate 7-7, *A*). This technique is essential when a continuous suture is used, to prevent torquing of the lamellarized graft in relation to the central penetrating portion fixed by radial interrupted sutures. Otherwise, interrupted sutures must be used. The wound is tested with fluorescein for leaks. Additional interrupted sutures are placed, if indicated.

The surgical keratometer is used again to verify that the continuous suture thread has been tensioned evenly (Plate 7-7, *B*).

Plate 7-7

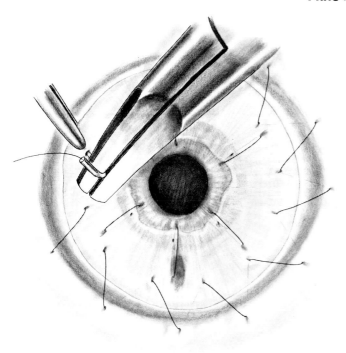

A. Completing the antitorque continuous suture.

B. Final appearance of mushroom graft in situ. Frontal view and cross section.

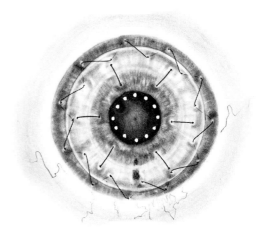

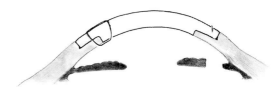

LAMELLAR FLANGED PENETRATING KERATOPLASTY

The penetrating graft with a lamellar flanged sector is sometimes used when the peripheral lamellar defect does not involve the entire periphery. Sometimes the flange may be used to cover a peripheral corneal defect and a contiguous scleral defect as, for instance, in scleral staphyloma.

One might ask why such combination grafts need be used when a better repair might be effected if lamellar and penetrating keratoplasties were performed at separate procedures. When a softened or degenerated peripheral area is removed and replaced by a lamellar graft, it often does not provide a good edge for suturing a penetrating graft in place. When the edge of the penetrating graft is contiguous to the lamellar graft, healing of that potentially weaker sector is ensured. A repeat penetrating graft, when necessary, is easier to perform and may be smaller.

It is mandatory to do the lamellar dissection of the recipient *before* preparing the donor. When outlining the recipient area in the case of a scleral staphyloma, care must be taken that a 2-mm edge of relatively normal lamellarized sclera surrounds the staphylomatous area. It is not always wise to unroof the staphyloma, since uvea can prolapse, vitreous may be lost, and closure can be made more difficult. The lamellar dissection of surrounding normal sclera provides the bed to which to suture the reinforcing lamellar flange. An optical penetrating graft can be included centrally, if required (Plate 7-8, *A*).

When the lamellar flange has been dissected, the central penetration of the recipient eye is made with an appropriately sized trephine (Plate 7-8, *B* and *C*).

Lamellar dissection of the donor will include cornea and sclera as necessary to repair the recipient. The dissection of the donor is made with the No. 1 corneal splitting knife to the edge of the area from which the penetrating portion of the graft will be prepared. The lamellarized flange, held by several loops of 8-0 silk suture, is then brought up into the barrel of the disposable trephine blade. The penetrating portion of the graft is cut just as is the mushroom graft.

The flange of the graft is sutured to the recipient using multiple interrupted sutures. The penetrating portion of the graft, connected to the flange at the periphery, is sutured at the penetrated lamellar edge of the recipient by one or more interrupted sutures, as previously described. The remainder of the periphery of the penetrating portion may be closed either with an antitorque continuous suture or with interrupted sutures (Plate 7-8, *D*). Particular care is taken to suture securely any angles or corners of the flange. If a mattress suture is used, the intracorneal loops are placed tangentially, proximal and distal to the angle. The overlying loops then will be positioned across the incisional line to either side of the angle. The suture is tied and the knot buried on the donor side (Plate 7-8, *E*). This technique avoids placing a suture directly across the joint angle.

Plate 7-8

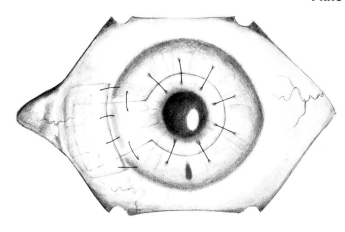

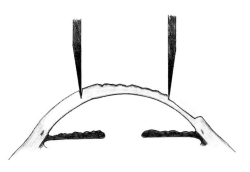

A. Flanged graft with central penetrating graft used to repair a scleral staphyloma.

B. Preparing the recipient for a lamellar flanged penetrating graft. Cross section.

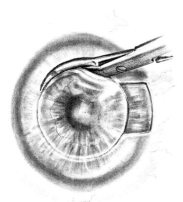

C. Completing the excision of the recipient.

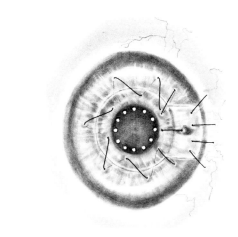

D. Final appearance of lamellar flanged penetrating graft. Frontal view and cross section.

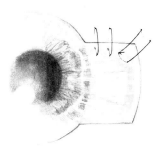

E. Detail of mattress suture closing a corner of the lamellar flange.

A midperipheral iridectomy is always performed in this, as in any other, penetrating keratoplasty.

LAMELLAR KERATOPLASTY IN KERATOMILEUSIS AND KERATOPHAKIA

These specialized optical lamellar keratoplastic procedures are done with the special instrumentation described briefly in Chapter 5. The reader is referred to the collected papers of José I. Barraquer.

KERATOPROSTHESIS

Keratoprosthesis is a complicated lamellar procedure similar in technique to the mushroom graft.

SUMMARY

Lamellar keratoplasty has been discussed in some detail in Volume I, Chapter 8. Lamellar dissection of the recipient, as well as some special procedures utilizing a combination of penetrating and lamellar grafts, have been described in this chapter. For these procedures, composite lamellar and penetrating grafts can be cut with the usual keratoplasty instrumentation. Such mushroom or flanged grafts are useful in pathologic situations in which circumferential or sector peripheral pathology may prevent adequate suturing of a simple penetrating keratoplasty. They are useful also in cases in which poor healing of a sector of the donor to the recipient is anticipated and edge-to-edge apposition may be difficult or not sufficiently secure.

CHAPTER 8

SIMPLE PENETRATING KERATOPLASTY

General considerations
Preparation for the surgical procedure
Exposure and fixation
Cutting the donor button
Cutting the recipient opening
Correction of preexisting astigmatism
   Oval recipient opening—round donor
      button
   Round recipient opening—single wedge—
      round donor button

Round recipient opening—oval donor
   button
Round recipient opening—double wedge—
   round donor button
Completing the trephine cut
Midperipheral iridectomy
Suturing the graft
Final suture adjustment using the Troutman
   surgical keratometer
Summary

GENERAL CONSIDERATIONS

Penetrating keratoplasty, in the absence of other-than-corneal anterior or posterior segment pathology or surgery, is referred to as simple penetrating keratoplasty. It involves primarily a combination of the keratoplasty technique on the donor and recipient corneas, as described in Chapters 4 and 6. Since success in penetrating keratoplasty is not only a clear graft, the indications for and techniques of concomitant refractive surgery, such as simultaneous wedge resection and ovaling the recipient opening or the donor button, are discussed. Though this may belie the description "simple," keratoplasty in the uncomplicated phakic eye is the easiest to perform and has the least postoperative complications; therefore, the importance of a good optical as well as anatomic result.

Prior to the surgical procedure, a careful preoperative evaluation is completed to determine whether the primary cause of vision loss is the corneal disease and whether keratoplasty alone will alleviate the vision problem. The operative plan is developed on the basis of the diagnosis and the extent of the pathology. The size to which the recipient opening will be cut and the donor button will be punched are determined not only on the basis of the extent of the pathology but also to avoid severe optical distortion in the healed, clear graft.

PREPARATION FOR THE SURGICAL PROCEDURE

Preparation for a primary penetrating keratoplasty need not be complicated. A routine admission work-up, to the standard of the surgeon's medical community, is done. The only preoperative local medication used is chloramphenicol (1%) eyedrops. These are instilled in both eyes four times, from admission to the time of surgery. Exceptionally, if a failed corneal graft is to be replaced, one dose daily of 100 mg of prednisone is prescribed, starting 72 hours preoperatively. If a bacterial infection of the eye or adnexa is suspected prior to surgery, but the culture is negative, a broad-spectrum systemic antibiotic such as cephaloridine, 2000 mg daily, is given prophylactically beginning 48 hours preoperatively. If the culture is positive, surgery is delayed. When one or both of these medications is administered preoperatively, it is continued postoperatively until all clinical signs of inflammation or infection have cleared completely. At the time of surgery, as an additional prophylaxis, gentamicin (Garamycin), 40 mg, 1 ml, may be injected subconjunctivally deep in the inferior cul-de-sac following preparation, exposure, and immobilization of the globe. When the patient is one-eyed, especially if a prosthesis is worn, stringent prophylaxis is mandatory. Since an orbit fitted with a prosthetic device often cultures *Pseudomonas* or *E. coli,* the artificial eye must be removed and the orbit cultured and treated intensively with specific antibiotics until a sterile culture is obtained. The patient is not permitted to wear the prosthesis for 6 weeks postoperatively, and an antibiotic ointment is used prophylactically in the orbit.

EXPOSURE AND FIXATION

The lids are separated with the Barraquer light-wire speculum. A superior rectus suture is placed and an appropriately sized titanium support ring is fixed to the sclera with a 6-0 silk continuous suture armed with a GS-9 needle (see Plate 6-4, *B*).

CUTTING THE DONOR BUTTON

The donor button is cut to a diameter that will ensure good circumferential anatomic apposition as well as an optimal optical result. For the phakic recipient eye with a normal corneal curvature at the mean, 43 diopters or 7.85 mm, the donor preparation is cut from its posterior surface on a Teflon backing block, with a trephine blade of a diameter 0.2 mm larger than the planned trephining of the recipient cornea (see Plates 4-14, *A*, and 4-15, *A*).

Since the optical curvatures of the donor usually are not known, it must be assumed that the donor cornea is anastigmatic and regular. A regular anastigmatic cornea is better ensured when cut on the Troutman spherical double-curve, Teflon backing block (see Plate 4-14, *A*) with a posterior-curve radius of 7.5 mm, purposefully made slightly steeper than the average corneal K. When the Troutman guided-piston trephine (see Plate 4-15, *A*) is used to cut the graft on this backing block, a vertical-edged, circular donor button is ensured. Should the donor cornea have an undetected astigmatic band, the meridional error in the donor button is minimized, since the cut is made inside the corneal ring. As the donor button is cut, unless it has a severe, undetected distortion, it will tend to conform to the spherical surface of the block. It is essential, therefore, that the backing block be cut and surfaced accurately, since any irregularity or asphericity in the block can induce a defective cut and an astigmatism in the donor button (Plate 8-1, *A*). The block should be discarded if it is etched by previous trephinings.

An aspheric or elliptical curve cut into the backing block can be used to cut an oval graft that can compensate astigmatism in the recipient (Plate 8-1, *B* and *C*). A uniformly deep, circular groove is cut in the aspheric surface. This permits an even, circumferential penetration of the trephine blade. The groove is filled with a backing material softer than Teflon. The blade penetrates first along the shorter axis of the ellipse and continues to cut through the softer backing material. When the cut is completed, the longer axis of the graft button is at a right (90°) angle to the longer axis of the Teflon block.

The resulting button will be oval rather than round in shape, with its longer axis corresponding to the shorter axis of the concavity of the backing block. This axis must be marked with the donor button in the block. A single suture loop of nylon is used to mark the axis.

The cut donor button is inspected and left on the backing block, covered by a few drops of the M-K tissue-culture medium. The backing block with the button is placed in an uncovered Petri dish and is transferred to the instrument table. Extreme care is taken to ensure that the endothelial side of the donor button does not come in contact with glass, plastic, fabric, or metal during any phase of cutting or during transfer to the recipient. The slightest contact between any of these materials and the donor endothelium will cause irreparable cell damage, which can compromise a technically successful procedure.

Plate 8-1

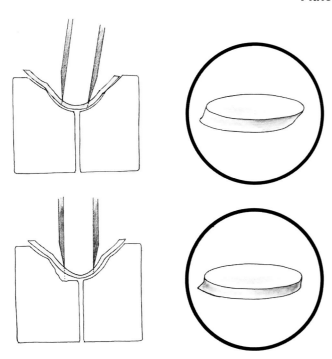

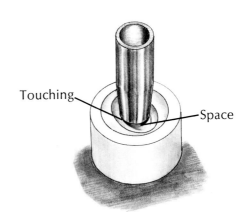

A. Irregularities of cutting, induced by side slipping of donor button or by irregularity of backing block surface.

B. Elliptic concavity used to cut oval donor button (cutting frame not shown).

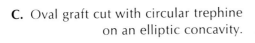

C. Oval graft cut with circular trephine on an elliptic concavity.

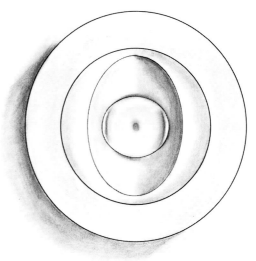

CUTTING THE RECIPIENT OPENING

The recipient eye should be protected from heat and drying by a piece of moistened cellulose sponge (Plate 8-2, *A*). At highest microscope magnification, the cutting edge of the selected trephine is examined (Plate 6-6). If the edge passes inspection, the obturator of the trephine handle is adjusted to the cutting depth. The sponge is removed, and the eye is fixated by grasping the Flieringa or titanium ring with an open-cupped MICRA-Pierse forceps (Plate 8-2, *B*). The trephine is centered on the cornea, and the cut is made as described in Chapter 6. A round recipient opening can be cut either with the manual or with a motor-driven trephine. If an oval-shaped recipient opening is to be made, a cam cutter, such as that designed by Lieberman (see Plates 5-2, *D,* and 6-8) is used.

Plate 8-2

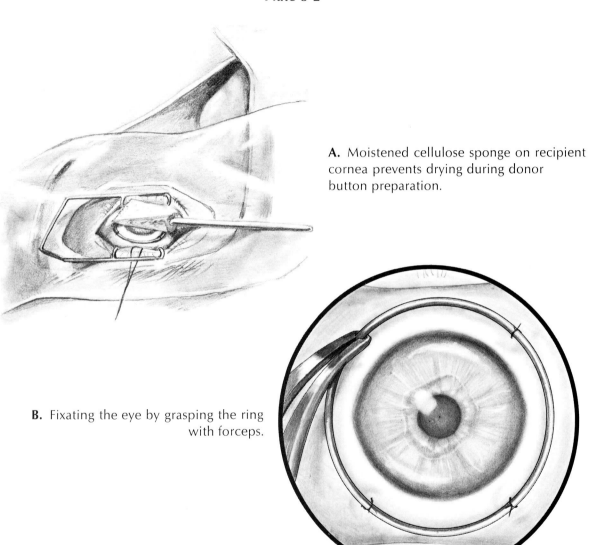

A. Moistened cellulose sponge on recipient cornea prevents drying during donor button preparation.

B. Fixating the eye by grasping the ring with forceps.

CORRECTION OF PREEXISTING ASTIGMATISM

When the preoperatively measured curvatures of the cornea are regular and normal, regardless of the pathology, there is no indication to vary the circular shape of the donor button or the recipient opening. However, if a marked astigmatic band is detected preoperatively by the keratometer or if a grossly distorted corneal ring is noted (Plate 8-3), either the donor button or the recipient opening is cut to an oval shape to compensate the meridional error. If no surgical adjustment is made, any meridional error in the recipient cornea will be induced in the graft. For example, if the corneal ring is elongated horizontally, the vertical meridian will be steeper (with-the-rule astigmatism) and can be compensated in one of four ways.

Oval recipient opening—round donor button

One way to correct a preexisting astigmatism is to cut an oval opening in the recipient cornea, using the Lieberman cam cutter. The longer axis of the recipient opening will correspond to the flatter meridian of the cornea (the elongated axis of the corneal ring) (Plates 8-3, A, and 8-5, A). When a round-cut donor button, equal in circumference to the oval-shaped recipient opening, is sutured in place, the longer dimension of the recipient opening is compressed centrally, steepening that meridian, while the shorter dimension of the recipient opening is expanded, flattening that meridian. The corneal ring becomes round (Plate 8-3, B). Therefore, if the circumference (and area) of the donor button is greater than that of the recipient opening, the cornea is steepened overall, thus becoming more myopic; conversely, if the circumference of the donor button is less than that of the recipient opening, the cornea is flattened overall, becoming more hyperopic, regardless of the astigmatism induced (see Plate 2-4). For example, to correct 10 diopters of a mixed astigmatism with a spherical equivalent approximating emmetropia, the donor button is punched from the posterior surface with an 8.2-mm diameter (25.8-mm circumference) trephine. The oval recipient opening is cut with the cam guide set to cut an oval opening measuring 8.25 mm on its longer axis and 7.75 mm on its shorter axis. This corresponds to the area of an 8-mm round graft (25.1-mm circumference).

Plate 8-3

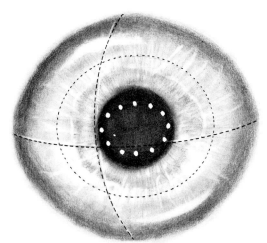

A. Horizontally elongated
corneal ring,
astigmatism with the rule

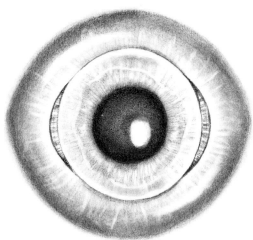

B. Astigmatism compensated
by placing round button
in oval recipient ring

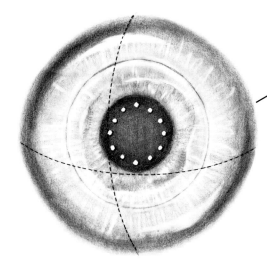

Ovaling of recipient opening compensates
distorted corneal ring.

Round recipient opening—single wedge—round donor button

A second way to correct a preexisting astigmatism is to follow a 7.5-mm circular trephine of the recipient with a wedge resection of one-fourth the recipient rim, centered on the longer axis of the distorted corneal ring (flatter corneal meridian) (Plate 8-4). The wedge should be crescentic, with its widest part, 0.5 mm, centered on the axis of the flatter meridian. In this instance, since tissue will be removed, the trephined area of the recipient will be increased by the area of the excised wedge. Therefore, in order to approximate the area of an 8-mm donor button, a 7.5-mm trephine is used for the recipient. After the wedge is excised, the total area of the 7.5-mm recipient opening will approximate the area of an 8-mm donor button, in the case of a single wedge, or an 8.2-mm donor button, in the case of a double wedge. If the trephine used for the donor button is the same diameter or less than 0.2 mm larger than the trephine used for the recipient opening, an excessively flat cornea will result.

Plate 8-4

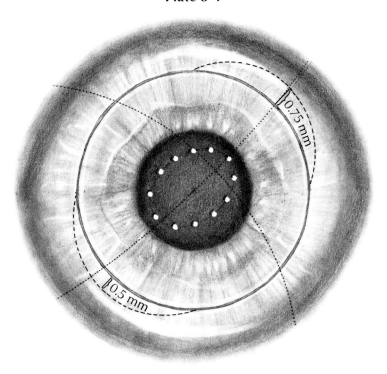

Positions of a single- or double-wedge resection
of recipient margin to correct
an astigmatic error.

Round recipient opening—oval donor button

Alternatively to ovaling by using the cam cutter, wedging, or double-wedging the recipient opening, an oval graft may be sutured in a round recipient opening to correct a preexisting astigmatism (Plate 8-5). The oval graft, corresponding in area to the round recipient opening, is cut on an elliptical-shaped concavity as described earlier. The ovaled donor button is placed with its longer axis corresponding to the shorter axis of the corneal ring centered on the steeper meridian.

Round recipient opening—double wedge—round donor button

As a fourth alternative, in the case of a larger astigmatic error, two 90° wedges can be resected opposite to each other, centered on the longer axis, or flatter corneal meridian, of the distorted corneal ring. Again, a larger donor button, 8.2-mm diameter, is used in a recipient opening cut originally to 7.5 mm in diameter, enlarged by the wedge resections (Plate 8-4).

The advantage of the wedge technique is that standard keratoplasty instrumentation can be used. These techniques are easier to perform if the initially 7.5-mm recipient trephining penetrates only partially. The wedge or wedges are more readily and accurately outlined and cut out before the recipient eye is finally opened. The diamond knife is used to outline and to excise the wedge, since the cut of the diamond knife is more regular and accurate. A Vannas scissors is used to complete the excision. Whether scissors or a diamond knife is used, a wedge is easier to cut if the two outer curvilinear incisions begin at either end of the crescent outline and join at the middle, or widest, portion.

COMPLETING THE TREPHINE CUT

When the trephined incision in the recipient penetrates only partially, the posterior lamella is opened with a razor knife or a diamond knife and is completed with the right and left corneal graft scissors. Great care is taken to maintain the vertical cut started by the trephine. If shelving should occur posteriorly, the rim of the shelf should be excised carefully, using Vannas scissors or corneal scissors. Care should be taken when fixating a fragment of the recipient rim with the MICRA-Pierse forceps, for excessive traction may cause the scissors to undercut the rim and have an optical effect similar to a wedge resection (see Plate 6-12, *B*).

MIDPERIPHERAL IRIDECTOMY

In all cases of simple penetrating keratoplasty, a midperipheral iridectomy is done as soon as the recipient opening is completed and before the donor button is sutured in place. This sequence prevents pupillary block during suturing or postoperatively.

Plate 8-5

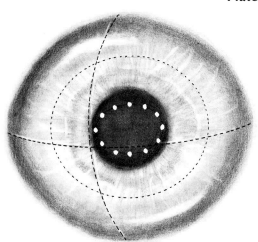

A. Horizontally elongated
corneal ring,
astigmatism with the rule

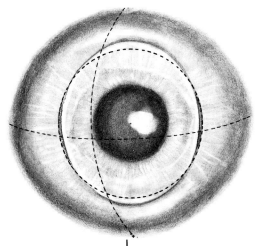

B. Astigmatism compensated
by oval corneal graft fit
to round recipient ring

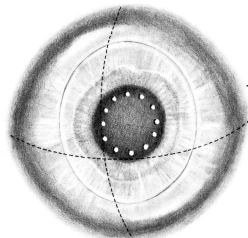

**Ovaling of donor button compensates
distorted corneal ring.**

211

SUTURING THE GRAFT

In simple penetrating keratoplasty in which no concomitant optical surgery is performed, six equally spaced and tensioned fixation sutures are placed through and through the donor and the recipient. The anterior chamber is inflated, and the accuracy of the positioning of the button by the sutures is checked with the surgical keratometer. A continuous suture (Plate 8-6, *A*) or a double continuous suture of 10-0, 22-micron, monofilament nylon or polypropylene thread is placed for definitive wound closure. Interrupted fixation sutures are always removed.

In a reoperation, in case of circumferential or sector peripheral vascularization, or in the event that the peripheral pathology cannot be removed in its entirety, a finer (16-micron) thread is preferred (Plate 8-6, *B*). When the finer thread is used, about one-third more suture bites are required than with a 22-micron single continuous suture. The 16-micron thread is more fragile and more elastic than the 22-micron thread. Greater care must be taken during suturing, particularly during the final stages of tightening and tying. When the suture loops are adjusted and tensioned to regularize the projection of the surgical keratometer, additional care must be taken not to overstretch the finer thread, or misleading results will be obtained. Although it is possible to overstretch 22-micron thread, it is less likely because of its greater strength, which lets it be manipulated with less probability of inducing an error.

It is important to note again that a continuous suture is not self-adjusting, but requires careful and accurate tightening or loosening of each suture loop, in turn, to obtain a circumferentially balanced suture tension. The use of a surgical keratometer is indispensable in ascertaining when a relatively ideal suture-tension balance is reached. This qualitative capability of the surgical keratometer is useful not only in checking appositional suture tension, but also in determining relative corneal curvatures, and in positioning and monitoring optical excisions, as well as in making final suture tension adjustments.

When the donor button and the recipient opening differ in shape, four or more additional interrupted fixation sutures are placed before placing the continuous suture or sutures (Plate 8-6, *C*). These temporary interrupted sutures ensure a better circumferential fit. Also, they maintain the apposition of the donor button and the recipient edge and facilitate placement of the continuous suture by preventing any distortion of the disparate-sized donor button in the recipient opening. The balanced suture tension is confirmed with the surgical keratometer.

Plate 8-6

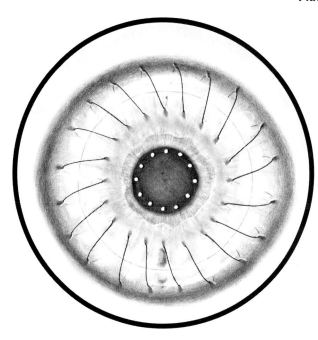

A. 22-micron continuous suture used for closure.

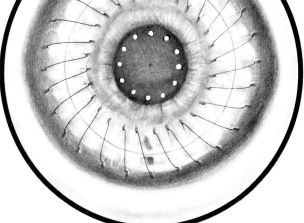

B. 16-micron continuous suture used for closure (one-third more bites).

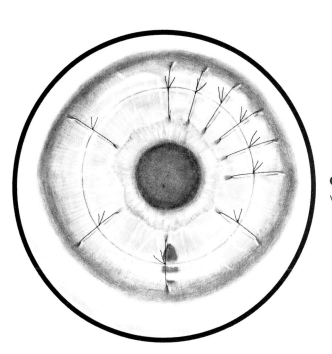

C. Additional interrupted sutures used to close wedge-resected sector.

Since a maximally secure, radial apposition is desirable when matching different shapes, the double-continuous suture (see Volume I, Plate 6-17) is used preferentially for final closure. A closely spaced, single continuous suture also may be used. Too wide a separation between the bites of a single continuous suture causes torquing between the overlying bites. The graft rotates in its bed, changing the relationship of the corneal curvatures of the graft and recipient, postoperatively. A single continuous, radially placed suture is undesirable when either an oval graft is used in a round recipient opening or a round graft is used in an oval recipient opening. The rotation of the graft periphery in relation to the recipient opening alters the corneal optics unpredictably. To maintain a constant relationship between the graft and the recipient opening in optical corneal surgery, the use of multiple interrupted sutures, an antitorque continuous suture, a combination of both, or a double continuous suture maintains better the constant radial appositional force. It is obvious that, when both the graft and the recipient opening are round, the optical effects of rotation are minimal.

The interrupted fixation sutures are removed as soon as the continuous suture or sutures have been placed, tensioned, and tied, and the knot or knots have been buried in recipient stroma.

FINAL SUTURE ADJUSTMENT USING THE TROUTMAN SURGICAL KERATOMETER

When the graft is sutured firmly into place, any residual air in the anterior chamber is removed, and the chamber is filled with balanced salt solution to approximate normal eye tension. The thread loops are adjusted so that the surgical keratometer projection is round, indicating that the donor button is essentially anastigmatic. The wound is tested with fluorescein dye for watertightness. The Flieringa titanium ring is removed. The superior rectus suture is released, and the lids are elevated from the eye by holding up the lid speculum. The surgical keratometer projection is again observed. The sutures are adjusted, as necessary, and fluorescein dye is again used to test for wound leaks. The superior rectus suture and the speculum are removed. Chloramphenicol drops are instilled and erythromycin ointment is applied over the closed lid margins. A unilateral protective dressing is applied.

The patient may be ambulatory, with no risk to the operative site, as soon as he has recovered from the anesthesia.

SUMMARY

Simple penetrating keratoplasty in the phakic eye, combining most of the technical skills of the corneal surgeon, usually produces the most satisfactory postoperative result. Often, this procedure is done in the younger patient and in patients with bilateral corneal pathologies, such as keratoconus and the familial dystrophies. Eventually it may be done in both eyes of the patient; thus, it is important that a uniform technique be followed to ensure approximately equal results, optical as well as anatomic. The technique may have to be altered in those cases in which the pathology cannot be excised completely or a monocular optical defect is present, which may induce disparate optical distortions from otherwise successful bilateral grafts. Radial suture apposition and a watertight closure are essential to ensure the anatomic integrity of the wound and the healing of the graft incision without inducing optical distortions.

Preoperative identification of severe optical defects enables the surgeon to attempt, with the help of the surgical keratometer, to compensate these defects during the initial surgical intervention. The surgical keratometer is essential also in minimizing surgically induced, optical distortions. It should be used successively during every keratoplasty to determine the relative amount and axis of the astigmatism prior to trephining, to guide in the correct placement of any indicated optical incision, and to monitor the positioning and suturing of the graft in order to ensure, insofar as possible, an essentially anastigmatic cornea at the close of the procedure.

Proper attention to these details will help the surgeon to achieve not only an anatomically well-apposed and well-positioned clear graft, but also a graft with minimal optical distortion postkeratoplasty.

CHAPTER 9

COMBINED CATARACT SURGERY AND KERATOPLASTY

General considerations
Simple cataract extraction with or without an intraocular implant
Keratoplasty in the presence of a minimal cataract
Cataract surgery following successful keratoplasty
Combined keratoplasty and cataract extraction
Technique of combined keratoplasty and cataract extraction
  Preparation for surgical procedure
  Exposure and fixation using the Troutman surgical keratometer
  Cutting the donor button
  Cutting the recipient opening
  Midperipheral iridectomy and radial sphincterotomies
  Fixing the donor button with interrupted sutures
  Intracapsular cataract extraction
  Closing the incision with interrupted sutures

Fixing the graft with a single continuous suture
Removing the interrupted sutures
Final suture adjustment using the Troutman surgical keratometer
Fluorescein leak test and the surgical dressing
Techniques for more extensive anterior segment surgery
Extracapsular cataract extraction
Intraocular lens implant
  Intracapsular technique
    Worst medallion lens
    Binkhorst four-loop intraocular lens
  Graft-to-recipient closure
Intraocular lens after extracapsular extraction technique
  Graft-to-recipient closure
Vitreous surgery
Iris surgery
Summary

GENERAL CONSIDERATIONS

It is not uncommon that an eye with vision-compromising corneal pathology will have also a moderate to severe cataract, especially in older people. Corneal endothelial-epithelial dystrophy with central corneal edema is often accompanied by a cataract. Even after successful penetrating keratoplasty, vision may be restored only partially. Steroid therapy, a strong miotic agent, or both may induce a secondary cataract that can nullify, in part, the vision result of a simple keratoplasty. The eye subjected to previous keratoplasty or to iris or glaucoma surgery is more prone to develop a cataract. Trauma causing corneal opacification may induce also lens changes either at the time of or subsequent to the injury. No matter what the cause, in order to restore maximum vision to the affected eye, the cataract must be removed eventually.

SIMPLE CATARACT EXTRACTION WITH OR WITHOUT AN INTRAOCULAR IMPLANT

Should the surgeon decide that the corneal opacity is so minimal that removal of the cataract alone combined with an optical iridotomy or iridectomy will suffice to restore functional vision, the added surgical trauma and potential complications of keratoplasty can be avoided.

Cases best treated by cataract extraction alone or in combination with an intraocular implant are those in which the discrete paracentral corneal opacities do not cause keratometric distortion or irregular astigmatism on the visual axis.

The surgeon must be very careful in making such a judgment, since the shift of the nodal point occasioned by removal of the cataractous lens and correction by a spectacle lens or contact lens may not provide the patient with the same vision as with the clear lens in the physiologic position. This is true particularly when faint nebulous corneal opacities are combined with a cornea of irregular thickness, as is seen in the older patient who has a history of a severe corneal disease early in life. These patients often see well for many years, without even needing to wear glasses for distance or for near vision. However, when the cataract is removed, the aphakic vision often is unsatisfactory, especially for reading. These patients achieve the best vision result by combined cataract extraction and graft and aphakic correction. Alternatively, a simple lens extraction combined with an intraocular lens implant, which does not change the nodal point appreciably, will restore vision to approximately the preoperative level without the need for keratoplasty.

The patient with minimal corneal guttata, relatively normal corneal thickness, and no visible stromal or epithelial pathology also may have good vision results from cataract surgery alone. In a small percentage of such cases, corneal changes typical of endothelial dystrophy will develop after cataract extraction and will require penetrating keratoplasty in the aphakic eye. Extracapsular cataract extraction, with or without an intraocular lens implant, or intracapsular cataract extraction, with the inclusion of an intraocular lens, may be used advantageously in these cases. Vitreous is retained behind the iris diaphragm or is supported by the intraocular lens, the intact posterior capsule, or both. Any secondary corneal surgery will be facilitated. *The additional manipulation necessary to perform extracapsular cataract surgery, to insert an intraocular lens, or both may accelerate endothelial-epithelial dystrophic changes.* Keratoplasty may be necessary more often as a result of the more traumatic and complex cataract procedure.

217

KERATOPLASTY IN THE PRESENCE OF A MINIMAL CATARACT

When keratoplasty alone is done in the presence of a minimal cataract, the trauma associated with the corneal surgery, the postoperative inflammatory reaction, and the use of steroids can accelerate the development of the cataract. In these cases, surgical judgment is critical. The surgeon must take into account not only the present pathologic situation but also the potential effect of the corneal surgery on subsequent cataract development. In doubtful cases, especially if the patient has relatively good vision in the other eye, it is better to delay surgery. The surgical decision may be that a cataract, though present, is not developed sufficiently to reduce the functional vision after successful keratoplasty, so keratoplasty alone is done. Later, when further vision loss makes it necessary, the cataract is extracted.

CATARACT SURGERY FOLLOWING SUCCESSFUL KERATOPLASTY

When cataract surgery must be performed following successful keratoplasty, the trauma of the second intervention compromises 10% to 15% of clinically clear grafts. A graft with a potential for failure subsequent to cataract surgery should be identified in advance of surgery by specular microscopy. If the graft endothelial cells show moderate to severe deficiency, any procedure known to cause moderate to severe endothelial depopulation, such as phacoemulsification, intraocular lens implantation, or both, should be avoided. It may be prudent even to plan the replacement of a borderline graft in conjunction with cataract surgery.

COMBINED KERATOPLASTY AND CATARACT EXTRACTION

I think the most effective way to deal with the problem of combined corneal pathology and a cataract is to perform the keratoplasty and the cataract procedure at one operative session. In suitable cases, the final result can be made optically more physiologic when the intraocular lens is placed at the combined procedure. This triple procedure is especially useful if the other eye still has functional phakic vision. In the older patient, over 65 years of age, with a functional fellow eye, an intraocular implant should be inserted in one eye only. The long-term risk is minimized by the shorter life expectancy. In the older patient, the early restoration of useful uncorrected vision, and often of binocularity as well, offsets the immediate risk of the additional surgery and the long-term risk of the implant.

Combined pathology of the cornea and lens can be accompanied by disruption or pathology of the iris, vitreous, retina, or all three. Surgery on these structures may be required at the time of the combined surgery.

The techniques for cataract extraction performed alone, either prior to or following keratoplasty, are not discussed. Extracapsular cataract technique, with or without intraocular lens inclusion, and intraocular lens inclusion after intracapsular surgery are discussed only insofar as they relate to the combined procedure.

TECHNIQUE OF COMBINED KERATOPLASTY AND CATARACT EXTRACTION
Preparation for surgical procedure

The preoperative preparation of the patient for combined cataract extraction and keratoplasty is modified to include the administration of 1.5 gm of mannitol per kilogram of body weight, given in 1000 ml of sterile water, to reduce vitreous volume. It is given rapidly, within 30 minutes, to be completed just prior to opening the globe. When vitreous surgery may be required, prednisone, 100 mg given daily in a single dose, is started 72 hours before scheduled surgery. For ease of administration, prednisone is available as Deltasone, 50 mg. Cephaloridine, 2000 mg daily, is started 48 hours preoperatively. When the patient is under deep general anesthesia, the eye is softened further by manual compression, 20 seconds on and 10 seconds off.

Exposure and fixation using the Troutman surgical keratometer

The light-wire speculum is used to expose the globe. Using the GS-9 spatula needle, the surgeon places a 6-0 silk traction suture intrasclerally just anterior to the insertion of the superior rectus. *The surgical keratometer reflection is observed, and any astigmatic band is noted and compared to the quantitative measurement recorded preoperatively.*

A 16-mm, wire-type Flieringa ring is sutured to the globe with four to eight 6-0 silk sutures (see Plate 6-3). Suture loops are left between the scleral bites, superiorly at 10 and 2 o'clock and inferiorly at 4 and 8 o'clock, to enable the surgeon or the assistant to manipulate the globe more readily. Alternatively, a 15-mm MICRA-Pierse titanium ring fixed with a 6-0 silk running suture can be used (Plate 9-2).

The reflection of the surgical keratometer is observed again. Any meridional distortion induced by the ring is corrected. The reflection should compare qualitatively to the quantitative measurements of the clinical keratometer.

Cutting the donor button

The operation proceeds to the cutting of the donor button from a tissue-culture preserved cornea. In the combined procedure, to obtain an exact fit and a steeper cornea, the donor button is cut 0.5 mm larger than the planned 7.5-mm recipient opening. The 8-mm trephine blade is fitted and is fixed on the adjustable stainless steel piston of the Troutman piston punch (see Plate 4-15). Care is taken not to decenter the donor tissue as the frame guide is placed. The surgeon rechecks the centering before introducing the piston into its sleeve in the cutting frame. This piston is advanced slowly until the edge of the trephine blade rests on the concave surface of the donor cornea. The centration is checked again. Then by exerting firm pressure on the top of the piston with the thumb, the surgeon cuts a centered, circular, straight-sided donor button. The button is retained in the concavity of the backing block, and the corneoscleral periphery adheres to the trephine blade as the guide and piston are removed. A few drops of tissue-culture fluid are used to cover the donor button. The block with the button is placed in a Petri dish, covered, and transferred to the instrument table.

Cutting the recipient opening

The surgeon fixates the globe by grasping the scleral ring with the MICRA-Pierse open-cupped forceps. This facilitates centering and maintains better vertical position of the trephine relative to the cornea (see Plate 6-5, A). A 7.5-mm trephine cut, centered in the recipient cornea, is made, using one of the several methods described in Chapter 6. Since the eye will be soft because of reduced intraocular pressure, resulting from the administration of mannitol and the use of digital pressure, it is important that the cut be effected only by the weight of the trephine and the sharpness of the rotating blade. If excessive pressure is exerted, the corneal dome will collapse under the knife and will invert, causing an irregular or sloping cut through the cornea (Plate 9-1). Full penetration of the cornea may be made inadvertently in a sector by the advancing trephine blade or, more selectively, at the depths of the partially penetrating trephine groove by the diamond or razor knife. The recipient corneal button is then excised with scissors. The surgeon may elect to do an incomplete excision, leaving the recipient button attached inferiorly.

Usually the pathologic button is excised completely, and any posterior tags of tissue are carefully trimmed, using the right or left corneal scissors or Vannas scissors.

Plate 9-1

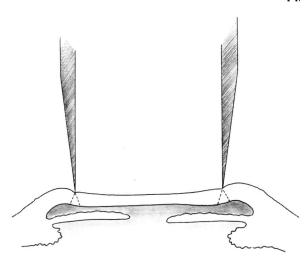

A. Effect of excessive vertical trephine pressure on soft eye. Cross section.

B. Sloping cut may be produced. Cross section.

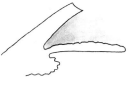
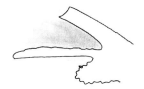

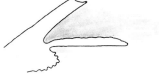
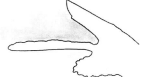

C. Bias cut may be produced. Cross section.

Midperipheral iridectomy and radial sphincterotomies

A midperipheral iridectomy is performed at the 12 o'clock meridian, using the MICRA-Pierse forceps and the Barraquer-de Wecker scissors.

The pupil, which was dilated minimally preoperatively with cyclopentolate, is dilated further, if required, by 2 or 3 drops of epinephrine solution, 1:1000.

If the iris is bound to the lens by synechiae, the 1-mm spatula is used to rupture the synechiae. If the pupil does not dilate sufficiently to permit removal of the lens, a short, 0.5-mm, radial sphincterotomy is performed at 3, 6, 9, and 12 o'clock (see Plate 6-14). These sphincterotomies should enlarge the pupil sufficiently to allow the cataractous lens to be delivered. This technique can be used also to open the fixed, small pupil often seen after prolonged administration of miotics. Alternatively, a radial sphincterotomy to the midperipheral iridectomy can be done, and, after lens extraction, the coloboma can be repaired with an iris suture.

Fixing the donor button with interrupted sutures

The donor button is fixed to the edge of the recipient cornea at 6 o'clock with a through-and-through interrupted suture of 22-micron nylon. Two additional interrupted sutures are placed at 4 and 8 o'clock to create an inferiorly hinged operculum (Plate 9-2, A). A running suture is placed with the through-and-through bites inserted at 2, 12, and 10 o'clock (Plate 9-2, B). The intermediate suture loops are retracted with the 1-mm spatula (Plate 9-2, C).

Plate 9-2

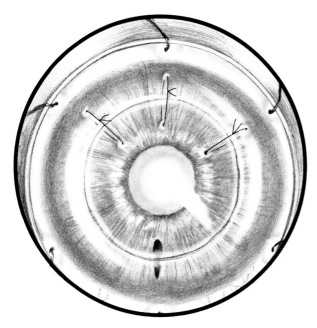

A. Three interrupted sutures placed to create inferiorly hinged, donor-button operculum.

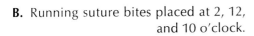

B. Running suture bites placed at 2, 12, and 10 o'clock.

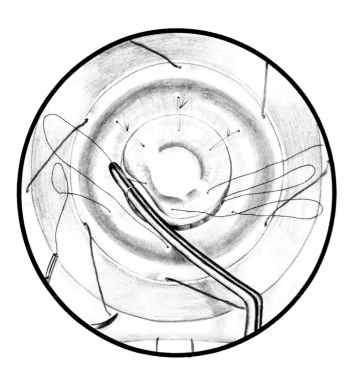

C. Intermediate suture threads looped out with 1-mm spatula.

Intracapsular cataract extraction

The donor corneal button is held away from the recipient opening by the threads on the donor button at 12 o'clock (Plate 9-3, *A*). Alpha chymotrypsin (0.2 ml of 1:5000 solution) is instilled beneath the iris with the Troutman olive-tipped irrigation needle (Plate 9-3, *B*). If necessary, the intermediate thread between the 10 and 2 o'clock donor-recipient suture bites is again retracted. The donor button is held by the assistant to prevent the corneal endothelium from coming in contact with the cryoprobe tip or the lens.

Plate 9-3

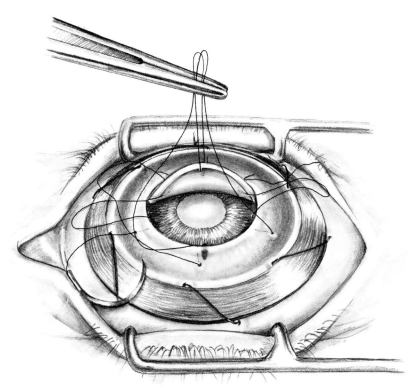

A. Retraction of donor button with 12 o'clock
donor thread loop.

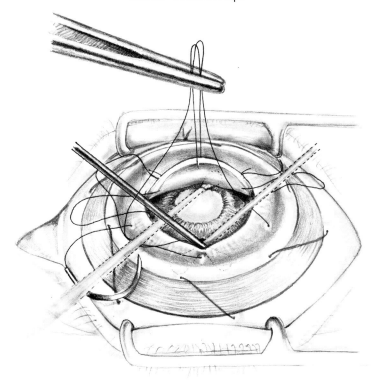

B. Alpha chymotrypsin being instilled
beneath the iris.

225

When the Amoils instrument is used, it is important to inspect carefully the silicone sleeve covering the cryoprobe tip. If the edge is found to be cracked or chipped, which often is the case, it should be trimmed with sharp scissors (Plate 9-4, *A*).

Before the probe tip is applied, the superior border of the iris should be retracted using the closed curved end of a tying forceps (Plate 9-4, *B*) or a cellulose sponge. The tip of the cryoextractor is applied to the anterior surface of the lens superiorly (Plate 9-4, *C*). The lens is rocked slowly back and forth to disengage any zonules still attached. The lens is then elevated into position to be extracted through the recipient opening (Plate 9-4, *D*).

Plate 9-4

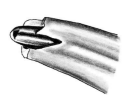

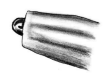

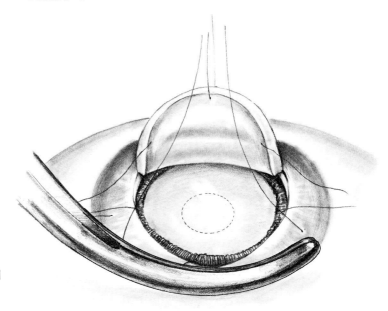

A. Chipped silicone sleeve (top) trimmed properly for cryoextraction (bottom).

B. Iris retracted, exposing the lens for application of cryoextractor tip.

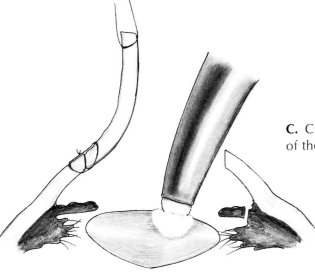

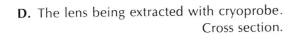

C. Cryoextractor tip applied to anterior surface of the lens. Cross section.

D. The lens being extracted with cryoprobe. Cross section.

227

If the upper edge of the lens tends to get caught internally on the rim of the recipient cornea, the lens is rotated downward by the cryoprobe, and the probe is released and reapplied more superiorly on the lens capsule. It may be necessary to repeat this maneuver several times until the upper pole of the lens can be disengaged (Plate 9-5, *A* and *B*).

As soon as the upper pole of the lens is in the recipient opening, the lens is rocked back and forth and is allowed to mold through the recipient opening (Plate 9-5, *C*). Great care should be taken, by both the surgeon and the assistant, to avoid any contact between the cryoprobe or the lens and the endothelium of the retracted donor button.

Plate 9-5

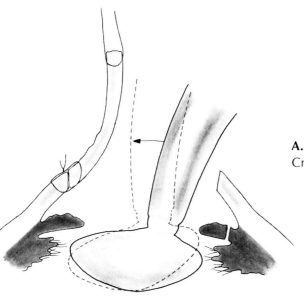

A. Elevating the upper pole of the lens. Cross section.

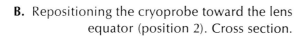

B. Repositioning the cryoprobe toward the lens equator (position 2). Cross section.

C. Sliding the lens through the pupil and recipient opening. Cross section.

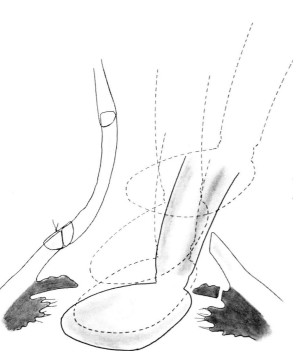

Closing the incision with interrupted sutures

As the lens is removed, the iris diaphragm retracts. The vitreous should remain behind the iris diaphragm. The continuous suture is drawn up to close the upper edge of the graft to the recipient edge (Plate 9-6, *A*). Usually an air bubble will be trapped, forming the anterior chamber. The suture loops between the three bites of the continuous suture are cut and the threads tied as three interrupted sutures (Plate 9-6, *B* and *C*). If not already formed, the anterior chamber is inflated with air to reposition the iris and to prevent the vitreous from coming forward while the continuous suture is being placed (Plate 9-6, *D*). Acetylcholine, 1:100 solution, can be used to constrict and center the pupil.

Fixing the graft with a single continuous suture

At 10× to 15× magnification, a closely spaced, single continuous suture of 22- or 16-micron nylon or polypropylene is placed, using the GS-14 or GS-19 needle. Between 20 and 30 through-and-through radial bites are taken to effect a watertight closure between the graft and the recipient.

As the slack in the continuous suture is taken up, the tension of each suture loop is adjusted with the tying forceps. The thread ends are tied together, and the knot is buried in the stroma of the donor button.

Removing the interrupted sutures

The six interrupted sutures will have been torqued from their original radial position in the direction of the overlying continuous loop. They will be loosened slightly because of the tighter wound apposition effected by the continuous suture. The interrupted suture loops are cut with the razor knife and removed with colibri-handled, suture-removing forceps.

Final suture adjustment using the Troutman surgical keratometer

The air is removed from the anterior chamber and replaced with basic salt solution. The projection of the surgical keratometer is then observed under highest power (22×), and the tension of each suture loop is adjusted with tying forceps to correct any meridional distortion indicated by the light reflexes.

The scleral support ring is removed by severing the fixing suture loops with a razor knife. The superior rectus suture is cut and removed. The speculum is used to lift the lids away from the globe. If the eye is hypotensive, basic salt solution is again introduced into the anterior chamber until the intraocular pressure is normalized. The surgical keratometer projection is observed under high power, and final suture adjustments are made, if necessary.

Plate 9-6

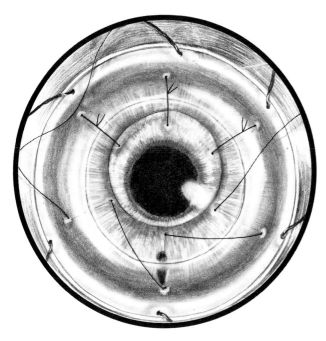

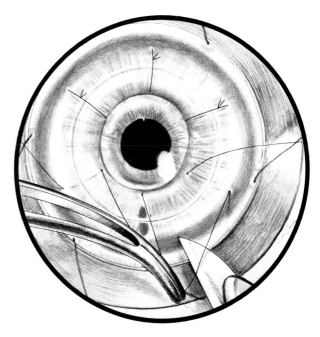

A. Continuous suture drawn up to close the superior graft edge to the recipient.

B. 10 o'clock suture loop being cut for tying as an interrupted suture.

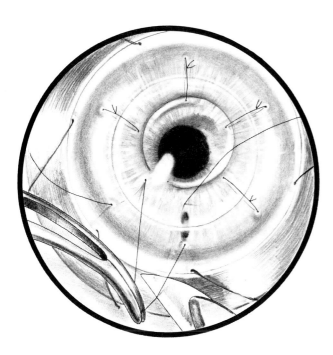

C. 10 o'clock suture tied; 12 and 2 o'clock suture loops being cut for tying.

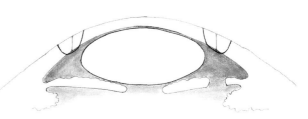

D. Air bubble maintains the anterior chamber. Cross section.

Fluorescein leak test and the surgical dressing

A drop of fluorescein dye is applied to ascertain that the final suture adjustment has not loosened a sector of the sutures (see Frontispiece). The light-wire lid speculum is turned 90° to slip easily from between the lids through the medial and lateral canthi.

A unilateral, minimal-pressure, protective dressing is applied. The patient may be ambulatory as soon as he is recovered from the anesthesia and is no longer under the influence of barbiturates or narcotics.

TECHNIQUES FOR MORE EXTENSIVE ANTERIOR SEGMENT SURGERY

If extracapsular cataract extraction is planned, if an intraocular lens is to be inserted, or if anterior segment reconstruction or vitreous surgery is to be performed, the trephined recipient button is not excised completely (Plate 9-7, A to C). A tag of tissue connecting the button to the recipient cornea is left at 6 o'clock.

If temporary closure of this flap is required, three interrupted suture bites are taken between the hinged pathologic button and the recipient at 9, 12, and 3 o'clock. These sutures are used during extracapsular cataract extraction when an infusion-aspiration unit (see Plate 5-4, B) is used to remove lens cortex or to tamponade vitreous after removal of the lens nucleus (Plate 9-7, D).

EXTRACAPSULAR CATARACT EXTRACTION

The operculum of recipient cornea is laid back and intraocular surgery proceeds. If a simple extracapsular cataract extraction is to be done, an anterior capsulectomy is performed, using a 6-mm disposable trephine blade to cut out the central portion of the capsule (Plate 9-7, A to C).

Plate 9-7

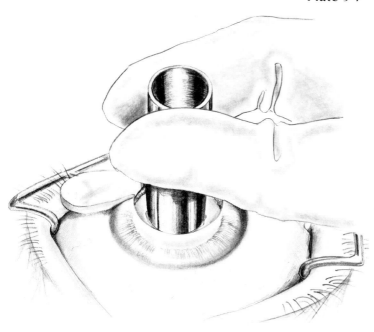

A. Trephining of anterior lens capsule.

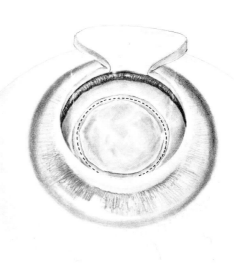

B. Circular section of anterior lens capsule after trephining. Hinged recipient flap retracted.

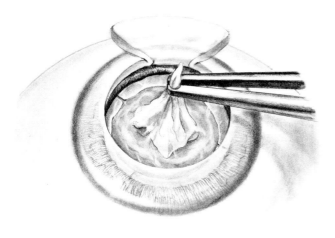

C. Removal of trephined anterior lens capsule.

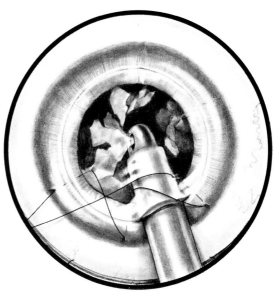

D. Tip of infusion-aspiration unit removing lens cortex. Hinged recipient flap closed with running suture.

Alternatively, a simple cystotome, made by bending the tip of a 25-gauge disposable needle, is used to puncture a pattern in the anterior capsule (Plate 9-8, *A*). The capsule is then opened along the pattern outlined (Plate 9-8, *B*). If an intraocular lens is to be inserted, an H-shaped or T-shaped opening is made. This opening maintains the fornix of the lens capsule so that, when inserted, the posterior haptics of the implant will be fixed firmly in the capsular bag postoperatively.

Plate 9-8

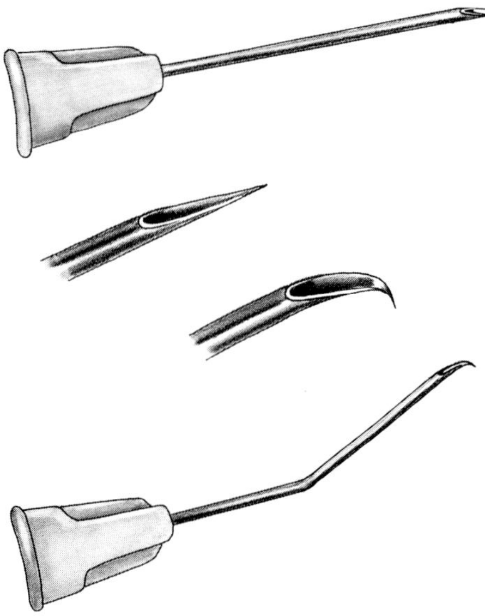

A. Cystotome made from 25-gauge disposable needle.

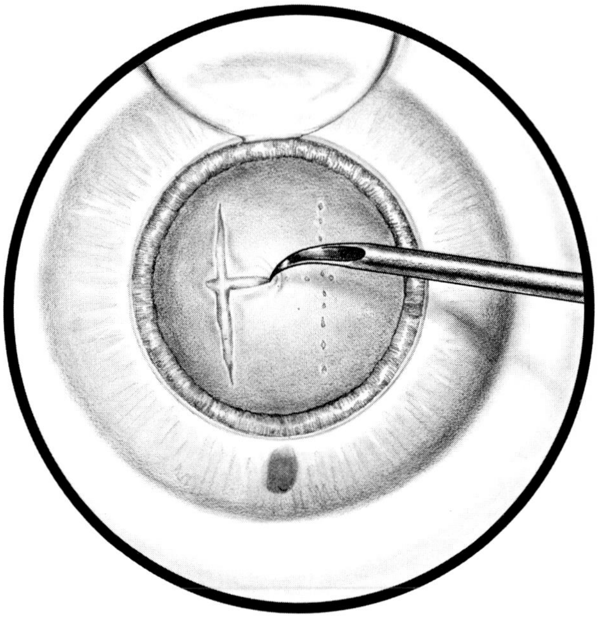

B. Cystotome ripping open punched-out pattern in anterior lens capsule.

The nucleus of the lens is expressed (Plate 9-9, *A*) or removed with the cryoextractor. A large nucleus may have to be broken into pieces before it can be expressed. Any cortical remnants are flushed from the lens fornix through the open wound, using the Troutman olive-tipped irrigator (Plate 9-9, *B*). Alternatively, a closed system, using an infusion-aspiration unit, may be preferred (Plate 9-7, *C*). When all free lens material is removed, the pathologic cornea is cut from its attachment, and the donor button is sutured in place.

Plate 9-9

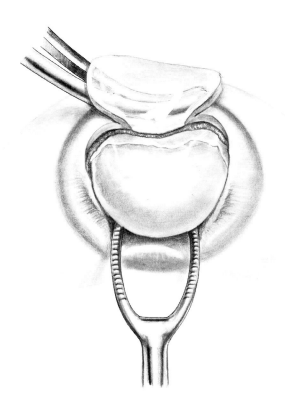

A. Expression of the lens nucleus.

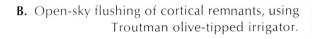

B. Open-sky flushing of cortical remnants, using Troutman olive-tipped irrigator.

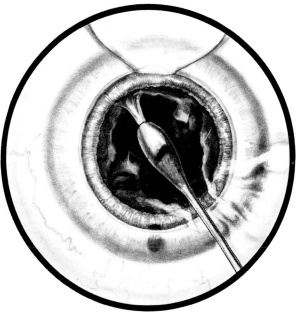

INTRAOCULAR LENS IMPLANT

If an intraocular lens implant is to be inserted, either after intracapsular or after extracapsular cataract extraction, it is done before the donor button is sutured in place. The endothelium of the donor button must not touch the methylmethacrylate lens surface or a Supramid loop. Because of their static electrical charge, the surface attraction of these materials can destroy endothelial cells. In a combined graft-intracapsular procedure with intraocular lens implant, the interrupted sutures that will fix the donor button to the recipient can be preplaced. The six suture loops are retracted or left loosely tied. When the cataractous lens is removed intracapsularly, the two-loop Worst medallion lens, a four-loop Binkhorst lens, or the Troutman neutral buoyancy lens is placed. The interrupted sutures are then drawn up to trap a protecting air bubble between the lens and the endothelium of the graft.

Intracapsular technique

Worst medallion lens. An iris-to-lens suture is used to fix the Worst medallion lens. The iris suture bite is passed in the iris midperiphery from right to left tangential to the pupil at the 12 o'clock meridian. The needle is then passed from the posterior, through the left hole of two small holes in the superior lens haptic. The needle is passed, in turn, from the front of the haptic through the second hole (Plate 9-10, A). The suture loop is then tied between the lens haptic and the iris.

The left posterior lens loop is inserted under the iris at 3 o'clock (Plate 9-10, B). As the left lens loop is held in position beneath the iris with the 1-mm iris spatula (Plate 9-10, C), a blunted iris hook is used to retract the pupillary margin of the iris at 9 o'clock, and the iris is allowed to slip between the left loop (behind) and the lens haptic (in front) (Plate 9-10, D). The 1-mm iris spatula is then withdrawn, releasing the lens (Plate 9-10, E).

Plate 9-10

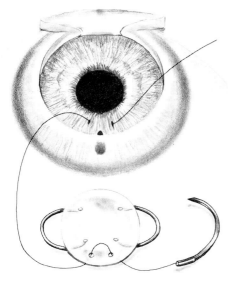

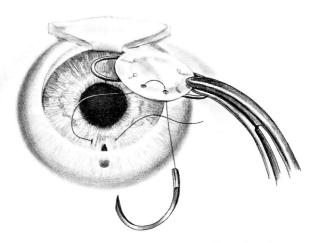

A. Iris fixation suture through iris and threaded through lens openings.

B. Lens held for insertion at the pupillary level.

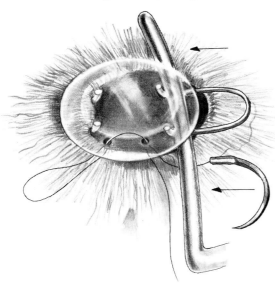

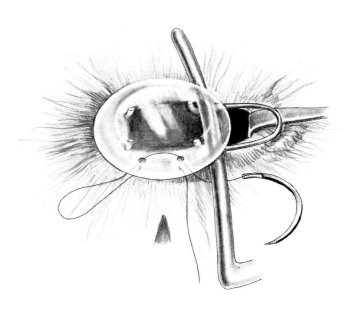

C. Left lens loop beneath the iris, using the 1-mm iris spatula.

D. Blunted iris hook retracting the iris to engage the second loop.

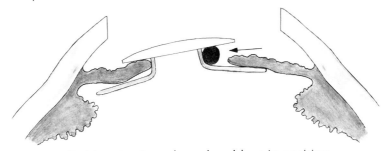

E. Iris retractor released and lens in position prior to removing 1-mm spatula.
Cross section.

When the lens is in position, the thread ends exiting behind the right lens haptic hole are tied together loosely to suspend the lens from the iris, as a pendant, hence the name medallion lens (Plate 9-11).

Plate 9-11

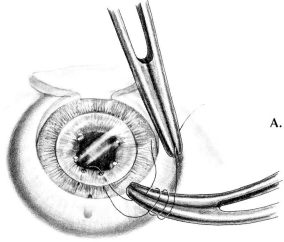

A. Lens suspension suture being tied.

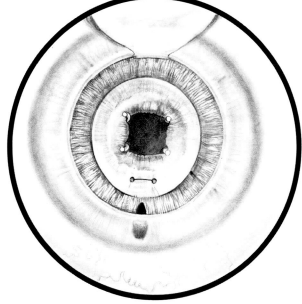

B. Detail of suture tied between lens and iris.

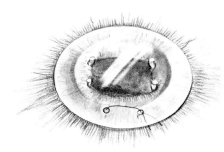

C. Final appearance of Worst medallion lens prior to suturing donor button.

239

Binkhorst four-loop intraocular lens. The Binkhorst four-loop lens with polypropylene haptics or the Troutman neutral buoyancy lens is introduced superiorly rather than laterally to engage the lower haptics or haptic across or under the inferior iris. As the lens implant is held to depress the iris slightly inferiorly, the superior iris is retracted with a small hook. The lens is released, and the iris slips around or over the upper haptics or haptic of the lens.

The Binkhorst lens is rotated until the posterior superior loop appears behind the midperipheral iridectomy. Using the GS-14 needle, the surgeon passes a polypropylene, 22-micron suture through the posterior and anterior superior loop apertures of the lens at the level of the iridectomy.

It is not always possible to pass the tip of the needle back through the recipient opening. In order to prevent excessive trauma, the tip of the needle can be driven up through the recipient cornea. The needle is retrieved, cut off, and discarded (Plate 9-12, A). The suture loop between the posterior surface of the cornea and the iris is brought into the recipient opening with a blunted iris hook (Plate 9-12, B). The distal end of the thread is pulled back through the recipient corneal ledge. The ends of the thread around the superior lens loops are tied to fix them together and to suspend the lens from the iris through the midperipheral iridectomy (Plate 9-12, C and D). This fixation prevents the total dislocation of the lens.

Several other types of lenses can be used, but those described and illustrated are the ones I usually use. The technique for inserting any pupillary lens, with minor variations, is essentially the same. Great care must be taken to avoid excessive trauma by the lens to the eye and, above all, to the endothelium of the donor button.

Graft-to-recipient closure

If the pathologic button has been left attached, it is cut free and removed when the lens implant is in place. The donor button is sutured in place with interrupted fixation sutures followed by a closely placed continuous suture.

The pathologic button, or its stripped-off Descemet's membrane, may be left temporarily between the lens and the endothelium of the donor button while interrupted fixation sutures are being placed and even as the continuous suture is placed and left untied. The pathologic button is then removed, the anterior chamber filled with air, and the sutures tied. This maneuver reduces the possibility of damage to the endothelium by the intraocular lens while the sutures are being placed. If the continuous suture is not yet placed, it can be inserted for final fixation of the donor to the recipient while the graft endothelium is separated from the intraocular lens by a bubble of air. The interrupted sutures are removed, the air replaced with solution, and the continuous suture adjusted finally with the use of the surgical keratometer.

Plate 9-12

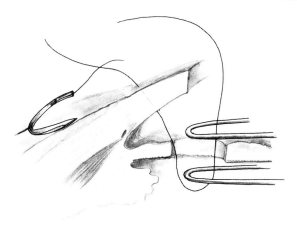

A. Needle cut off after passing through recipient ledge.

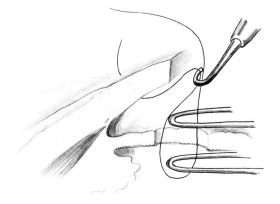

B. Retrieving thread in preparation for tying together lens loops.

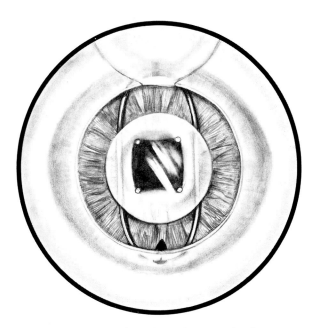

C. Binkhorst four-loop intraocular lens with polypropylene loops in situ with superior loops tied through iridectomy.

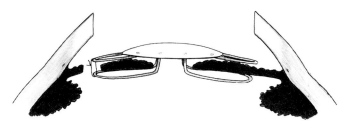

D. Four-loop lens in situ with superior loops sutured through iridectomy. Cross section.

It is essential, in any keratoplasty, but particularly when an intraocular lens is used, to have a watertight closure of the eye. This is best assured by a closely spaced continuous suture.

INTRAOCULAR LENS AFTER EXTRACAPSULAR EXTRACTION TECHNIQUE

If an intraocular lens is used after extracapsular surgery, the posterior loops of a neutral buoyancy Binkhorst two-loop or four-loop lens are inserted into the fornix of the capsular bag (Plate 9-13) following expression of the nucleus and removal of the residual cortical contents of the lens bag. Only lenses with polypropylene haptics are used as metal loops make the lens too heavy and can result in eventual lens disinsertion.

The posterior lower loop is inserted first into the inferior capsular fornix. As the lens is depressed inferiorly, the anterior superior edge of the capsule and the iris are slipped over the upper posterior loop of the lens implant with a small blunted hook. Miosis of the pupil with 1:100 acetylcholine solution centers the lens. The lens is rotated so that the posterior polypropylene loop of the iridocapsular lens is visible within the upper capsular fornix in the midperipheral iridectomy.

A suture is inserted through the midperipheral iridectomy, through the anterior capsule, and beneath the posterior lens loop. The needle continues up through the iris bordering the edge of the peripheral iridectomy to the opposite side. The needle passes directly through the recipient opening or the recipient cornea, whichever is less traumatic, to be retrieved externally. If the needle has been passed through the cornea, the internal thread is cut free from the needle, retreived, and the ends tied. This maneuver fixes the lens to the edge of the iris at the midperipheral iridectomy, preventing lens haptic dislocation until it is fixed by the lens capsule.

Graft-to-recipient closure

Once the lens is in place, the tag connecting the operculum of trephined recipient cornea is cut, and the pathologic button is removed. The donor button is sutured in place, first with interrupted sutures, then with a closely spaced, single continuous suture. The six or eight interrupted fixation sutures are removed, having fulfilled their role of ensuring that the anterior chamber remained filled and the endothelium of the donor button was clear of the intraocular lens during placement of the continuous suture. As an added precaution against endothelial damage to the donor button, the pathologic button can be left in place during suture placement, as described.

Plate 9-13

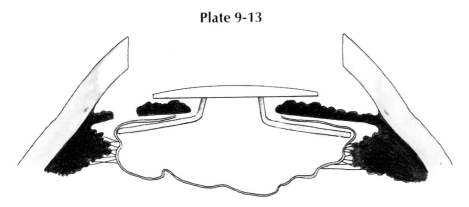

Binkhorst two-loop intraocular lens in position
in the fornix of the capsular bag. Cross section.

VITREOUS SURGERY

Vitreous surgery may follow or accompany the removal of the lens. Vitreous can be lost unexpectedly at the time of the cataract extraction or can be removed deliberately because of obstructive opacities. Extraction of vitreous by vitreous sucking-cutting technique is described in more detail in Chapter 10.

Formerly, when sponges were used for vitrectomy, if vitreous loss occurred unexpectedly when the donor was partially sutured in place, it was necessary to cut the sutures and put the graft aside to do the vitrectomy. With a vitreous sucking-cutting instrument, however, vitrectomy following accidental vitreous loss is potentially less traumatic. The graft is merely retracted carefully, and damage to endothelium during vitrectomy can be prevented by a careful assistant and an alert surgeon.

IRIS SURGERY

When the iris diaphragm has been disrupted as a result of previous or present surgery, it should be repaired. Usually this is not done until after the lens is removed. If an intraocular lens is to be used, repair of the iris diaphragm may be done, incorporating the suture used to fixate the lens. Coreoplasty is described in Chapter 6. The circumstance and the ingenuity of the individual surgeon determine the procedure for reconstruction of the iris diaphragm and for recentering of the pupil. A disrupted iris diaphragm, when possible, should be reconstructed, since an intact, taut diaphragm is less likely to come into contact with, and thus damage or adhere to, the internal aspect of the graft or the incision. Also, it prevents the vitreous from impinging on, and possibly adhering to, the healing internal aspect of the graft incision.

SUMMARY

In the management of cataract coincident with corneal pathology, I prefer, when possible, to perform keratoplasty and cataract extraction at the same intervention. The intraocular lens may be used to advantage in the older patient but at greater long-term risk to the outcome of the keratoplasty procedure.

Removing the cataract following successful keratoplasty presents an additional hazard, especially when an intraocular lens is used. Removing the cataract prior to keratoplasty adds a second operative procedure and increases the probability of complication.

The variations in technique for more or less complicated interventions, involving intracapsular or extracapsular removal of cataract during the keratoplasty procedure, the insertion of an intraocular lens, and additional surgery of the vitreous or iris, have been described in detail.

CHAPTER 10

APHAKIC KERATOPLASTY

General considerations
B-scan tomography for surgical indications
Avoiding unnecessary surgery
Preparation for surgery
Exposure and fixation
Cutting the donor button
Cutting the recipient opening
Management of additional anterior
   segment pathology

Suturing the donor to the recipient
The fluorescein leak test
Adjusting the sutures using the Troutman
   surgical keratometer
Vitreous loss
Coreoplasty
Summary

GENERAL CONSIDERATIONS

The prognosis of keratoplasty in the aphakic eye has been improved greatly by microsurgery and by the concomitant use of elastic monofilament suture material. By the time a graft is performed on an aphakic eye, the eye has had at least one and often several previous surgeries or traumatic incidents. In the case of previous surgery, operative or postoperative complications often have occurred, contributing to the corneal pathology. In the case of traumatic injury, damage may have occurred to anterior segment or posterior segment structures other than the lens and cornea. These complications not only contribute to the technical difficulty of the keratoplasty procedure but also increase the morbidity. In addition, they reduce the opportunity to obtain a clear graft and an optimum optical result. Though technical perfection does not always ensure a perfect result, perfect technique is essential to obtain the best possible result in the more anatomically and surgically complicated aphakic eye. Perfection of technique, preceded by careful planning and preparation for the surgical procedure and followed by meticulous postoperative care, is the hallmark of successful penetrating keratoplasty in the aphakic eye.

B-SCAN TOMOGRAPHY FOR SURGICAL INDICATIONS

Nowhere is it more important to employ the Bronson B-scan ultrasound unit (Plate 10-1) than in the preoperative planning for and the postoperative follow-up of aphakic keratoplasty. As in phakic corneal pathologies, often it is not possible to visualize the posterior segment. Even when it can be seen or when indirect ophthalmoscopy is used, one or more sectors can be obscured from view. B-scan tomography should be done routinely on any aphakic eye with corneal opacification sufficient to prevent adequate visualization of the retina. This probably includes every eye with corneal pathology sufficiently dense to require keratoplasty. Thus, a patient may be spared unnecessary surgery or may have a procedure more appropriate to the condition.

Plate 10-1

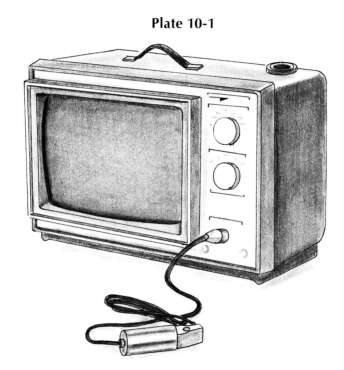

Bronson B-scan ultrasound unit.

The surgeon may be spared a postoperative "surprise" if the B-scan indicates the presence of posterior segment or retinal pathology that might nullify or modify an anticipated result of keratoplasty (Plate 10-2, B to F). For example, the ravages of a long-standing glaucoma, including severe cupping of the nerve, can be detected by ultrasound. This additional information may enable the surgeon to advise against surgical intervention or to give the patient a more realistic prognosis. On the other hand, sometimes in a very severely disrupted anterior segment, where one expects to find severe posterior pathology, the posterior segment may be found sonically to be clear (Plate 10-2, A).

AVOIDING UNNECESSARY SURGERY

Often, the aphakic penetrating keratoplasty is done on the patient's only seeing eye. The more detailed the information obtained in advance of the surgery, the more exact the prognosis can be and the better the patient is able to accept the outcome realistically, especially when the results may be limited. Every nonsurgical means should be sought to restore useful vision to the one-eyed patient. Even following technically successful surgery, the incidence of delayed postoperative complications, such as glaucoma, vitreous opacification, or vitreous retraction and retinal detachment, is high. The possibility that minimum functional vision could be reduced to blindness demands a very conservative approach. As an example, in severe aphakic bullous keratopathy, a therapeutic contact lens not only can control pain but also may improve vision.

In a patient with useful vision in the other eye, especially when that eye is phakic or if the patient is of advanced age, keratoplasty in the aphakic eye should be deferred since, even when the aphakic eye is operated on successfully, the patient usually does not use it. An exception would be when there is evidence that failure to do immediate surgery would result in loss of the vision potential of the eye because of untreated secondary pathology, such as retinal detachment, glaucoma, or uveitis controllable only by surgical intervention.

Plate 10-2

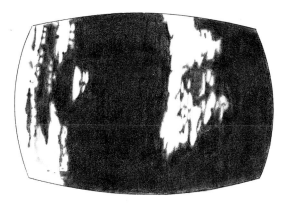

A. Normal B-scan.

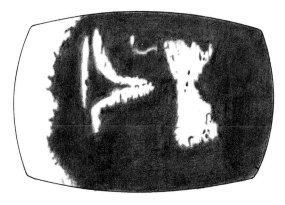

B. Morning glory (total) retinal detachment.

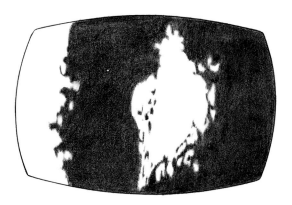

C. Tumor in posterior segment.

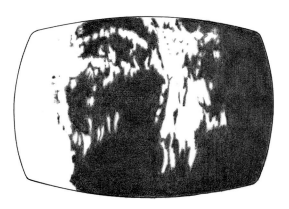

D. Resolving intravitreous hemorrhage.

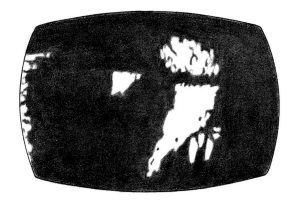

E. Intravitreous foreign body.

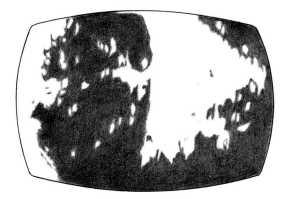

F. Vitreous opacifications.

Representative B-scan Polaroid reproductions.

PREPARATION FOR SURGERY

In aphakic keratoplasty, once the decision to operate has been made, the preoperative preparation of the patient is more critical than in phakic keratoplasty. Glaucoma should be controlled or its control included in the surgical plan, as is discussed in Chapter 12. Postoperatively, the primary threats to a successful outcome of aphakic keratoplasty, aside from glaucoma, are uveitis and vitreitis. Corneal vascularization, formerly a feared complicating factor, usually recedes after microsurgical keratoplasty, since the 16- or 22-micron suture material used does not induce neovascularization, as does silk or gut thread.

When possible, the eye should be free of inflammation when surgery is performed. However, it is not always possible to control uveitis. It may be counterproductive to allow an extensive vitreitis to resolve spontaneously, for vitreous retraction and detachment may result. Preoperatively, immunosuppressive agents should be used to effect temporary control of or as a prophylactic agent against anticipated early postoperative uveitis or vitreitis.

Since the pathology already may involve the vitreous at the time of surgery—in a large proportion of cases the vitreous becomes involved during the surgical procedure—the prophylactic dose of prednisone is routinely given orally. Since more extensive surgical trauma is anticipated, for example, vitrectomy or coreoplasty, the eye is more susceptible to postoperative infection. Prophylactic cephaloridine, 2000 mg daily, is given beginning 48 hours preoperatively. When the patient's medical condition permits, mannitol, 1.5 gm per kilogram of body weight, is given intravenously half an hour prior to the surgical procedure. Administration should be completed before the globe is opened.

When a chronic local inflammatory reaction is present or when there is a history of recurrent local infection threatening intraoperative bacterial invasion, the prophylactic systemic antibiotic is reinforced at surgery, prior to opening the globe, with a sub-Tenon's capsule injection of 20 mg of gentamicin deep in the inferior cul-de-sac.

EXPOSURE AND FIXATION

The speculum is inserted, and the globe is immobilized with a 16- or 18-mm Flieringa ring, as described in Chapter 9. If a massive scleral collapse is anticipated, a LeGrand ring or a Girard scleral expander (Plate 10-3) may be used. A moist cellulose sponge is placed on the eye to protect the exposed cornea while the donor button is cut.

Prior to preparing the donor button, the surgeon should partially penetrate a vascularized cornea by trephining. This will provide sufficient time for bleeding to stop while the donor button is being prepared and facilitates the final excision of the pathologic button.

Plate 10-3

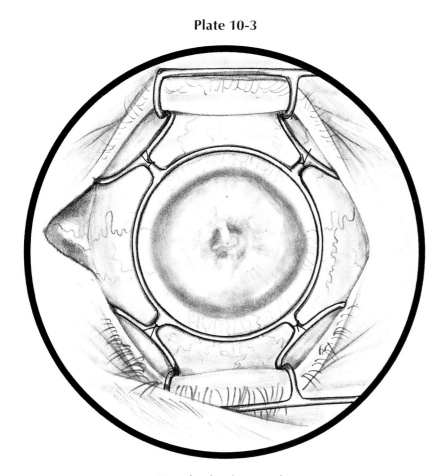

Girard scleral expander.

CUTTING THE DONOR BUTTON

In aphakic keratoplasty, the donor button is always cut with a trephine blade 0.5 mm to 1 mm larger than that used to cut the recipient opening. This ensures a tighter fit of the graft in the recipient opening and tends to reduce the aphakic hyperopia. Each 0.1-mm increase in the graft diameter will induce about 0.5 to 1 diopter of myopia. *In addition, the anterior chamber angle is deepened and postoperative aphakic glaucoma is decreased significantly.* When a graft 9 mm or larger is used, a trephine 1 mm larger in diameter is used to cut the donor button. However, if the other eye also is aphakic but has a normal cornea or has had a successful keratoplasty with the same-diameter graft as recipient opening, anisometropia can result if now the donor button is cut larger than the recipient opening. In this instance, the trephine used to cut the donor button may be the same size as or no more than 0.2 mm larger than that used for the recipient opening for optical purposes, but only if glaucoma has not complicated the course of the fellow eye.

The donor button of appropriate size is cut and is immersed in tissue-culture fluid in the hollow of the Teflon cutting block—ready for use in the recipient.

CUTTING THE RECIPIENT OPENING

The recipient eye is trephined. Occasionally, the recipient eye is so soft it may collapse when the trephine is applied. In this event, the trephine is withdrawn, and a puncture is made obliquely, with a sharp needle or a Ziegler-type knife point, through the cornea at the limbus. Basic salt solution and air are introduced through a No. 30 blunted needle to normalize the tension of the eye. The trephine is again placed on the eye, and the cut is continued. To trephine the aphakic eye, the trephine stop should be set for partial penetration. With the thumb and second finger, the trephine handle is turned through 360°; then the direction of the rotation is reversed, as described for other procedures. With minimal pressure a sharp blade should cut evenly until it reaches the stop, at which point it is withdrawn.

It is best not to penetrate the full thickness of the cornea with the trephine blade because when the eye is opened, the weight of the trephine causes the globe to collapse and may result in loss of vitreous. Also, too-rapid decompression may cause a subchoroidal, or even an expulsive, hemorrhage from new-formed vessels in the anterior segment.

The trephine cut should be made to as deep a level as possible. From the depth of the trephined incision, the anterior chamber is entered between 9 and 11 o'clock with a diamond or razor knife (Plate 10-4, *A*). From this position, the right and left keratoplasty scissors can be introduced more easily to complete the circumferential incision.

252

Plate 10-4

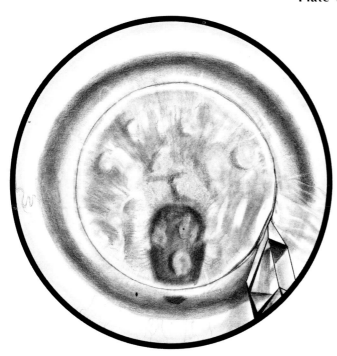

A. Completing the trephine cut with the diamond knife.

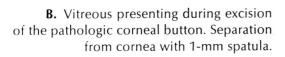

B. Vitreous presenting during excision of the pathologic corneal button. Separation from cornea with 1-mm spatula.

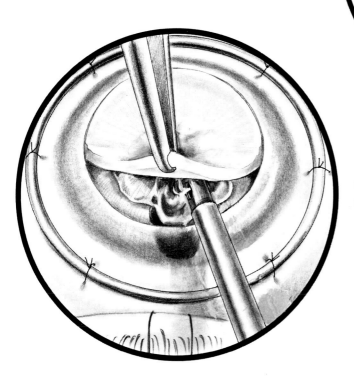

C. Tip of vitreous sucking-cutting instrument excising vitreous in the anterior segment.

MANAGEMENT OF ADDITIONAL ANTERIOR SEGMENT PATHOLOGY

Iris or vitreous attached to the corneal endothelial surface or to a previous graft incision should be separated carefully with the 1-mm spatula. If the hyaloid face ruptures or is not intact, vitreous will present at this point. If possible, the button should be first separated completely from underlying structures and then excised to provide better visualization for subsequent coreoplasty or vitrectomy.

If vitreous loss is severe and continues to interfere with visualization and to jeopardize the routine completion of the incision, a vitreous sucking-cutting instrument is introduced to cut the vitreous from the wound area and from the anterior segment before the button is excised (Plate 10-4, C). When the hyaloid face remains intact, and the vitreous body retracts behind the pupil, the pathologic button can be excised without the need for vitreous surgery.

If the iris cannot be separated readily from its attachment to the corneal endothelial surface, it can be cut free with the Vannas scissors (Plate 10-5, A). Corneal tissue remaining attached to the iris or any residual iris tissue adhering to the cornea is then dissected as the pathologic cornea is being removed or immediately following its removal (Plate 10-5, B). Scar tissue remaining on the sphincter or adjacent iris is excised (Plate 10-5, C). Iris sutures are used, when necessary, to close a resulting coloboma or to recenter the pupil (Plate 10-5, D).

Plate 10-5

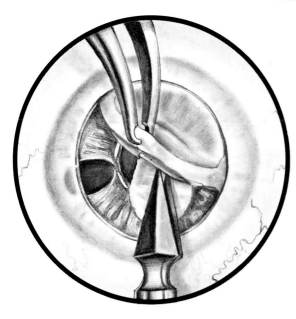

A. Vannas scissors used to split cornea that is adherent to iris.

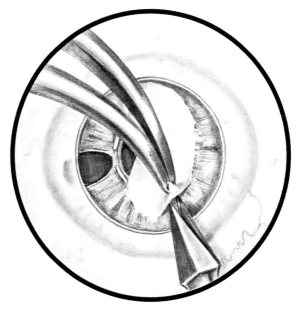

B. Vannas scissors used to dissect carefully the remaining adherent cornea from the iris.

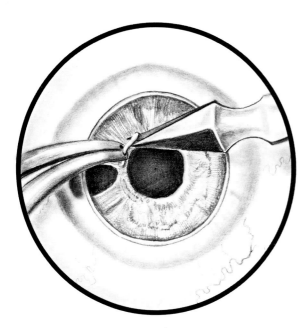

C. Vannas scissors used to excise scar tissue from the sphincter.

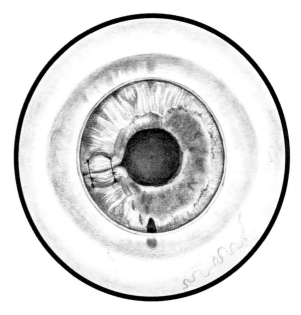

D. Coloboma closed with two iris sutures.

SUTURING THE DONOR TO THE RECIPIENT

The donor button is sutured in place immediately, using six or eight cardinal fixation sutures followed by a closely spaced, single continuous suture. The loops of the continuous suture are adjusted, and the closing knot is tied and buried in the needle tract on the donor side. Any air in the anterior segment must be removed and the normal tension of the eye restored with saline before a reliable reading can be taken with the surgical keratometer. A single air bubble is removed readily with a syringe attached to a 30-gauge angled needle (Plate 10-6). The needle is introduced through the wound between two adjacent suture loops. The blunted tip of the needle is passed into the air bubble and gentle suction is applied. If the needle tip is kept within the bubble, the air is withdrawn easily. Care is taken not to back-flush small bubbles into the anterior segment, since these are difficult to remove. The fixation sutures are removed. The anterior chamber is filled from the exterior with basic salt solution forcefully directed around the circumference of the incision (see Plate 6-28, *A*). Sufficient fluid is forced between the lips of the incision to normalize the tension without distorting the incision or stretching the suture loops.

THE FLUORESCEIN LEAK TEST

The watertight integrity of the wound is tested with fluorescein (see Frontispiece).

ADJUSTING THE SUTURES USING THE TROUTMAN SURGICAL KERATOMETER

The surgical keratometer projection is viewed at highest magnification, and the tension of the suture loops is adjusted, as necessary, to round out the projected pattern.

The fixation ring and the superior rectus suture are removed. The speculum is lifted to elevate the lids away from the eye, and, if indicated, a final adjustment of the continuous suture is made under surgical keratometer observation. The intraocular pressure is checked by scleral and corneal depression. Additional basic salt solution is injected, if necessary, before the final surgical keratometer–monitored suture adjustment.

Plate 10-6

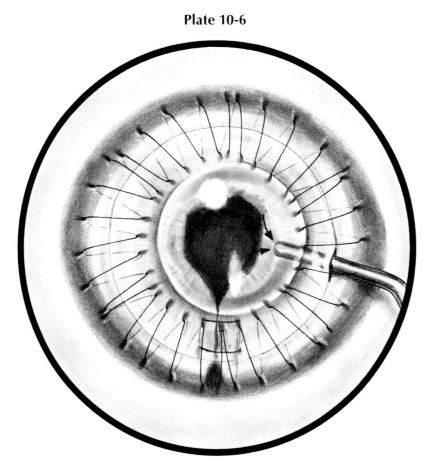

Removing air from the anterior chamber
in preparation for adjustment of
continuous suture, using surgical keratometer.
Cardinal sutures still in place.

VITREOUS LOSS

In the event of vitreous loss, a shallow anterior vitrectomy, extending about one-third of the way into the vitreous body (Plate 10-7), is performed prior to suturing the donor button in place. A vitreous sucking-cutting instrument, such as that of Douvas, is used. If a more sophisticated instrument is not available, the Kaufman vitrector can be used. However, this unit is not easily controlled and can be traumatic. The sponge technique is my second choice.

Plate 10-7

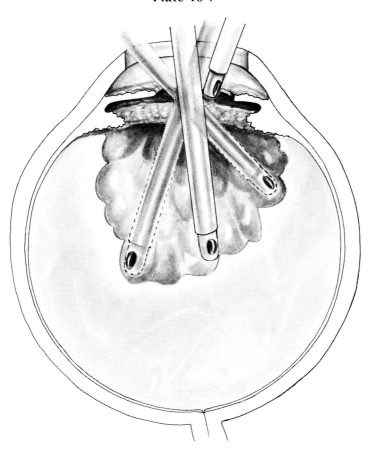

Shallow anterior vitrectomy and
marginal iridectomy using
Douvas rotoextractor.

When the vitrectomy is completed, the iris surface is cleaned of adherent vitreous strands with the tip of a moistened cellulose sponge (Plate 10-8, *A*). This maneuver serves also to position the pupil or to align iris fragments for coreoplasty.

COREOPLASTY

If synechiae are present, the pupil will not center, and the iris is distorted. The restricting tissue bands and their points of adhesion are identified and evaluated with the 1-mm spatula (Plate 10-8, *B*). Sometimes these adhesions can be separated gently by blunt dissection with the spatula, but usually they have to be cut free with Vannas scissors (Plate 10-8, *C*). Care must be taken, however, not to dissect too deeply into the angle, since sharp bleeding can occur. Often, sufficient iris tissue can be mobilized to reconstruct a disrupted iris diaphragm and to form a new pupil (Plate 10-8, *D*). An intact iris diaphragm tends to prevent residual vitreous from moving into the anterior segment and attaching to the graft incision. The reconstructed pupil reduces glare and diffraction from the scar of the successful graft. The possible disadvantage of the reduced visualization of the peripheral fundus is compensated partially by the postoperative use of the B-scan. One or several interrupted polypropylene sutures are used to close the iris colobomas.

If it is not possible to reconstruct the pupil, additional iris tissue may have to be resected, either with Vannas scissors or with the rotoextractor, to prevent the possibility of a flap of iris adhering to the internal graft incision or blocking the angle.

Should the globe retract or collapse during any phase of the surgical procedure, particularly during vitrectomy, the suture loops fixing the scleral ring are lifted to expand the globe. The vitreous falls back, and the anterior-posterior segment relationships are reestablished (see Plate 6-2, *A*).

Plate 10-8

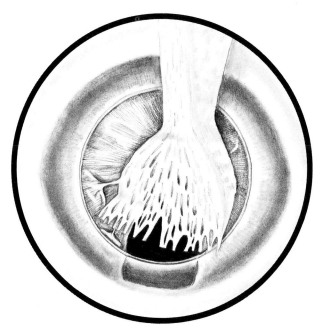

A. Cleaning vitreous strands from iris following anterior vitrectomy.

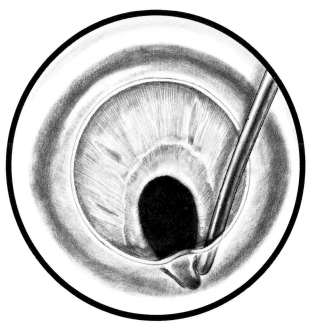

B. Identifying and testing strength of iris adhesion to angle.

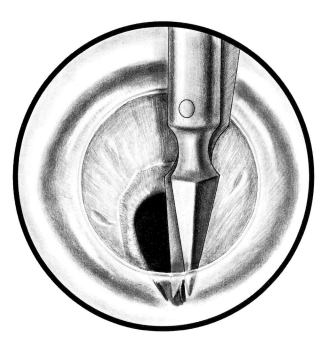

C. Cutting resistant iris adhesion with Vannas scissors.

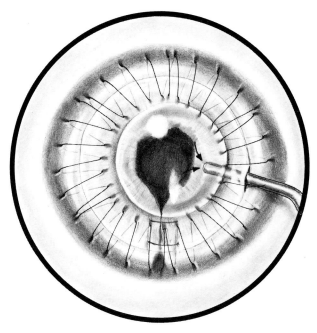

D. Reconstructed pupil. Superior coloboma closed with two iris sutures.

SUMMARY

Aphakic keratoplasty is among the more difficult, varied, and challenging corneal graft procedures. The slightest technical error may compromise the repair of these often seriously damaged eyes. In aphakic keratoplasty, more than in phakic keratoplasty, the surgeon's work does not begin or end in the operating room. Often the most significant contributions are made prior to surgery, medically during the postoperative period, or by a subsequent surgical intervention to control a medically unresponsive complication.

Nevertheless, with the use of the surgical microscope, microsurgical instrumentation, and elastic monofilament suture materials, the prognosis in aphakic keratoplasty has improved significantly in recent years. When relative integrity and function of the posterior segment can be ascertained preoperatively, the surgeon should not hesitate to perform keratoplasty in the aphakic eye. More often than not, the effort may be rewarded by a functional graft and a grateful patient.

CHAPTER 11

TROUTMAN CORNEAL WEDGE RESECTION FOR CORRECTION OF ASTIGMATISM

General considerations
Principle of wedge resection
General theory—membrane equation
    Effect of altering the shape of the
        corneal ring
    Practical application of theoretic
        considerations
    Clinical application
Surgical technique
    Timing

Preparation
Selection of the sector to be wedge-
    resected
Cutting the wedge
Suturing the edges of the resection
Summary of the technique
Repair of edge elevation
Postoperative care
Troutman relaxing incision for lower
    degrees of corneal astigmatism
Summary

GENERAL CONSIDERATIONS

Residual postoperative astigmatism, in an otherwise successful, clear, corneal graft, remains the major unsolved complication of corneal microsurgery. This astigmatism, usually averaging about 4 diopters, is almost always functionally annoying. It can be of such magnitude that the patient may see less through an optically clear corneal graft than preoperatively through the pathologic cornea. Many patients who anticipated enjoying good vision without spectacles following keratoplasty have been forced to wear either unsightly astigmatic spectacle corrections or to return to contact lenses. Nevertheless, this "complication" has been virtually ignored by corneal surgeons, who, until very recently, have understandably been preoccupied with obtaining a good anatomic, surgical result and a clear graft. As a consequence, not only is astigmatism not included in most lists of complications, it is not quantified in most reported results of keratoplasty.

As microsurgical techniques for keratoplasty have improved its performance and outcome, the possibility of technical and tissue failure has diminished. My previous, overriding concern regarding physiologic and anatomic results has given way to a concern regarding the optical results of penetrating keratoplasty, with particular emphasis on astigmatism. The first line of attack in the correction of preexisting or in the prevention of surgically induced ametropia is at the primary procedure (see Chapter 8).

My first attempt, made in 1963, at primary surgical control of astigmatism using an equal-sized circular donor button and recipient opening, began with a 7-mm diameter graft. The diameters were increased in 0.5-mm steps up to a diameter of 9 mm. Larger-diameter grafts—until then subject to a higher rate of complication—became possible as a result of the use of microsurgical technique and, in particular, elastic monofilament nylon suture. Using this approach, spherically equivalent myopia, then occurring routinely with the smaller-sized graft, was controlled successfully when a graft with an 8-mm diameter was used. However, the postoperative astigmatism, which I had hoped to control as well, was not decreased significantly.

Before 1967, when I developed and put into practice the operation of corneal "wedge" resection for correction of astigmatism postkeratoplasty, there was no mention in the literature of the systematic use of this technique.

The desire to correct corneal astigmatic ametropia, however, has preoccupied several other authors, notably Sato, who was the first to publish a paper on the use of an optical incision. His incision was made into the posterior cornea through a paracentesis incision to flatten a steeper corneal meridian. His technique was abandoned, since it produced minimal and somewhat random results, and when it succeeded it often induced myopia as well as an irregular astigmatism.

Another investigator, J. I. Barraquer, has concentrated on the spherical optical modification of resected corneal segments on a lathe—keratomileusis and keratophakia. His operation, though technically complicated, is relatively safe and effective and will probably come into wider use.

The Troutman corneal wedge resection to correct astigmatism is used, in most instances, following an otherwise successful penetrating keratoplasty; in some cases, at primary keratoplasty; and, in a few cases, at or following cataract surgery. The operation consists of the removal of a crescentic wedge-profiled sector of cornea across the axis of the flatter meridian (the minus cylinder). This has the effect of steepening the flatter meridian, flattening the steeper meridian at 90°, and decreasing the overall corneal spherical equivalent power.

The first patients on whom such correction was attempted were those who, after successful penetrating keratoplasty, had residual astigmatic bands in excess of 10 diopters. More recently, as the accuracy and reliability of the corneal procedure have been improved with the use of the Troutman surgical keratometer and, in particular, with the Troutman relaxing incision technique (see p. 286), correction for as little as 5 diopters of astigmatism postkeratoplasty has been performed successfully. In the average case, the Troutman corneal wedge resection technique has been consistent in reducing the preoperative excessive astigmatic band by 75%. In every case attempted, the astigmatism has been reduced in power in the desired meridian, though not always in the amount anticipated. This is in contrast to attempts to control astigmatism at primary keratoplasty. Deliberate ovaling of the recipient bed by a wedge resection at the preoperatively measured flatter meridian (at primary keratoplasty) was demonstrated to reduce a preexisting astigmatic band. However, sometimes a marked under- or overcorrection occurred. In early cases, the results were so random that the technique was temporarily abandoned. More recently, with the use of the surgical keratometer, the primary control of astigmatism has been more successful. Nevertheless, it is necessary to have available a technique to correct postoperatively those cases with excessive errors following routine keratoplasty or in which the attempted control of an anticipated error at the primary procedure failed.

PRINCIPLE OF WEDGE RESECTION

Though the principle of the Troutman corneal wedge resection is not complicated, if it is poorly understood, serious errors in its surgical execution may be committed. We will again consider, therefore, the anatomic and optical bases of astigmatism and how a meridional error can be corrected by corneal wedge resection. In addition, a mathematical basis will be given to approximate the amount of tissue resection required to achieve a desired result.

Surgically induced ametropia results from, and its correction is accomplished by, accidental or deliberate resection or incision of or addition to the corneal tissue. Sutures, even when inaccurately positioned or deliberately misplaced, have only a secondary influence.

First, we will examine the physical structure of the cornea and its geometric optics without considering the effects of incisions, excisions, or sutures. Physically and optically, the external coat of the eye is made up of overlapping segments of two spheres of different diameter (Plate 11-1). The larger spherical segment, the sclera, consists of randomly arranged, fibroelastic tissue and is contiguous to the smaller, spherical segment, the cornea, which consists of transparent, more linearly arranged, elastic tissue. The junction of these two spherical segments, the limbus, is a ring-like structure that is assumed, for purposes of our calculations, to be 12 mm in diameter. This composite-tissue ring is not only an anatomic boundary but also an optical boundary, limiting the secondary effect of an anatomic distortion of either spherical segment on the other. For practical purposes, the scleral hemisphere has no primary optical function. However, the function of its anterior limit at the posterior border of the cornea, the limbal ring, is of great importance in the production or control of meridional corneal errors.

The cornea is both plastic and elastic, capable of assuming and maintaining a curvature or of taking a different one. A meridional distortion, or astigmatism, occurs as the result of alterations in the shape of the limbal ring with a corresponding change in the curvature of the corneal dome. Inversely, a change induced in the curvature of the corneal dome will alter the shape of the limbal ring. The shape of the limbal ring or the corneal dome is determined by genetic or pathologic factors and is maintained by the intraocular pressure.

GENERAL THEORY—MEMBRANE EQUATION

In theory, if the elastic modulus of the cornea were a known quantity, we could solve its membrane equation, and we would be able to describe exactly, in mathematical terms, the corneal shape. However, this membrane equation, which derives from the elastic theory of plates and shells and is

266

Plate 11-1

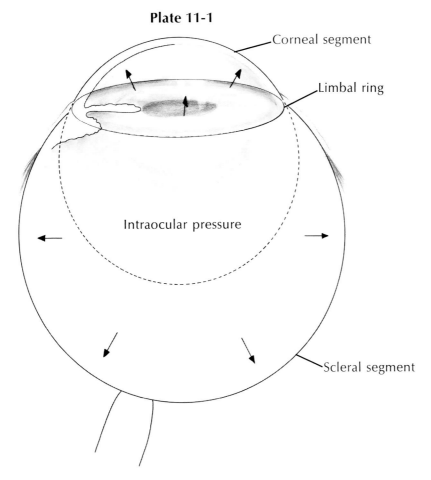

Corneal segment

Limbal ring

Intraocular pressure

Scleral segment

Optical, anatomic structure of the globe.

used in the design of deep-diving craft, has a form similar to Einstein's general field equation. For our purposes, unfortunately, it cannot be defined precisely. The inability to solve the membrane equation to modify the corneal configuration does not prevent us from attacking this problem from another, more practical and accessible route. The corneal wedge resection—initially an empiric surgical approach—has been shown to yield a reasonably accurate mathematical solution.

Effect of altering the shape of the corneal ring

The resection of a crescentic wedge of tissue from the corneal dome induces, in turn, an alteration in the shape of the limbal ring. The shortening of the corresponding corneal diameter produces a steepening of that corneal meridian, which results in the reduction or elimination of the flat (minus) astigmatic band. The opposing diameter (at 90°) is lengthened correspondingly. This effect is the same as that demonstrated in Chapter 2. When the limbal ring is made oval, the corneal dome (meridian) is steepened across the shortened diameter, whereas the meridian corresponding to the lengthened diameter (90° to the shortened one) flattens. This effect can be accomplished temporarily, by external compression, or permanently, by ovaling the donor cornea or ovaling the recipient opening by wedge-resecting a sector of the recipient edge (see Plate 2-9). In the present example, however, it is assumed that the limbal ring initially is oval, not round, and that the resection is done to correct, rather than to create, an error.

When a section of the meridional plane (corneal dome) is excised and the edges of the resected area held firmly apposed by sutures, the corneal geometry is altered in two ways. First, it shortens the arc length (anatomic curvature of the corneal dome). Second, the chord length (diameter) is shortened (Plate 11-2).

This second point requires some clarification. First, the circumference of the limbal ring remains constant and is not affected when a section of the corneal dome (meridional plane) is removed and the resected edges are apposed by sutures. Furthermore, it follows that the shape of this fixed-circumference ring, whether round or distorted originally, is altered by the wedge resection of a meridian of the corneal dome.

In mathematical terms, the shortened chord length or diameter of the wedge-resected meridian becomes the minor axis. The simultaneous shortening of the arc length (corneal curvature) and the chord length (corneal diameter) in the resected meridian steepens the cornea in this meridian and has the concomitant effect of lengthening the chord (but not the arc length) in the meridian perpendicular to the resected meridian. This results, therefore, in a flattening of the corneal curvature at 90° to the steepened meridian, enhancing the wedge resection effect.

Corneal wedge resection, therefore, changes the curvature of not just one but of two meridians, the resected meridian and that meridian at right angles to it. Therefore, to predict any optical or refractive result from a corneal wedge resection, one must consider not only the primary steepening effect, but also the concomitant secondary flattening effect on the opposing meridian.

Plate 11-2

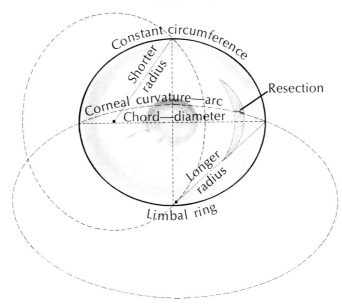

A. Three-quarter view of elliptic corneal ring:
astigmatic cornea.

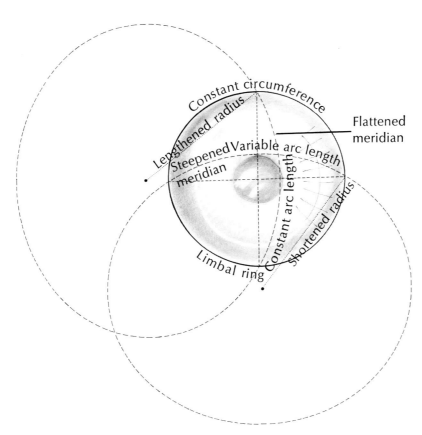

B. Three-quarter view of circular corneal ring:
anastigmatic cornea.

For example, consider a hypothetical case based on findings from a number of my actual surgical results. Preoperatively, the keratometer reads a steeper 48 diopters (radius 7.03 mm) at 90° and a flatter 42 diopters (radius 8.03 mm) at 180° (Plate 11-3, *A*). The limbal ring preoperatively is oval, the chord lengths measuring 12.95 mm at 180° and 12.05 mm at 90°. The goal of the planned corneal wedge resection procedure is to achieve, finally, an almost spherical cornea and a circular limbal ring.

It should be noted that in ophthalmic terminology, as translated from the mathematical, in the cornea the diameter (d) is the same as chord length, and the curvature (c) is the same as arc length.

The circumference of the limbus is derived from the equation for the circumference of an ellipse:

$$C_e = \pi \, [(1.5) \, (a+b) - \sqrt{ab}\,]$$

where

a = ½ major chord (lengthened diameter)
b = ½ minor chord (shortened diameter)

and is found to be 39.28 (Plate 11-3, *A*).

In the hypothetical example given above, in order to steepen the flatter horizontal meridian, the correcting wedge resection is centered at the 180° meridian. If the resection is performed at the flatter meridian, in this case the 180° meridian, our clinical results suggest that to effect a correction, the radius of that meridian needs to be reduced by *approximately* two-thirds the difference between the preoperative dioptric meridional powers [(48 − 42) (⅔) or 7.67 mm], or to about 44 diopters, steepening the cornea in that meridian (Plate 11-3). In order to calculate the amount of resection required to accomplish this steepening, the arc length of the flatter meridian at 90° to the steeper meridian must be determined trigonometrically, and it is calculated to be 15.04 mm (Plate 11-3, *A*).

The mathematical problem now is to determine the width of the resection (w). Though w can be calculated for each case, a nomogram may be prepared to determine it more readily. It is important to note that only one value of w satisfies the requirements for the individual case. Solving the transcendental equation that arises, one finds w to be equal to 0.47 mm (Plate 11-3, *A*).

After suturing, the limbus will be more circular in shape, and the radius of the 180° meridian correspondingly decreased (Plate 11-3, *B*). The chord (diameter) of this shortened (minor) axis will be 12.95 − 0.47 = 12.48 mm (Plate 11-3, *B*). (The width of the resection is subtracted from the chord length rather than from the arc length to simplify the calculation.) For a smaller wedge resection, 1 mm or less, the increase in the length of the shorter chord (at 90°) is equal to the decrease in the resected opposing chord. In this example, the lengthened vertical chord (vertical corneal diameter) will then be increased from 12.05 mm to 12.52 mm (Plate 11-3, *B*).

Using the lengthened chord and the original arc length on the steeper

Plate 11-3

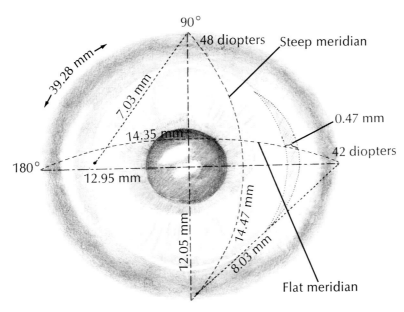

A. Dimensions of flatter and steeper
meridians before wedge resection.

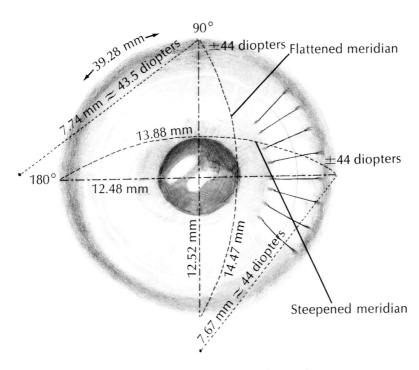

B. Dimensions of corneal meridians after
corneal wedge resection.

(preoperative) meridian (14.47 mm) (Plate 11-3), one can repeat the calculation so that the final radius (R) rather than w is the unknown, since both arc length and chord length are now known. One then finds R = 7.74 mm, confirming the previous calculation of the width of resection, (w) = 0.47 mm, necessary to produce an essentially spherical corneal shape (less than 0.5 diopter residual corneal astigmatism).

It should be pointed out again that the corneoscleral junction, the limbal ring, acts as the optical boundary. It is at this level that the optical elastic properties of the corneal tissue essentially terminate. There will be, of course, some differences between this hypothetical example and the results obtained by the actual procedure, especially since corneal wedge resection is an asymmetric procedure. Indeed, it might eventually be possible, with more sophisticated instrumentation, to achieve better symmetry. An elliptical wedge could be removed from the flatter meridian of the cornea, be reduced to a circular section, and then be inserted in a contiguous groove in the cornea at the steeper corneal meridian, 90° to the original flatter meridian, as a deep lamellar autograft (Plate 11-4). Though this approach has been attempted surgically using current microsurgical instruments and should have provided more symmetry and a more predictable result, it was not as accurate as the asymmetric single wedge resection. With the surgical keratometer and more refined instrumentation to permit the accurate cutting of circles and ellipses, which need to be sized within fractions of a millimeter, it should be possible to eliminate completely any meridional error.

Plate 11-4

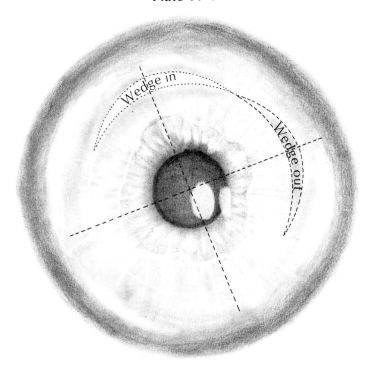

Wedge resection used as symmetrical lamellar autograft
in hypothetical example.

Practical application of theoretic considerations

Recognizing that all ophthalmic surgeons are not necessarily mathematicians, the theoretic calculations must be reduced to more practical terms, especially as they might apply to a surgical procedure. As a general rule, an 0.1-mm resection will induce about 0.67 diopter of steepening in the meridian of the resection and a corresponding flattening of 0.33 diopter in the meridian at 90°, to achieve a net correction of 1 diopter. A 1-mm wedge resection, therefore, should correct approximately 10 diopters of corneal astigmatism and a 1.5-mm wedge resection should correct 15 diopters. Because of anatomic and elasticity factors and our present technical inability to cut the cornea precisely to within 0.1 mm, the ultimate correction obtained will vary slightly in the individual case. Correspondingly less effect will be obtained with a resection of less than 0.5 mm, whereas a resection of more than 1.5 mm not only will produce a variable result but also can cause an irregular astigmatism. Though an initially irregular astigmatism will usually regularize with time, the final result of a large resection may vary significantly from the intended correction.

A wedge resection following penetrating keratoplasty is done not only inside the limbal corneal ring but also contiguous to a second ring created by the graft scar. This inner ring can have a variable and often a more than negligible effect on the outcome of the procedure. The variability of the thickness and density of the graft scar, as well as its shape and the circumference, has an unpredictable and incalculable effect on the final outcome of a given wedge-resection procedure. Nevertheless, on the basis of our clinical results, it would appear that on the average the graft-recipient scar ring has not had a significant effect.

On the other hand, it has been noted that the closer the wedge resection to the limbal ring, the less the effect of a given width of resection. This is the case when a wedge resection is done outside the usual graft-recipient scar ring, as in a wedge resection for excessive astigmatism following cataract surgery.

Clinical application

The wedge resection technique has been used most often in cases of high astigmatism following otherwise successful keratoplasty. As has been inferred, corneal wedge resection at the limbus or just inside the limbus, done usually in conjunction with cataract surgery, requires a relatively larger resection and produces less consistent results. It should be stated also that the preceding mathematical discussion assumes that the tissue factors are constant. In addition to variations in tissue in the individual case, clinical results depend on other factors, such as the amount of astigmatism requiring correction, the configuration and tightness of sutures, the intraoperative surgical keratometer interpretation, and the time required or allowed for healing before suture removal. Of primary importance, however, is the fact that the foregoing factors, either individually or in combination, can contribute to correction of the meridional error only if resection of corneal tissue is done. Nevertheless, the secondary factors, in particular the depth of suture placement, the security of wound closure, and the time of suture removal, are important to an optimal result.

SURGICAL TECHNIQUE
Timing

Clinical keratometer readings are taken periodically for 3 months prior to a corneal wedge resection. Surgery should not be performed while there is evidence of continuing change in the astigmatism, especially if that change tends to reduce the error. Though in rare cases, there may be measurable changes in corneal astigmatism for up to 6 months following suture removal, usually there is no significant alteration after 2 or 3 months. Nevertheless, corneal wedge resection should not be done until the corneal astigmatism has been stable for at least 3 months.

In the case of an elevation of the graft edge that can occur because of too-early suture removal and results, too, in severe astigmatism, a corneal wedge resection usually is not indicated. If performed, it may cause separation or stretching of the wound at the side opposite the resected meridian, not only nullifying the result but also complicating future refractive surgery. In the case of wound separation, immediate anatomic suture repair should be done, and the wound allowed to heal completely. Wedge resection may be done secondarily 6 months after suture removal, should a residual astigmatism make it necessary. The technique for immediate repair of a graft edge elevation or separation requires an approach (see Chapter 13) different from wedge resection.

Preparation

The eye is prepared as for penetrating keratoplasty except that a scleral support ring usually is not used. Instead, a superior rectus fixation suture and an inferior rectus fixation suture are inserted and used to center the cornea and to steady the globe during the procedure.

Selection of the sector to be wedge-resected

The projection of the Troutman surgical keratometer is centered on the astigmatic cornea under highest magnification (22×). The qualitative surgical keratometer reading is compared to the last recorded preoperative quantitative reading, and the axis and approximate amount of the astigma-

275

tism are verified. The axis of the flatter meridian is indicated by the longer diameter of the oval-shaped keratometer projection (Plate 11-5, *A*).

A wedge resection sector of 90° is outlined and centered on the axis of the flatter meridian (Plate 11-5, *A*). The selection of which of two possible sectors should be resected depends on the corneal effect of the apparent cause of the meridional elongation, usually the result of wound slippage or a poorly cut or misshapen graft or recipient cornea. In the former case, the resection is made in the sector of the slippage, usually identifiable by a wider, denser scar (Plate 11-5, *B*). In the latter case, either sector across the flatter meridian may be chosen. The resection may be done inside, to encompass, or outside the graft scar. Usually the resection is done outside the scar, as illustrated, unless the limbus is directly adjacent to the scarred area, whereupon it is done to encompass the scar or inside it.

Plate 11-5

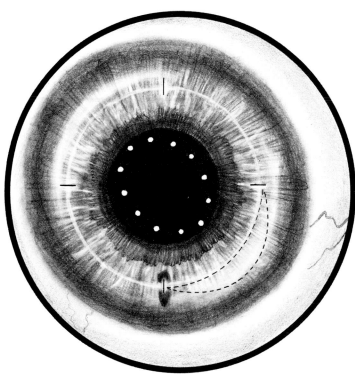

A. Surgical keratometer projection indicating the meridian of resection. Resection area is outlined.

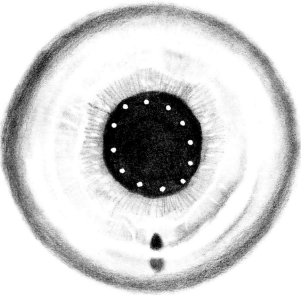

B. The wide, dense sector scar (3 to 6 o'clock) in the flatter corneal meridian.

Cutting the wedge

The assistant holds the globe fixed by the two rectus sutures. With the diamond knife, the surgeon makes a vertical, curvilinear incision to coincide with the edge of the graft scar. The length of the incision, centered on the axis of the flatter meridian, is approximately 90° of the graft circumference. This incision is usually made as a continuous cut starting 45° to one side of the axis of the flatter meridian and continuing for an equal distance to the other side (Plate 11-6, A). The blade of the diamond knife makes the most regular, accurate incision, which, however, must not be made so deeply as to penetrate the full thickness of the cornea. A second pair of elliptical incisions is made, each one-half the length of the first, slanted to meet the first incision at its maximum depth. These cuts start from the ends of the first incision, forming curved lines to meet at the axis of the flatter meridian (Plate 11-6, B). A single cut is avoided since there is a tendency to widen the resection as the cut is extended to its distal end (Plate 11-6, C). The width to which the center of the ellipse is cut depends on the dioptric power of the astigmatic band to be corrected. In the illustration, the width at the center of the ellipse is 1 mm wide to correct an astigmatic band of approximately 10 diopters. The sector outlined by the diamond blade should be crescent-shaped.

Since the first cut will have been made vertically and the second cut angulated toward the posterior limit of the first incision, the cross-section of the excised segment of tissue will be a right-angled triangle, or a wedge shape, with the base at the corneal surface and the apex at the deepest part of the wound, hence, the derivation "wedge" resection. A wedge, rather than a full-thickness crescent with parallel vertical edges, is cut, since the alteration of the anterior corneal surface provides the greatest power correction.

Plate 11-6

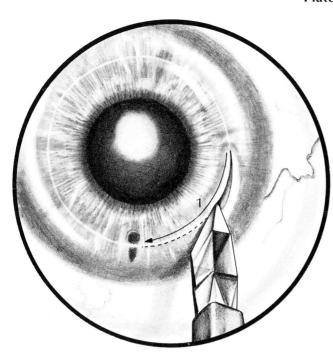

A. Step 1. Single continuous cut along 90° of the graft scar, centered at the axis of the flatter meridian.

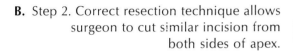

B. Step 2. Correct resection technique allows surgeon to cut similar incision from both sides of apex.

C. Incorrect cutting of second slanted incision. It is difficult to guide knife accurately on the projected incision line.

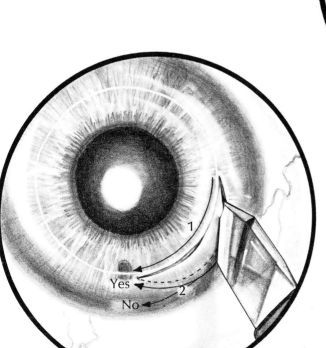

Troutman corneal wedge resection.

The two outlined incisions are deepened as necessary to meet at about the level of Descemet's membrane. When the excision of the wedge is completed, the anterior chamber is entered, and some aqueous is allowed to escape. This planned loss of aqueous is necessary in order to reduce ocular volume sufficiently to approximate the edges of the resected area. If aqueous is lost too soon, it may not be possible to complete the incision accurately with a diamond knife, and the excision of the wedge must be completed using Vannas scissors (Plate 11-7, *A*). The resected wedge and the resected sector of cornea are inspected, and the length, depth, and width of the excised wedge and the corneal excision are measured. Any irregularities of the edges of the resected area are trimmed with Vannas scissors. The paracentesis is done at this point if the chamber has not already been entered (Plate 11-7, *B*).

Plate 11-7

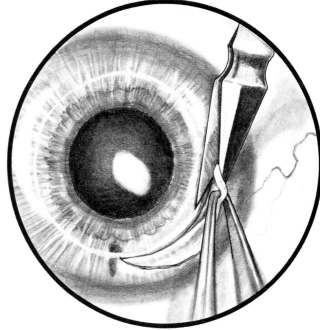

A. Step 3. Incomplete diamond knife excision being completed with Vannas scissors.

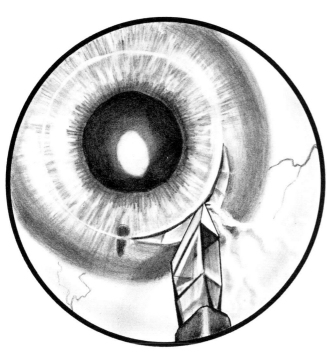

B. Step 4. Excision completed with diamond knife alone. Chamber is entered to allow escape of aqueous.

Suturing the edges of the resection

With the eye softened from the paracentesis done at the depth of the resection, the incision is easily closed with eight to ten closely spaced interrupted sutures. The suture bites are inserted to the level of Descemet's membrane or, when possible, passed through and through the cornea to assure firm, full-thickness apposition of the vertical edges of the wedge-resected sector. The sutures are tied to appose firmly the edges of the incision (Plate 11-8).

The surgical keratometer projection is observed as each suture is placed, tightened, and tied successively, in pairs, from each end of the crescent and continuing to its center. The ring of lights of the surgical keratometer changes from its original direction and shape to a less pronounced oval with its longer axis at 90° to the original flatter meridian axis.

When the suturing is completed, the ring projection of the surgical keratometer should be distorted to indicate approximately one-half the dioptric power of the original astigmatic error.

The interrupted suture knots are retracted into the proximal needle tracts to the donor-tissue side of the incision. If a knot cannot be buried easily on the donor side, it is pulled into the tract on the recipient side. It is important to bury the knots of the interrupted sutures since the loops may be left in place for as long as 6 months, and not less than 3 months, to effect firm healing. Too-early removal will result in wound slippage and recurrence of the astigmatic band.

Summary of the technique

1. Identify the flatter meridian with the surgical keratometer.
2. Outline a 90° crescent, centered on the axis of the flatter meridian. For each diopter of correction desired, 0.1 mm of corneal tissue is removed at the widest point of the crescent.
3. Cut a vertical incision along the graft scar.
4. Cut two angulated opposing incisions to meet each other and the first incision at the level of Descemet's membrane.
5. Complete wedge resection with Vannas scissors, and remove the wedge.
6. Do a paracentesis.
7. Close the wound with paired through-and-through interrupted sutures of monofilament elastic threads.
8. Confirm the steepening effect with the surgical keratometer.

Plate 11-8

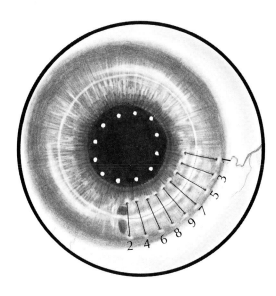

A. Step 5. Sutures are tied to appose the incision. The flatter meridian of the keratometer projection is rotated 90° from its preoperative direction.

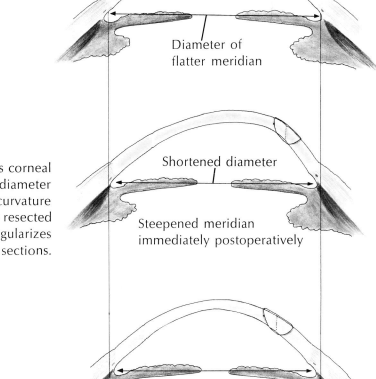

B. The wedge resection shortens corneal curvature (arc length) and reduces diameter (chord length), steepening curvature (increasing dioptric power) of wedge resected meridian. Initial sector distortion regularizes postoperatively. Cross sections.

Asymmetric wedge resection

Diameter of flatter meridian

Shortened diameter

Steepened meridian immediately postoperatively

Steepened corneal curvature regularized later postoperatively

Effect of asymmetric wedge resection of a flatter meridian

REPAIR OF EDGE ELEVATION

If an astigmatic distortion results from sector edge elevation (Plate 11-9, *A*), or if it seems that a sector of the graft-recipient scar ring has not healed well or is stretching, modified incision and suture techniques are used.

A partially penetrating circumferential cut is made on the graft scar with a trephine of the same diameter used for the primary procedure (Plate 11-9, *B*). The trephine opens the scar circumferentially for one-third to one-half of the corneal thickness. If the edge elevation is uneven, the diamond knife is used to incise the elevated edge along its border. Eight to ten interrupted sutures are placed around the circumference to appose the gaping, partially penetrating incision and to close the site of the edge elevation. Suture bites are inserted closer together across the elevated sector. Then an antitorque continuous suture is placed. The suture bites in the sector of the edge elevation are spaced more closely (Plate 11-9, *C*). When the continuous thread has been tightened and tied and the knot buried, the interrupted fixating sutures are removed. The continuous suture is adjusted, monitored by the surgical keratometer. The continuous individual loops are loosened or tightened to induce a slight overcorrection of the preoperatively flatter meridian. The flatter meridian should be always slightly overcorrected, since it tends to become less steep postoperatively. When this technique is followed, astigmatism will be minimal, and subsequent corneal wedge resection rarely will be necessary.

I have used the corneal wedge resection with consistently good results in more than 50 eyes. On the average, 75% of the power of excessively high astigmatic errors (greater than 10 diopters) is corrected. The maximum correction obtained was 28 diopters. The average residual astigmatism after wedge resection, about 2.5 diopters, is less than the average astigmatism I have obtained in routine keratoplasty cases (about 4 diopters). Because of the tissue resection, which induces an overall flattening of corneal K, reducing corneal power, the eye becomes less myopic or more hyperopic. Since astigmatism postkeratoplasty is usually myopic, the patient has less astigmatism and also is less myopic following successful surgery.

POSTOPERATIVE CARE

When a circumferential suture is used to correct an edge elevation, it is essential that the suture not be removed for 6 months following the repair. Sufficient time must elapse to permit the disrupted corneal edges to heal together well enough so they will not tend to separate or to stretch when the sutures are removed.

When interrupted sutures are used in corneal wedge resection, the sutures are removed 3 to 6 months postoperatively, in pairs, one to one side and one to the other side of the apex of the now steeper meridian. As each pair of sutures is removed, the keratometer reading is taken. If the astig-

Plate 11-9

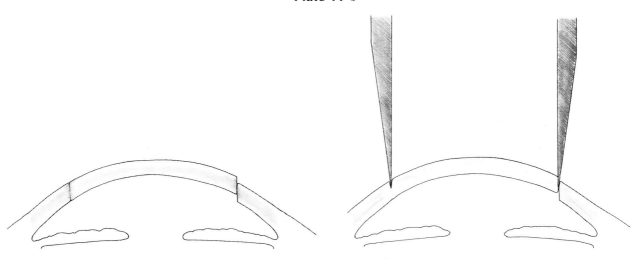

A. Sector elevation of graft edge.
Cross section.

B. Partially penetrating trephining
in preparation for suturing of edge elevation.
Cross section.

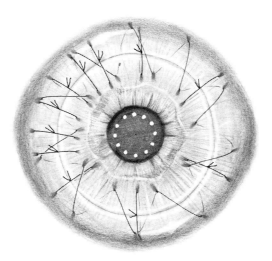

C. Typical suture pattern for repair
of edge elevation before removal of
temporary interrupted sutures.

matism tends to reduce rapidly toward an anastigmatic state after removal of less than half the sutures placed, the remaining sutures are left in place. An even longer period, 1 year or more, may be necessary to achieve sufficient healing for a satisfactory final correction before they can be removed.

When polypropylene thread is used, the closing sutures may be left in place indefinitely. In contradistinction to nylon, which will dissolve eventually, polypropylene should remain in situ virtually forever and may better ensure that the planned optical correction will be maintained. It is important always to explain to the patient the prolonged postoperative period necessary to ensure a favorable result. The patient must be made aware of the fact that the cornea will be distorted temporarily and that there will be a significant astigmatic band in the opposite meridian. The patient should be told that, for the operation to be successful, there eventually will be a period during which he will be visually handicapped almost to the same degree as before the correction was made.

TROUTMAN RELAXING INCISION FOR LOWER DEGREES OF CORNEAL ASTIGMATISM

Sometimes a residual astigmatism of lower degree, 4 to 8 diopters, persists after suture removal in penetrating keratoplasty or following a partially successful wedge resection. In this instance a partial penetrating relaxing incision can be made across one or both axes of the steeper meridian. Each incision is made for about one-half corneal thickness, into or directly adjacent to the graft recipient scar, with a razor blade knife. The incision is extended for about 15° to either side of the meridian axis. The procedure is performed in the office under the biomicroscope. The anterior chamber should not be penetrated. Local topical anesthesia is used, and a firm pressure dressing is applied for 48 hours.

Only about a one-half correction of the band should be attempted initially since the incision will tend to spread further apart over several weeks. From 3 to 5 diopters of correction can be obtained without unduly weakening the corneal scar. The correction remains stable after 4 weeks. Normal corneal thickness is regained within 6 to 10 weeks. A slight increase in myopia or decrease in hyperopia can be anticipated as a result of the secondary increase in axial length and in corneal curvatures.

SUMMARY

It is now possible, by means of the Troutman corneal wedge resection or relaxing incision, to correct an often visually crippling degree of astigmatism occurring postkeratoplasty. This unfortunate problem occurs to an unpredictable and still essentially uncontrollable degree following otherwise successful corneal grafts. An excessive astigmatic band can be almost fully corrected by the accurate and meticulous application of the corneal wedge resection technique. The mathematical computations derived from clinical experience confirm the results. Together with more sophisticated instrumentation, these determinations may lead eventually to improved predictability and quantification of optical results, at either primary or secondary corneal wedge resection. Edge elevation is treated as a separate problem, requiring a different surgical approach. Success in penetrating keratoplasty is not just a clear graft; it is also the control of preoperative or surgically induced ametropia, in particular, astigmatism, as a final result.

CHAPTER 12

GLAUCOMA SURGERY AND KERATOPLASTY

General considerations   Trabeculotomy
Transient ocular hypertension   Cyclocryothermy
Surgical indications   Summary
Trabeculectomy and keratoplasty

GENERAL CONSIDERATIONS

In aphakic keratoplasty in particular, the presence of or the postoperative occurrence of glaucoma can nullify an otherwise perfect technical result. The usual glaucoma effect is on the optic nerve, with subsequent visual field loss. In addition, continued increased intraocular pressure can compromise the clarity of a graft by damaging the endothelium or by delaying healing as the result of stretching or disrupting the wound. Specular microscopy may aid the surgeon in deciding when to operate to relieve the pressure, should endothelial cells begin to be compromised.

Clinically, an increase in intraocular pressure may be difficult to detect even by scleral tonometry. Vision and fields often are unreliable indicators of the severity of the disease process. Thus the surgeon is forced to rely on other clinical signs and symptoms.

TRANSIENT OCULAR HYPERTENSION

Though intraocular hypertension often may occur following aphakic keratoplasty as well as after combined cataract surgery and keratoplasty, it is often a transient phenomenon that can be controlled medically. The surgeon may be placed in a dilemma, since increased intraocular pressure may be initiated or exacerbated by steroid medication sometimes essential to survival of the graft. For example, a postoperative inflammatory reaction, following anterior segment reconstruction and vitrectomy, can induce ocular hypotonia. This is often followed by transient hypertension before a normotensive state is reached. The surgeon should be constrained from attempting surgical control during the hypertensive phase since an operative intervention would only compound a self-limiting medical problem. It has been my experience, especially in the use of a larger donor button than

287

the recipient opening, that most cases of postkeratoplasty intraocular hypertension will respond to intensive medical therapy and a watchful, "hands off" attitude.

SURGICAL INDICATIONS

When surgery is indicated, trabeculectomy or trabeculotomy is preferred to cyclocryothermy or cyclodiathermy. The last two procedures not only are less effective in the long-term control of aphakic glaucoma following keratoplasty but also seem to result more often in corneal decompensation and clouding of the graft.

Though control of glaucoma by trabeculotomy tends to be somewhat transient in nature, rarely does it compromise the graft, nor does it preclude other surgery or render it less effective.

An operative procedure performed too early in the postoperative course may appear to effect control only because the natural course of the ocular hypertensive phase is toward resolution. The disease would have been controlled even *without* surgery.

Trabeculectomy is currently the procedure I prefer for both phakic and aphakic glaucoma. If glaucoma accompanies corneal and other anterior segment pathology, necessitating keratoplasty, the overall surgical plan must include either a preliminary glaucoma procedure or an attempt at surgical control at the time of keratoplasty.

When the anterior chamber is badly disrupted—particularly when there are extensive anterior synechiae and lens and vitreous pathology—a trabeculectomy is performed in combination with the keratoplasty procedure. When it appears that the angle is open and the iris, lens, and vitreous essentially are not involved in the corneal process, either a trabeculotomy or a trabeculectomy is performed simultaneously with the primary keratoplasty.

In my opinion, the glaucoma procedure, performed in preparation for keratoplasty in the aphakic eye, offers no advantage over the combined procedure. When keratoplasty is done as a secondary procedure, as often as not the glaucoma filtration area is compromised.

Extensive anterior segment reconstruction and vitrectomy performed at the time of the keratoplasty may suffice to control postoperative glaucoma. The addition of a filtering procedure, in fact, may produce intractable hypotension and may even lead to phthisis bulbi.

When an extensively damaged anterior segment is seen for the first time in the late posttraumatic state, there is the probability that glaucoma may have been present between the time of injury and the consultative examination, even though the intraocular pressure was not elevated at the time of the initial examination. In this event, severe nerve damage may exist even in the presence of good light perception and projection and an essentially normal B-scan. If an atrophic optic cup is visualized by B-scan, it must be presumed that the glaucoma damage is severe. If, preoperatively, the posterior segment cannot be visualized directly, the patient or a responsible member of the family must be informed of the possibility that a glaucomatous optic atrophy may exist and that, even with successful repair of the anterior segment and a clear graft, the vision result may be less than anticipated.

In the relatively rare situation in which glaucoma exists in a phakic eye prior to keratoplasty, the glaucoma should be treated as a separate entity. It is important that it be controlled, either medically or surgically, prior to keratoplasty. Keratoplasty alone will not control phakic glaucoma postoperatively, and uncontrolled pressure, subsequent glaucoma surgery, or both can compromise graft clarity.

One would expect that an eye with severe corneal disease also might be more prone to other diseases of the anterior segment, such as a cataract and glaucoma. Though it is true that a cataract is more common in some corneal pathologies—for example, in endothelial-epithelial dystrophy—in the phakic eye, glaucoma usually does not accompany the commonly encountered corneal pathologies.

It is essential that the corneal surgeon be aware of and be constantly on the lookout for glaucoma, which—similar to homograft reaction but more subtly and irreversibly—can compromise an otherwise perfect technical result.

TRABECULECTOMY AND KERATOPLASTY

A trabeculectomy performed under a protecting scleral flap is the filtering procedure preferred in aphakic keratoplasty, since the danger of early loss of the anterior chamber is minimized. Although the prevention of a flat chamber is important to the success of the filtering procedure, the prevention of peripheral anterior synechiae in the glaucomatous eye with an abnormal cornea or a keratoplasty is doubly important.

The procedure to be described and illustrated is as performed on an aphakic eye simultaneously with a penetrating keratoplasty. A thorough knowledge of the anatomy of the angle especially as it pertains to trabecular surgery is essential (Plate 12-1).

Plate 12-1

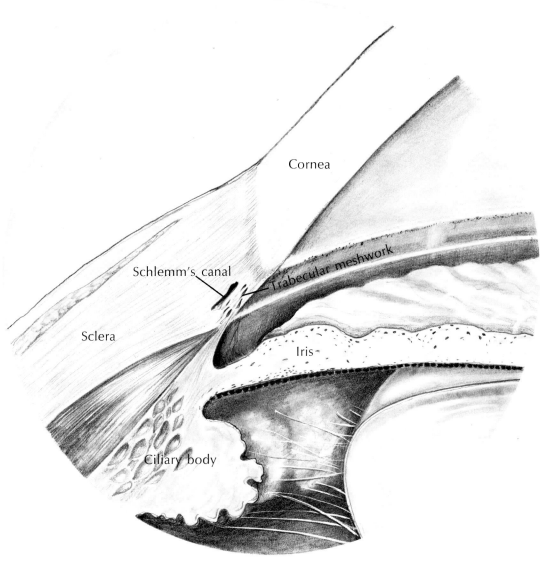

Cornea

Schlemm's canal

Trabecular meshwork

Sclera

Iris

Ciliary body

Anatomy of the angle pertinent
to trabecular surgery.

The corneal procedure is basically as described in Chapter 10, but differs in several respects. The eye is prepared as for aphakic keratoplasty. Before the scleral support ring is sutured in place, a broadly based, deep conjunctival flap, approximately 1.5 cm by 1 cm, is outlined and dissected to the surgical limbus. Care is taken not to thin the conjunctiva excessively as the episcleral tissue is stroked away from its tenuous scleral attachment (Plate 12-2, A). The superior tangential conjunctival incision is extended radially from its extremities toward the limbus so that the flap may be retracted easily.

With the flap prepared, the scleral support ring is fixed with four 6-0 silk interrupted sutures. The thin-wire, support ring should be 18 or 20 mm in diameter and placed slightly eccentrically superiorly, to encompass the area where the scleral flap of the trabeculectomy is to be performed. Three sides of a 4-mm square—the base left intact at the surgical limbus so the flap can be turned back at the surgical limbus—are outlined with a razor knife or a diamond knife (Plate 12-2, B). The two radial incisions are equidistant from the extremities of the conjunctival flap. They are made to a depth two-thirds of the scleral thickness. Using the No. 1 corneal splitter, the surgeon dissects a lamellar scleral flap, beginning at one corner of the outlined incision (Plate 12-2, C). The dissection is continued to the limbus. As the limbus is approached, the full width of the flap is mobilized.

Plate 12-2

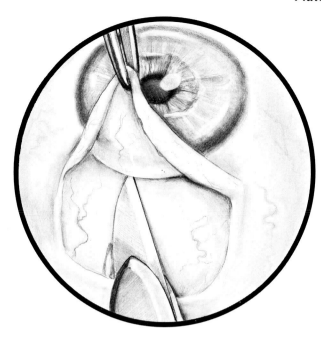

A. Conjunctival flap everted. Limbal dissection in progress.

B. Outlining the lamellar scleral flap.

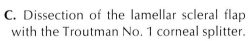

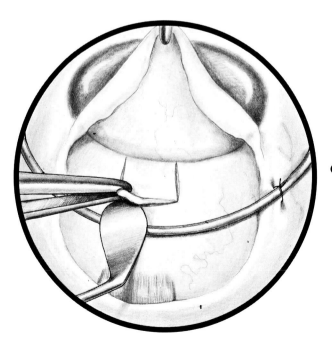

C. Dissection of the lamellar scleral flap with the Troutman No. 1 corneal splitter.

At this point, extreme care must be taken not to deepen the plane of dissection (Plate 12-3, *A*). The scleral curvature changes abruptly at the limbus, and the plane of the lamellar incision must be directed more anteriorly to correspond to the corneal curvature in order not to penetrate the anterior chamber. The junction of the sclera and the clear corneal tissue, at the spur, is crossed at about two-thirds the corneal thickness. The demarcation line between the scleral tissue and the corneal tissue identifies the position of Schlemm's canal and the underlying trabecular meshwork.

The surgeon must consciously avoid the tendency to dissect too deeply. At the proper depth of dissection, Schlemm's canal can be seen in faint outline. To verify its position, a partially penetrating radial incision (see Plate 12-7, *A*) is made directly across the line of demarcation. When the canal is opened, a Mackensen trabeculotomy probe (Plate 12-3, *B*) can be passed readily 2 mm to 3 mm into the canal to verify its patency (Plate 12-7, *B* and *C*).

Plate 12-3

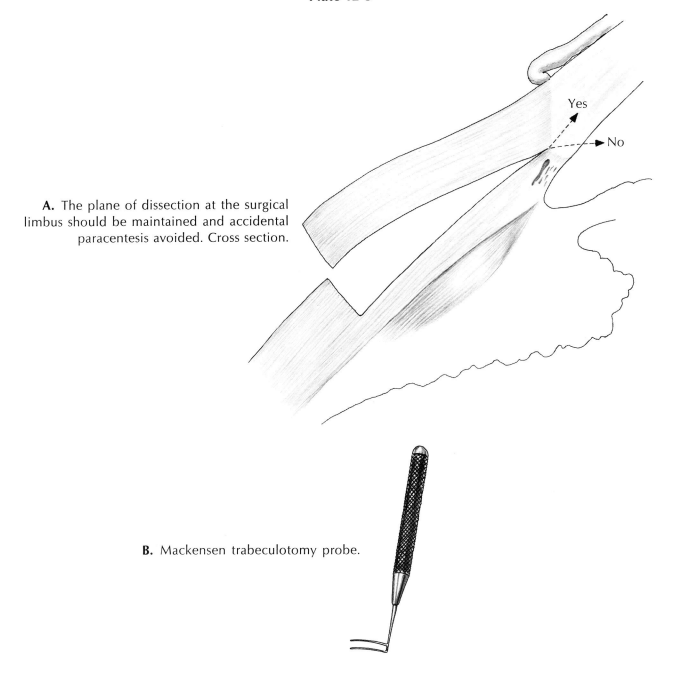

A. The plane of dissection at the surgical limbus should be maintained and accidental paracentesis avoided. Cross section.

Yes

No

B. Mackensen trabeculotomy probe.

295

At the limbal extremity of the scleral lamellar bed, a partially penetrating rectangular incision, 3 mm long by 1.5 mm wide, is made (Plate 12-4). The two longer sides are cut equidistant to each side of the spur and are connected to the shorter sides across the demarcation line. This outline should encompass a sector of Schlemm's canal and trabecular meshwork and occupy about one-fourth of the area of the lamellar scleral dissection. The scleral and conjunctival flaps are pulled back temporarily from their retracted positions to cover the scleral defect.

Plate 12-4

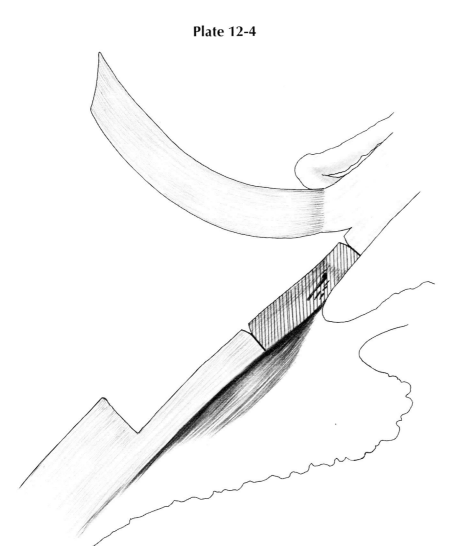

Partially penetrating trabeculectomy excision.
Cross section.

The keratoplasty and any other necessary related surgery of the anterior segment are performed. Any dissection of the cornea or anterior segment adjacent to the trabeculectomy site is done at the time of the keratoplasty. However, if the area is obscured by the pathology, it is better to delay any dissection until it can be performed through the trabeculectomy opening. It is essential to have a rotoextractor or similar vitreous sucking-cutting instrument available for use during keratoplasty, especially when keratoplasty is combined with trabeculectomy. A major reason for failure of trabeculectomy in the aphakic eye is the presence of formed vitreous in the vicinity of the internal orifice of the trabeculectomy or failure to do a vitrectomy when vitreous loss occurs as a complication of the keratoplasty procedure. Other surgery necessary to ensure that the fistula is not blocked includes iridectomy, iridotomy, or iris suture. When vitreous obstructs the trabeculectomy site, an anterior vitrectomy must be performed.

When the keratoplasty procedure has been completed, it is ascertained that there is no leak; then the eye is filled with basic salt solution and air, as necessary, to restore the globe to about normal intraocular pressure. The previously prepared conjunctival and scleral flaps are retracted to expose the outlined trabeculectomy site. The partially penetrating incision distal and parallel to the spur is deepened with the diamond knife to enter the subchoroidal space just behind Schlemm's canal at the insertion of the trabeculum. Using Vannas scissors, the surgeon extends forward, full thickness, the two short radial incisions of the rectangular outline to form an anteriorly attached lamellar flap. As the trabeculum is crossed, some aqueous will escape. The deep scleral lamellar flap is grasped firmly with the MICRA-Pierse cupped forceps, and the flap is excised with the Vannas scissors by cutting along the anterior demarcation line. As the flap is excised, it is separated gently from its trabecular attachment. The iris periphery is seen to prolapse into the incision where it is grasped at the anterior extremity of the incision with the tips of the MICRA-Pierse cupped forceps and is gently pulled up through the wound. The iris is cut proximal to the forceps tips with the 5-mm Barraquer-de Wecker iris scissors (Plate 12-5, A). Only the tissue included in the forceps teeth is excised. Thus accidental cutting of the ciliary process, which may cause intractable bleeding, is avoided. Should bleeding occur, the wound is held open to allow the area to bleed externally until controlled. Gentle lavage is combined with spatulation with the 1-mm iris spatula to verify that the posterior pigment layer of the iris is dislodged and that the posterior as well as the anterior chamber communicates with the trabeculectomy opening (Plate 12-5, B).

298

Plate 12-5

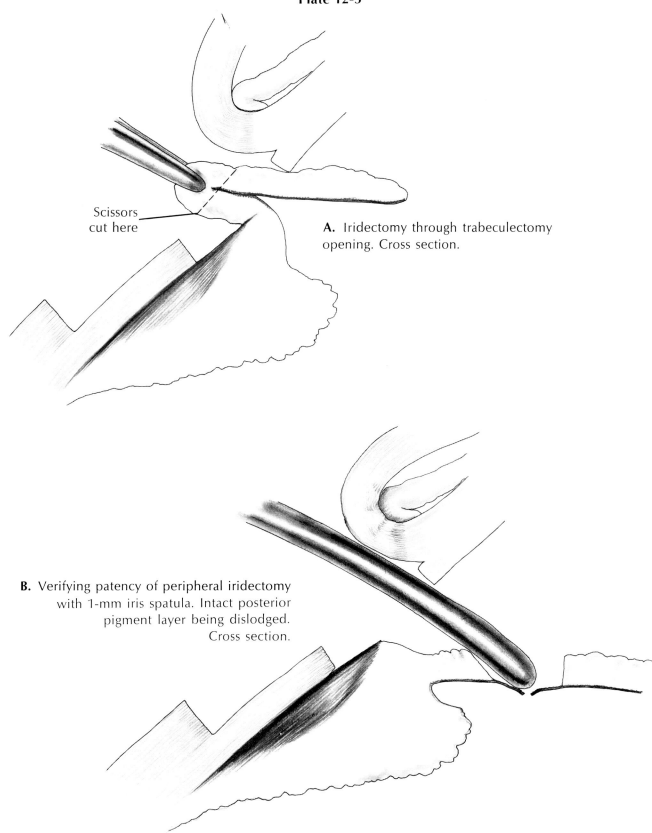

Scissors
cut here

A. Iridectomy through trabeculectomy
opening. Cross section.

B. Verifying patency of peripheral iridectomy
with 1-mm iris spatula. Intact posterior
pigment layer being dislodged.
Cross section.

With coaxial illumination, a red fundus reflex, viewed through the iridectomy opening, confirms patency (Plate 12-6, *A*). It is impossible to determine in every case whether or not vitreous is present behind the excised area. Even after careful vitrectomy from the traditional anterior route, a thin sheet of the vitreous base can remain across the trabeculectomy site. Any residual formed vitreous is removed with the rotoextractor directly through the trabeculectomy fistula. The wound area is flushed; the eye is refilled with basic salt solution; and a Weck-cel sponge is applied at the trabeculectomy opening to determine whether or not any residual vitreous strands are present. If no vitreous attaches to the tip of the sponge as fluid is absorbed and the eye softens, the scleral trabeculectomy flap is closed to complete the operation. However, should vitreous adhere to the tip of the cellulose sponge, further vitrectomy must be performed.

Before being closed, the globe is filled with basic salt solution and air. The scleral flap is brought across to cover the trabeculectomy opening and lamellar defect. The posterior edge of the flap is approximated to the posterior edge of the lamellar scleral dissection with two, 22-micron nylon interrupted sutures, placed one at each corner. The conjunctival flap is closed with a monofilament nylon running suture locked by a knot at each end of the incision (Plate 12-6, *B*).

The reformed anterior chamber is inspected with slit-lamp illumination to verify that the iris is well away from the posterior aspect of the graft incision and trabeculectomy site. Any remaining bubble of air is removed and is replaced with basic salt solution. The fluorescein dye test is performed to detect possible leaks in the graft incision. The Troutman surgical keratometer is used to detect any suture-induced meridional errors, and the continuous suture loops are adjusted accordingly. The scleral support ring and the superior rectus fixation suture are removed; the speculum is elevated to release the pressure on the lid, and the cornea is again observed with the surgical keratometer. Final suture adjustments are made, as necessary.

Immediately following the surgery, a unilateral protective dressing is applied. It is removed on the following morning. A flat conjunctival bleb should begin to develop within 5 days, and the anterior chamber depth should be maintained.

An eye subjected to multiple surgical procedures has a greater tendency to postoperative inflammatory reaction than does an eye subjected only to a penetrating keratoplasty. In addition to routine local steroid and antibiotic medications, a systemic immunosuppressive agent, prednisone (100 mg daily), is prescribed until all signs of postoperative inflammatory reaction have subsided.

When vitrectomy is performed, the risk of infection increases, and a prophylactic dose of cephaloridine, 2000 mg daily, is given for 5 days postoperatively. If extensive surgery is anticipated preoperatively, it is useful to prescribe these dosages daily, beginning 48 hours prior to surgery.

300

Plate 12-6

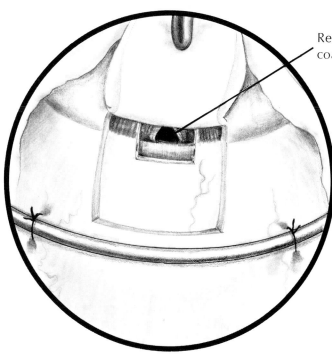

Red reflex visible with coaxial illumination

A. Completed trabeculectomy prior to suturing the flap.

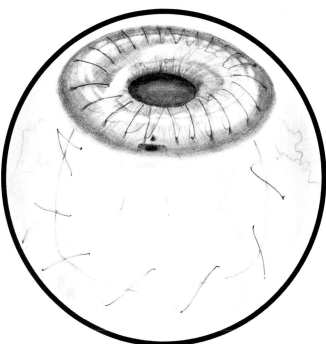

B. Trabeculectomy completed. Scleral and conjunctival flaps sutured in position with 22-micron nylon interrupted and running sutures, respectively.

TRABECULOTOMY

Trabeculotomy can be performed either in a phakic or an aphakic eye, when the anterior chamber angle is open and the iris configuration is relatively normal. The operation for trabeculotomy proceeds exactly as that for trabeculectomy, except that the limbus-based conjunctival flap is smaller, approximately a 1-cm square. Since the anterior chamber is not lost during a well-performed trabeculotomy, the procedure can be completed immediately prior to the keratoplasty. Since rupture of the trabeculum almost always results in some bleeding, the clots then can be flushed out during the keratoplasty procedure. At 10× to 15× magnification, a 3-mm square, two-thirds depth scleral flap is dissected to the limbus over the area of Schlemm's canal. It is important not to dissect into the anterior chamber. Under maximum magnification, the diamond knife or a razor knife is used to make a shallow, 2-mm radial incision across the spur over the canal (Plate 12-7, A). As the incision is deepened gradually, the tissue to either side of the cut is pushed gently to the right and to the left with the flat of the knife blade until the canal is seen to be unroofed just behind the spur.

When the canal is identified positively, the tip of a Vannas scissors is slipped, in turn, into each orifice, and the roof of the canal is opened about 1 mm to either side (Plate 12-7, B). This provides a more oblique entrance of the probe tip for the canalization.

The tip of the Mackensen trabeculotomy probe is then slipped gently into the canal, where it should meet slight resistance (Plate 12-7, C). If there is no resistance, the cannula probably is behind the canal in the suprachoroidal space. If the resistance is more marked, the probe is probably above or in front of the canal in a false passage in the sclera or cornea (Plate 12-7, D). The initial dissection should be made at 12 o'clock. Should the surgeon fail to find the canal, another dissection can be done at 10 or at 2 o'clock.

Plate 12-7

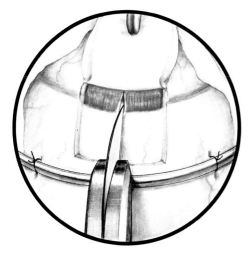

A. Radial incision over Schlemm's canal.

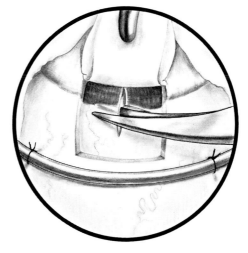

B. Incising the roof of Schlemm's canal with Vannas scissors.

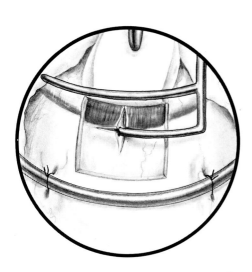

C. Probe entering Schlemm's canal.

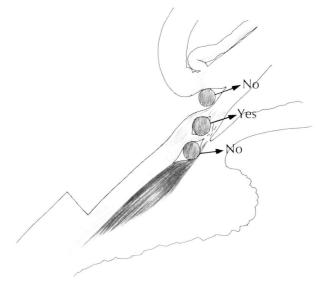

D. Correct position of probe in Schlemm's canal (center); making false passage in sclera (top); dialyzing iris root (bottom). Cross section.

Once it is ascertained that the probe is in the canal, it is advanced slowly up its full length to the right angle where the probe wire turns to join the handle. The tip of the probe is pressed lightly anteriorly against the outer wall of the canal as it is advanced along the curvilinear course of the canal. This prevents the probe from accidentally penetrating the internal wall of the canal before its full length is traversed. With the probe fully in the canal—that is, up to the right angle at the handle—the handle is rotated so that, starting with the tip, the full length of the probe in the canal tears progressively through the trabecular meshwork (Plate 12-8, A). As the probe tip enters the anterior chamber, the surgeon confirms, at high magnification (15×), under slit-lamp aperture, that the tip does not pass interlamellarly or posteriorly to the iris root.

Some sharp bleeding usually occurs as the trabeculum is ruptured. This bleeding lasts only a few moments, but occasionally it is necessary to do a paracentesis and to wash the blood from the anterior chamber to prevent pupillary block or blood-staining of the cornea. When trabeculotomy is done just prior to keratoplasty at a combined operation, the anterior chamber is washed after trephining.

The same maneuvers are repeated to rupture the trabecular meshwork to the opposite side.

The scleral lamellar flap is sutured with six monofilament Ethilon interrupted sutures in order to pull the flap tightly to close as well as to cover the canal incisions (Plate 12-8, B). The radial incision is sutured only if isolation of the canal required extensive dissection.

The conjunctival flap is repositioned and sutured with a continuous thread of monofilament nylon locked by knots at each extremity of the incision.

The keratoplasty then proceeds as outlined in Chapters 8 to 10. Since no iridectomy will have been performed at the trabeculotomy, and if none is present from a previous surgery, a midperipheral iridectomy is performed at the time of the keratoplasty. In this instance, the function of the iridectomy is not to prevent blockage of the filtering cicatrix, as is the case in trabeculectomy, but rather to prevent pupillary block during or following the keratoplasty. A blood clot, if present, is washed gently from the anterior chamber. Minimal clotting in the angle at the site of the trabecular rupture is not disturbed, since it absorbs within a few days postoperatively and does not interfere either with the function of the glaucoma procedure or with the keratoplasty procedure. To disturb this minimal clotting at the time of keratoplasty could initiate additional sharp bleeding from the trabeculotomy site.

Plate 12-8

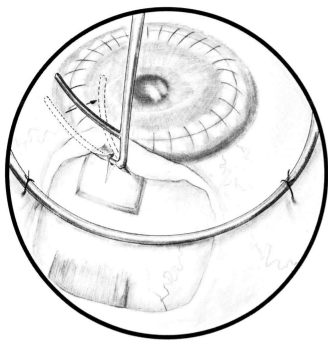

A. Mackensen probe being turned through inner wall of Schlemm's canal.

B. Trabeculotomy completed. Scleral and conjunctival flaps sutured in position with 22-micron nylon interrupted and running sutures, respectively.

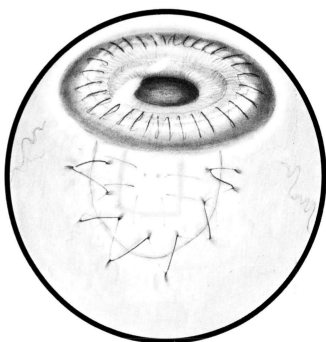

CYCLOCRYOTHERMY

Cyclocryothermy is usually performed at a separate procedure. Cyclocryothermy is used to effect temporary control of glaucoma, before attempting keratoplasty or following a successful keratoplasty, when medically uncontrolled glaucoma threatens survival of the graft and the optic nerve. I have not performed cyclocryothermy in combination with keratoplasty. The technique is described in Chapter 13.

SUMMARY

Glaucoma, even more than homograft reaction, is one of the more compromising problems complicating keratoplasty, especially in the aphakic eye. As in the case of cataract surgery combined with surgery for corneal pathology, I would rather combine the glaucoma procedure—preferentially trabeculectomy or trabeculotomy—with keratoplasty in the aphakic eye than do these as two separate procedures. Combined glaucoma surgery and keratoplasty can be done only when the presence of glaucoma is known in advance of keratoplasty or can be anticipated as a postoperative complication. Microsurgical technique is essential not only for the precise location of Schlemm's canal required in trabeculotomy but also for the best performance of the technically less demanding trabeculectomy.

When glaucoma occurs postkeratoplasty, after surgical precautions have been taken or after simultaneous surgery has been performed, it is often transient in nature and may be managed medically with no need for surgical intervention.

Glaucoma that is present soon after a cornea-compromising injury or its repair can burn itself out without medical or surgical intervention. Nevertheless, it may have been established long enough to cause a severely damaged nerve that can compromise the visual result of keratoplasty. The surgeon must be aware and the patient informed of the possibility of a negative functional result even after a successful surgical result when glaucoma accompanies the corneal pathology.

CHAPTER 13

SURGICAL MANAGEMENT OF POSTOPERATIVE COMPLICATIONS

General considerations
Glaucoma
Homograft reaction
Donor tissue failure
Dehiscence of the wound

Hemorrhage
Infection
Keratoconjunctivitis and blepharitis
Trauma
Summary

GENERAL CONSIDERATIONS

A number of postoperative problems that can arise following keratoplasty have been mentioned or discussed in some detail. Emphasis has been placed on meticulous microsurgery technique and fresh, healthy, homograft tissue, which, after all, are the main deterrents to postoperative complications. Nevertheless, complications do occur, and additional medical or surgical management, or both, are required to resolve them. In the approximate order of incidence and probable significance in delaying or preventing the successful outcome of the primary procedure, these complications include: glaucoma; homograft reaction; donor tissue failure; minimal to marked wound dehiscence resulting in delayed reformation of the anterior chamber; anterior synechia to the wound; prolapse of the iris, lens, or vitreous; hemorrhage; and infection. Postoperative excessive astigmatism, myopia, or hyperopia are not included in this list since the mechanism and management of each are discussed in previous chapters.

GLAUCOMA

The pre- and postoperative occurrence of and surgery for glaucoma is discussed in Chapter 12. It has been stated that glaucoma is primarily transient in nature, responding usually to medical therapy or watchful waiting. Definitive surgical therapy rarely is necessary. A period of sustained elevation of intraocular pressure often is observed postoperatively, especially following aphakic keratoplasty. The hypertension is usually followed by moderate to marked hypotension, after which the eye recovers to a normotensive state.

However, rather than a persistent elevation in pressure, which responds better to a trabeculectomy or to a trabeculotomy, the eye sometimes suffers a series of intermittent pressure elevations that eventually result in severe nerve damage. In the management of intermittent glaucoma postkeratoplasty, medical therapy is preferred to surgical therapy.

Cyclocryothermy may be used to normalize the pressure curve. When circumstances dictate the use of cyclocryothermy in preference to trabecular surgery, which may have been tried unsuccessfully, it is important not to overdo the operation. Excessive surgery not only may compromise the clarity of the graft but also can result in eventual loss of the eye from excessive ciliary body destruction.

A maximum of two quadrants is treated at the first surgical session. A retinal cryoprobe (Plate 13-1, A), cooled to −79° C, is applied to each of the selected scleral quadrants for a period of 2 minutes, for a total of three applications to each quadrant. The probe is applied to the sclera directly over the ciliary body, at a point within an area no less than 2 mm and no more than 4 mm from the surgical limbus (Plate 13-1, B). Three slightly overlapping freezing points are made in each quadrant. From 3 to 5 minutes should elapse between each application of the probe to allow the circulation of the eye to recover.

Should the initial cyclocryothermy fail to control the intraocular pressure, the remaining two or three quadrants can be treated, one quadrant at a time, at intervals of no less than 4 weeks between treatment of successive quadrants. Care should be taken not to apply the probe directly over the long ciliary vessels at 3 and 9 o'clock, especially in the case of a severely damaged eye, since intraocular bleeding, intractable ocular hypotonia, or both—leading ultimately to phthisis bulbi—may result.

Plate 13-1

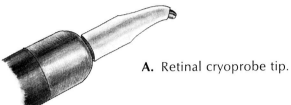

A. Retinal cryoprobe tip.

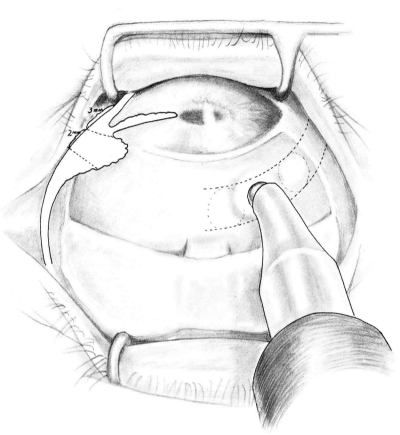

B. Position for application of retinal cryoprobe over ciliary body for cyclocryothermy.

HOMOGRAFT REACTION

With microsurgery and, in particular, with the use of fine, minimum-reaction suture material, such as monofilament nylon or polypropylene, the incidence of homograft reaction as a complication of lamellar or penetrating keratoplasty has been reduced markedly. Nevertheless, homograft reaction continues to occur in isolated instances in pathologies such as keratoconus and the corneal dystrophies and more often in pathologies that have induced a greater degree of peripheral corneal vascularization, such as herpetic keratitis, ulcerations, and caustic or acid burns.

Most important to the management of homograft reaction is prompt recognition and intensive early treatment. Each patient, therefore, must be told the early signs of a reaction so that the symptoms will be recognized should they occur. Because blurring or haziness of vision is one of the earlier signs, the patient is in the best position to protect the eye if there is some functional vision in the operated eye early postoperatively. For this reason, it is important, at the end of the procedure, to have the least amount of astigmatism in the graft and only enough axial error to compensate eventual steepening of the grafted cornea at the removal of the sutures. *With a clear graft, the eye should be not only correctable but corrected during the postoperative period so that the patient can check daily the vision of the operated eye and can report immediately any subjective change in acuity.*

An early homograft reaction causes little or no photophobia or inflammatory reaction; rather, it is manifested primarily by slight thickening and microcystic edema, which in turn cause hazy vision. Although there is no time relationship between surgery and the occurrence of a homograft reaction, it is more likely to occur during the intermediate postoperative period, that is, between the second and the fourth month; at the time of suture removal, the sixth to the eighth month; or during the second year postoperatively. Its onset often is preceded or accompanied by a severe upper respiratory infection; a family crisis, particularly one that evokes frequent or continuous crying; prolonged exposure to wind, dust, or pollen; or an irritative, localized lid infection, such as an untreated hordeolum or chalazion.

All my patients are requested to have the currently recommended influenza vaccine yearly. The patient who contracts a severe febrile upper respiratory infection within 3 to 5 years postkeratoplasty is instructed to increase the dosage of, or to resume the use of, hydrocortisone (1%) drops to a frequency of every 3 to 4 hours until the upper respiratory infection is resolved.

The patient is instructed also to increase or to resume hydrocortisone drops should there be a family crisis that may be sufficiently upsetting emotionally to cause eye irritation from crying.

The patient is cautioned to avoid prolonged exposure to wind, dust, or dirt and to wear protective glasses in the event of unavoidable exposure.

If a patient is subject to allergies, which seems to be especially the case in keratoconus, antihistaminic medication should be taken regularly, under the direction of an allergist, during allergic seasons. During the period of highest sensitivity, it may be necessary to increase the dosage of corticosteroid drops.

Should any local eye irritation or infection occur, the patient is told to seek ophthalmologic help immediately.

If, during any of these occurrences, there is the slightest blurring in vision or change in visual acuity, the patient should seek an immediate ophthalmologic examination. A suspected early graft reaction can be diagnosed readily biomicroscopically, and intensive, appropriate therapy can be instituted immediately. In doubtful situations, the corneal specular microscope is a more sensitive means of assessing the early subtle endothelial cell changes of homograft reaction before frank biomicroscopic evidence exists. The patient who comes in with an obvious and well-advanced reaction presents no problem in diagnosis.

When homograft reaction is diagnosed or suspected, either earlier or later in the course of rejection, intensive local steroid therapy is instituted immediately. Hydrocortisone (1%) or dexamethasone (0.1%) drops are prescribed every hour during the patient's waking hours. Methylprednisolone sodium succinate (Solu-Medrol) (40 mg) is given subconjunctivally biweekly if the reaction is an early one. If there is no response after three or four doses, methylprednisolone acetate (Depo-Medrol) (40 to 80 mg) is injected subconjunctivally. If severe circumciliary injection is present, particularly in an aphakic eye, and there is evidence of vitreitis, systemic steroids are given in a single dose daily in the form of prednisone (100 mg). Vitreitis may indicate a widespread ocular inflammatory reaction with only secondary corneal involvement that will clear as the vitreitis is resolved by the steroid. Uveal and vitreous inflammation can be suppressed readily by systemic medication.

If there is no response to local steroid drops, a mydriatic may be used, but this is of little value in a primary homograft reaction.

The surgeon should not be discouraged by the lack of an immediate response. The prognosis is considerably better, if, at the onset of treatment, less than one-third of the endothelium is involved in the reactive process (Plate 13-2, A and B). Nevertheless, an almost completely cloudy cornea (Plate 13-2, C and D) can clear after several weeks of intensive therapy.

If the eye fails to respond to therapy, the graft should be replaced with fresh tissue while the patient is still on local or systemic steroid therapy.

Should the patient refuse surgery at this time, medication should be discontinued as soon as the eye is quiet, even though the cornea remains cloudy, even bullous, otherwise secondary drug effects may complicate the situation. Some period of time, usually 6 months to 1 year, may be allowed to elapse before a second procedure is considered. Should the inflammatory reaction resume and the process appear to spread or to increase, immediate surgery is indicated.

A common error in the management of homograft reaction is to continue the patient on massive local or systemic steroids long after any reasonable hope of recovery of the graft can be expected. In addition to a cloudy cornea, the patient then develops glaucoma, a cataract, or both. Several surgeons have reported reasonable success with the use of tissue-matched donor material, immunosuppressive drugs, such as azathioprine, or both, in intractable cases. Drug therapy, however, should be used only at the dosages recommended by and under the careful medical supervision of an immunotherapist, for the systemic effects can be devastating to the patient's general health.

Plate 13-2

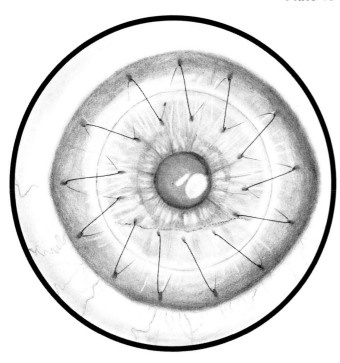

A. Appearance of early graft reaction. The graft reaction (line) extends to the inferior third of the cornea.

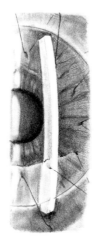

B. Slit-lamp view of early graft reaction, showing stromal and epithelial thickening and extent of endothelial reaction (line).

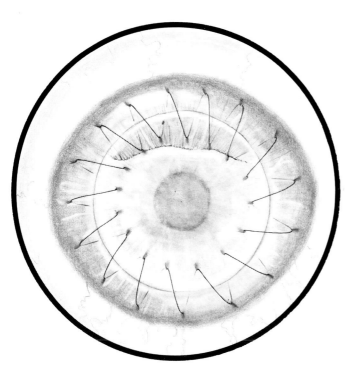

C. Late graft reaction. The process has extended to involve most of the cornea.

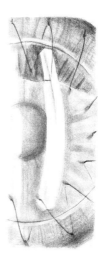

D. Slit-lamp view of late graft reaction.

DONOR TISSUE FAILURE

Donor tissue failure often may be confused with early graft reaction. The surgeon should remember, however, that early graft reaction is extremely rare. In the early stages postkeratoplasty, a cloudy cornea almost always represents donor tissue failure. Should the graft thicken and become cloudy from the first day postoperatively, donor tissue failure is almost certainly the case. Should the graft remain clear for a few weeks and then thicken and become cloudy throughout, again primary endothelial failure of the donor is more probable than graft reaction.

Specular microscopy can aid in the differential diagnosis, since the type and numbers of endothelial cells can be seen directly (Plate 13-3, *A*). It is useful, however, only when the cornea is still relatively clear. The corneal pachymeter also may be of help is assessing response to medication.

Increasing corneal thickness while on maximum immunosuppressive therapy indicates progressive decompensation and the need for early graft replacement. Nevertheless, it is always worth a few days of watchful waiting, while prescribing an increased dose of corticosteroids. However, if clearing does not take place, the graft should be replaced with fresh donor tissue before the necrotizing process involves the recipient cornea. Regrafting then becomes more difficult, and the subsequent development of a true graft reaction more probable. Furthermore, the degenerating defective donor button induces reaction and vascular response from the recipient cornea.

When monofilament suture has been used in the primary procedure, replacement of a defective homograft is easier. When the nylon or polypropylene sutures are cut and removed, the defective graft button usually can be separated easily from the recipient cornea without damage to the latter. This is done by using the razor knife for blunt dissection along the donor-recipient edge and then stripping away the graft using traction with MICRA-Pierse corneal forceps (Plate 13-3, *B* and *C*). Suturing the replacement graft in the recipient follows the same technique as described and illustrated in previous chapters.

The recipient cornea will not suffer the necrosis and softening adjacent to the suture tract points commonly encountered when silk sutures or absorbable sutures are used. Nevertheless, postkeratoplasty, the replacement graft is more prone to homograft reaction and to inflammatory postoperative complications, and so it is followed closely. With modern eye-bank techniques, especially with the use of tissue-culture preserved cornea and specular microscope screening of donor tissue, early graft failure is encountered infrequently. Nevertheless, graft failure undoubtedly will always be a problem, if only as the result of defective surgical technique. Its differential diagnosis from homograft reaction is important to its rational therapy.

Plate 13-3

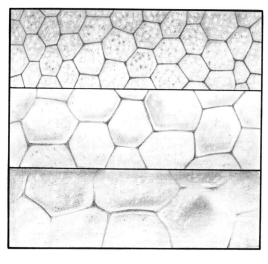

Normal
endothelium

Expanding cells in early
tissue failure

Endothelial cells
approaching limit
of viability—
tissue failure imminent

A. Endothelial cell appearance
(specular microscopy).

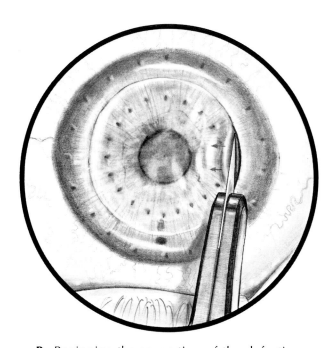

B. Beginning the separation of the defective
homograft from the recipient after sutures
have been removed.

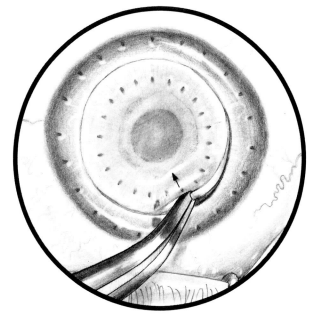

C. Forceps are used to complete the
separation by stripping the defective homograft
from the recipient edge.

315

DEHISCENCE OF THE WOUND

A dehiscence of the surgical wound may vary from a suture tract leak to the opening of a sector of the wound or, indeed, of the entire incision. It is caused by defective suture placement, an untied knot, or too-early suture removal. Depending on its extent, a wound separation results in a variety of problems, ranging from a transient delayed reformation of the anterior chamber to peripheral or wound anterior synechiae, prolapse of the uvea, and loss of the lens or the vitreous. A dehiscence of the wound, even when the anatomic problems it causes are not severe, can often induce severe optical problems (Plate 13-4, *A*). Elevation of a sector of the edge of a graft may produce no loss or only transient loss of the anterior chamber, but a high astigmatic error commonly results (Plate 13-4, *B*).

Any alteration in wound apposition allowing the interposition of iris, lens, or vitreous tissue between its lips has as a secondary effect the creation of a severe meridional optical error (Plate 13-4, *C*).

Repair of a wound dehiscence involves not only wound apposition and restoration of the normal anatomy of the anterior segment but also restoration of the normal corneal curvatures.

The surgical keratometer, therefore, is as essential as the surgical microscope to the repair of a wound dehiscence. The surgeon must take into account two factors in the repair of a wound dehiscence. The first is the need to restore the normal anatomic relationship of the disrupted wound and the anterior segment. The second is to place the sutures and to adjust the approximated wound so that the projection of the surgical keratometer indicates that the optical curvatures of the cornea have been normalized.

Though the repair of a dehisced sector of the wound may solve the anatomic problem, wound slippage or excessive tension on a poorly healed incision in another, previously uninvolved sector can compound the optical problem. To effect an optical as well as an anatomic repair, it is necessary to use a balanced, antitorque, continuous suture either in conjunction with or in place of sector interrupted sutures (see Plate 11-9). Otherwise, a radially placed continuous suture will cause torquing of the healed edge and further graft dislocation.

Plate 13-4

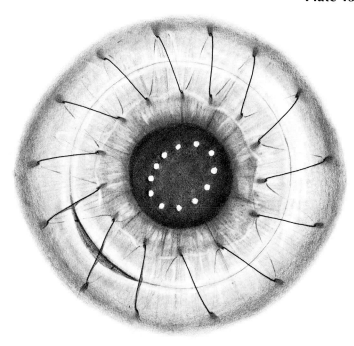

A. Wound separation without prolapse induces high astigmatic error.

B. Sector elevation of graft induces high astigmatic error.

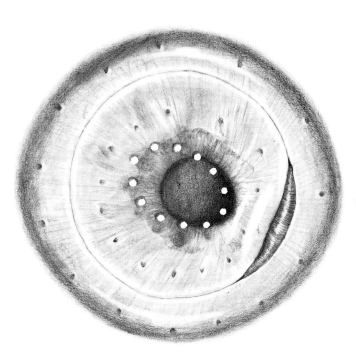

C. Iris prolapse induces high astigmatic error.

HEMORRHAGE

Hemorrhage may sometimes occur in aphakic keratoplasty when extensive resection or reconstructive surgery of the anterior uvea, a vitrectomy, or both accompany the keratoplasty procedure. It can occur also following excessive cyclocryothermy or when such therapy is applied accidentally over the long ciliary vessels. Severe postoperative trauma is one of several even more serious occurrences that can cause hemorrhage.

Usually, a hemorrhage that fills less than one-half to two-thirds of the anterior chamber volume but does not involve the vitreous is treated surgically only if the bleeding increases or the intraocular pressure remains elevated. However, a corneal graft is more susceptible to blood staining than is normal corneal tissue. Also, blood under pressure may be forced into the incision, delaying or complicating healing. Therefore, earlier surgical intervention may be required.

To remove clotted blood from an eye that has recently undergone penetrating keratoplasty is a hazardous procedure, at best, and the graft may well be compromised. Nevertheless, if the tension remains high or if the wound is involved, surgical removal of the clot and lavage of the chamber are necessary. The use of enzymes to soften or to dissolve the clot should be avoided because of possible damage to the graft endothelium. Because of the potentially greater damage that can be inflicted to the endothelial cells, as demonstrated by corneal specular microscopy, phacoemulsification should not be used. One of the vitreous sucking-cutting instruments, such as the Douvas or Peyman unit, often can be used to advantage. However, should the surgery needed to remove the clot compromise the graft, the graft can be replaced at a later date without the eye having been compromised, in turn, by glaucoma, cataract, or uveal atrophy resulting from prolonged inaction in removing the clot.

INFECTION

In all my experience as a corneal surgeon, I have seen only one presumptive case of endophthalmitis immediately following keratoplasty. No positive culture was obtained, and the eye cleared promptly with the administration of local and systemic steroids and antibiotics. Often, eye-donor tissue is removed under less-than-ideal sterile conditions, following a prolonged and debilitating illness. It must be presumed that numerous organisms flourish in the vicinity of such an eye. At the Eye Bank for Sight Restoration, Incorporated, no eye is utilized if there is a positive culture. Often, however, the eye is used so quickly that microorganisms cannot be cultured until after the surgery. Even in cases where positive cultures are subsequently obtained, complicating infections are rare. Minor infections do occur, probably more often than detected or treated. These can result in stitch abscesses with softening of the adjacent tissue and loosening of the affected suture loop, creating a potential for separation of the wound, with its resultant problems.

A stitch abscess about an interrupted suture is resolved readily by removal of the offending stitch and curettage of the infected, softened, necrotic tissue, followed by frequent instillation of an appropriate antibiotic solution or ointment. When a nylon continuous suture has been used, it will not be possible to remove the offending stitch. Nevertheless, one or two loops may cut through partially without separating a sector of the incision. Though there may not be an actual wound dehiscence, there can be a significant alteration in corneal curvature, with resultant excessive astigmatism. In this event, which can occur after loss of a sector of a continuous suture, secondary interrupted sutures should be placed once the infection is cleared. The surgical keratometer should be used to monitor the corneal curvatures as these secondary sutures are being placed.

KERATOCONJUNCTIVITIS AND BLEPHARITIS

Mild to severe keratoconjunctivitis and blepharitis, which are most often a result of inflammatory reaction incited by the healing incision and the suture material, also occur. When the eye remains irritated, the upper lid should be everted and carefully examined with the slit lamp. Severe proliferative blepharitis can occur as a result of an exposed knot or knots. If the offending suture cannot be removed, it may be necessary temporarily to separate the lid from the cornea with a therapeutic contact lens to allow the blepharitis and keratitis to clear. Though such inflammations can prolong the period necessary for epithelialization of the cornea and so cause some discomfort, they are rarely dangerous if treated promptly. Bacterial superinfection responds to the instillation of a specific local antibiotic.

Because of the frequent and prolonged use of steroids, the possibility of a fungous infection should not be overlooked. In case of an intractable abscess or conjunctivitis, fungous cultures should be taken and, if found positive, appropriate therapy instituted.

Idoxuridine, or adenine arabinoside, used in the early postoperative management of keratoplasty for active herpetic keratitis or as a prophylactic against its recurrence, can cause a chronic irritation and stippling of the corneal epithelium resembling superficial punctate keratitis. For this reason, we do not use antiviral agents prophylactically. Signs and symptoms usually disappear promptly on discontinuing the medication.

TRAUMA

Since many individuals undergoing keratoplasty are young and male, the incidence of ocular trauma is higher than, for instance, in older postoperative cataract patients. For this reason, the patient is required to wear a protective shield or spectacle in front of the operated eye day and night, for 6 months following penetrating keratoplasty. The patient is cautioned also to attach both seat and shoulder belts when in a motor vehicle, either as the driver or as a passenger, and to avoid heated arguments or contact sports. I have never had a patient report serious damage to a graft during sexual activity. All degrees of damage—from transient loss of the anterior chamber without significant sequelae through complete rupture of the graft incision with loss of ocular contents—can ensue. Appropriate medical and surgical measures, as are explained in Volume I and in the preceding chapter, must be applied as they are indicated by the nature and extent of the injury.

SUMMARY

The postoperative complications of keratoplasty can vary with the initial pathology, the extent of surgery, and the activity and age of the patient. They can be anticipated, or they may occur spontaneously and unexpectedly. When possible, medical measures should be used first to control the problem, but if wound integrity and the optics of the final graft are compromised, surgical intervention is mandatory.

CHAPTER 14

POSTOPERATIVE MANAGEMENT OF THE SUCCESSFULLY GRAFTED EYE

General considerations
Immediate postoperative period—from
  surgery to hospital discharge
Second postoperative period—from hospital
  discharge through the sixth week
Third postoperative period—from the sixth
  week through the sixth month

Late postoperative period—after the sixth
  month
Specular microscopy and pachymetry
Summary

GENERAL CONSIDERATIONS

When keratoplasty is performed using the surgical microscope, micro-surgical instruments, and microsurgical suture techniques, the majority of cases will be technically successful. On the other hand, because of the relatively atraumatic nature of the surgical technique and the minimal tissue irritation from monofilament suture fixation, a long healing period is required. This slow healing occurs as a predominately keratocytic, rather than fibroblastic, proliferation of cells across the incisional area. Thus, the formation of a dense, fibrotic scar is prevented. A more physiologic and optically clear graft-recipient junction not only is anatomically more secure but also produces and maintains a more regular optical surface in the healed clear graft. Such a desirable result depends also on proper diagnosis and the selection of an individualized surgical plan, meticulously executed, using viable, optically regular donor tissue. Following a technically successful graft, the postoperative period is as critical to the initial success and final outcome of the intervention as any preoperative or surgical step.

Postoperative management is divided into four time periods: first, the immediate postoperative period, from surgery to hospital discharge; second, from hospital discharge through the sixth week postoperatively; third, from the sixth week to the sixth month postoperatively; and fourth, the late postoperative period, after 6 months.

IMMEDIATE POSTOPERATIVE PERIOD—FROM SURGERY TO HOSPITAL DISCHARGE

Following the successful grafting of either the phakic or aphakic eye, from 4 to 7 days of close observation in the hospital are required. Immediately after surgery, the operated eye will have been lightly patched and further protected with a Fox-type metal shield (see Plate 6-31, C). The patient may experience varying degrees of discomfort during the immediate postoperative period. The dressing is not disturbed unless discomfort is severe and prolonged and not substantially relieved after one or two administrations of a mild narcotic agent, such as pentazocine lactate. Meperidine and morphine are to be avoided because of their frequent systemic side effects.

Routine postoperative orders include bed rest until the patient is recovered from the anesthesia or until the eye is dressed on the day following surgery. The male patient is allowed to stand at the bedside to void, if necessary, as soon as he is recovered from the anesthesia. If the operated eye is the patient's only seeing eye or if vision in the other eye is poor, private duty nurses are ordered for the first 24 to 48 hours postoperatively. In these instances, both eyes are patched so that personnel automatically treat the patient as being temporarily without vision.

On the morning following surgery, at the first dressing, the degree of postoperative reaction is noted; the clarity of the graft is ascertained; the integrity of the closing suture or sutures is determined; and the depth of the anterior chamber is noted, using the slit lamp if necessary. From the first dressing, no patch is used. The patient is cautioned to wear spectacles or a taped-on Fox shield over the eye at all times. The patient is informed that the eye may tear profusely and that any tears should be wiped away from the cheek, not from the lid margin.

Following the first dressing, the patient is allowed to be ambulatory at will, provided he has recovered fully from the anesthesia and from any depressant or narcotic postoperative medications and provided his general physical state permits. He is allowed to comb his hair, shave, brush his teeth, tub bathe (no showers), and wear a contact lens on the other eye, if this is required for best correction. Hydrocortisone (1%) drops are instilled three times daily and chloramphenicol (1%) drops are instilled twice daily. No mydriatic is used unless there is a greater than 2+ anterior segment flare and cells. The eye is examined biomicroscopically daily until discharge. The patient with a graft in a phakic eye, such as for keratoconus, is discharged on the third or fourth postoperative day. The patient with a graft in an aphakic eye or with a combined graft and cataract extraction is discharged between the fourth and seventh day, depending on the extent of the surgical procedure and when the condition of the posterior segment can be ascertained.

Following keratoplasty the aphakic eye is more prone to develop inflammatory reaction of the uvea or vitreous, whether or not vitrectomy is performed. In the combined operation without vitreous loss or the necessity for vitrectomy, uveitis is rare. However, when vitrectomy must be performed, both uveitis and vitreitis occur commonly and are treated vigorously until the conditions are resolved. Only then is the patient allowed to leave the hospital. Especially in the case of anterior segment reconstruction involving extensive uveal surgery as well as vitrectomy, large daily doses (100 mg) of prednisone or prednisolone together with a prophylactic antibiotic, such as cephaloridine (500 mg), four times daily, are given. Usually the steroid, and sometimes the antibiotic, is continued into the second postoperative period, as indicated.

SECOND POSTOPERATIVE PERIOD—FROM HOSPITAL DISCHARGE THROUGH THE SIXTH WEEK

At discharge, the patient is given a printed instruction sheet, outlining permitted activities and detailing medications. An appointment is made for a return office visit in 5 to 7 days. The patient is instructed to call at any time, day or night, in the interim, if there is any change in the feeling or appearance of the eye, if there is decreasing vision, or if there is any question about the prescribed medication or eye care. Often, a patient can return immediately to part-time home or business activities during the first week after discharge.

At the first postoperative office examination, the thickness and clarity of the graft and the integrity of the wound closure are determined. Endothelial specular microscopy is performed if corneal clarity permits, and a photographic record is made of the donor endothelium.

A clinical keratometer reading is taken, and, on the basis of that reading and by trial and error, an initial refraction is done. At this stage, retinoscopy is of limited value for determining axial or astigmatic errors. With the approximate correcting lenses in place, the vision is taken using a pinhole. Vision results will vary widely, and the patient is almost always apprehensive and must be reassured that the vision will continue to improve, regardless of the level found initially.

If the vision cannot be improved or if the fundus cannot be visualized adequately, a B-scan tomography is performed. This is important, especially in the aphakic eye in which there has been vitreous or uveal surgery. Resolution of vitreitis may be monitored, or early detachment may be discovered and treated.

Tonometry should be performed if there is persistent epithelial edema or mild pain. A carbonic anhydrase inhibitor is prescribed when increased intraocular pressure can be measured or is suspected, even if tonometry is unsatisfactory.

Local medication given in the hospital and renewed at discharge is continued. Steroid drops may be increased if there is any evidence of redness of the eye or persistent cloudiness of the graft.

Systemic medication usually may be decreased gradually or discontinued. In the absence of signs of infection, antibiotics are not given for more than 7 days. Systemic steroid dosages are reduced progressively, as soon as a reversal of the inflammatory process is noted. Usually, at least 2 to 3 weeks of therapy are required, and small dosages (5 to 20 mg daily) may be continued for as long as 6 weeks.

Patients vary not only in their responses to a given medication but also in their reliability and the facility with which they apply local medication. Therefore, the therapeutic response to a standard dosage and frequency of use may vary considerably. One should not hesitate to increase medication well above the usual therapeutic level when the desired or anticipated therapeutic response is not obtained. This is true particularly in the treatment of early postoperative glaucoma, in which case it may be necessary to use two or three times the usual dosage of a carbonic anhydrase inhibitor; for example, as much as 2000 mg of acetazolamide every 24 hours, provided there are no medical contraindications.

On the second visit, 2 or 3 weeks postoperatively, a clinical keratometer reading and refractive vision are again taken, and the eye is examined with the slit lamp and specular microscope. If the graft remains clear, is of normal thickness, and shows no decrease in endothelial cell population, the medication is reduced. The corticosteroid drops are prescribed once or twice daily. If the fluorescein dye indicates that the epithelium is intact over the incision and sutures, chloramphenicol is discontinued. If intraocular pressure is increased, appropriate medications are prescribed.

At the third visit, 6 weeks postoperatively, if the graft remains clear, the sutures are in place, vision continues to improve, and intraocular pressure is normal, medication is reduced to, or maintained at, 1 drop of corticosteroid daily. The intraocular pressure may be elevated because of the local steroid, which should be discontinued completely if this is suspected. If the keratometry and refraction have stablized and there is useful corrected vision, a temporary correcting lens may be prescribed, especially if the vision in the other eye is diminished or absent.

THIRD POSTOPERATIVE PERIOD—FROM THE SIXTH WEEK THROUGH THE SIXTH MONTH

The patient with a normotensive eye and a clear, well-positioned graft returns at 6-week to 2-month intervals for a period of 6 months postoperatively. At each evaluation of the graft and suture line, a clinical keratometer reading is taken, refraction is done, and the spectacle lens is modified, as indicated. Specular microscopy is performed if, at the slit-lamp examination, the graft shows any sign of thickening or of epithelial edema. Changing cell morphology or decreasing numbers of viable endothelial cells may indicate an impending graft reaction or tissue failure and the need to increase or to institute immunosuppressive therapy. Corneal pachymetry may be performed separately or with the specular microscope. In particular, the patient is instructed to call or visit the office should he contract a severe febrile upper respiratory infection or note any haziness or blurring of corrected vision.

Approximately 6 months after surgery, the sutures are removed. *The time for removal of sutures depends on many factors and must be individualized for each case.* It is always better to remove sutures a few days after healing has occurred rather than a few days before. There is no certain way, other than experience, to know when healing is complete. Removal of sutures should be delayed in certain diagnoses, such as advanced bullous keratopathy, endothelial-epithelial corneal dystrophy, or any case with a soft or degenerating avascular recipient cornea. Conversely, in a vascular recipient, firm healing may occur in 3 to 4 months, and sutures should be removed as they loosen. If vessels tend to cross the incision into the graft, it may be presumed that healing has occurred in that area.

In almost every case, removal of the sutures is performed under the biomicroscope as an office procedure, using topical anesthesia. Sutures are removed in the operating room under the operating microscope only in special circumstances, such as in a mentally retarded patient, in a child, or in the rare instance of an uncooperative adult. In these instances, general anesthesia is used.

Sutures are removed under slit-lamp or surgical microscope magnification of $10\times$ to $20\times$. When local anesthesia is used, three applications of benoxinate drops are instilled at intervals of 2 minutes. The surgeon holds the lids open with the thumb and index finger of the nondominant hand (Plate 14-1). Two instruments, a razor knife with a blade cracked to a sharp point and the Troutman colibri-handled suture forceps with angulated jaws, are used alternately to cut and to elevate and to remove isolated suture loops (see Volume I, Plates 2-7, 5-16, and 5-17). When possible, sutures are cut over the donor cornea, which, of course, is insensitive.

Plate 14-1

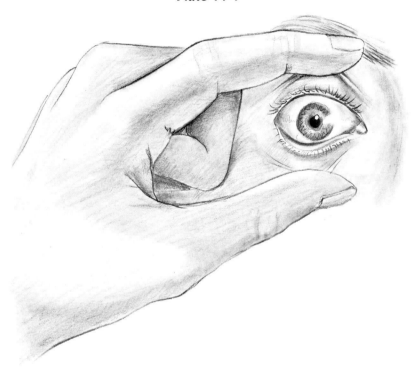

Lids being held open for suture removal.

With a continuous suture or double continuous suture, the loop or loops containing the knot or knots are first isolated by cutting the subepithelial monofilament thread anteriorly at the middle of the loop to either side of the knot to be removed. This is done with the razor knife. The point of the cracked blade, its sharpened edge directed slightly away from the corneal surface, is passed under the suture loop. With a slight upward direction of the blade, the suture is cut (Plate 14-2, *A* and *B*). Since the nylon thread is under elastic tension, the cut thread ends separate.

If the suture loop is loose, it is exposed and can be cut more readily with the blade directly. When the suture loop is taut, the thread almost always lies subepithelially, on top of Bowman's membrane, where it is approached through the epithelium.

When the knot has been isolated, the loose end of the suture over the donor cornea is elevated from beneath the epithelium by the point of the razor blade, so that the thread end proximal to the knot can be grasped firmly with the pointed suture-removal forceps. With a slight jerking motion, the surgeon pulls up the thread end centrally, radial to the needle tract. The knot should pull free from the tract so that the suture loop, including the knot, is removed (Plate 14-2, *C*). Should the thread break, the knot catch, or the cut thread ends fail to disengage as the thread end is pulled toward the donor side, the recipient end of the thread is isolated and grasped, and the knot is pulled through the needle tract in reverse to exit to the recipient side (Plate 14-2, *D* and *E*).

Occasionally, the knot will be untied by the pulling or jerking motion; the two ends are then removed separately. Sometimes, however, the knot will stick within the needle tract and cannot be removed by tugging from either end. In this instance, the loose thread ends should be cut flush to the cornea with the razor knife or scissors, and the portion of the loop containing the knot left buried in the stroma.

Plate 14-2

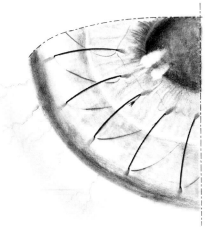

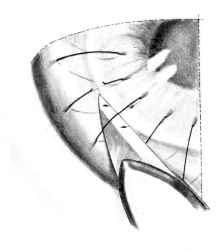

A. Continuous suture loops.

B. Cutting the second suture loop adjacent to the knot.

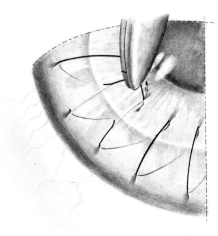

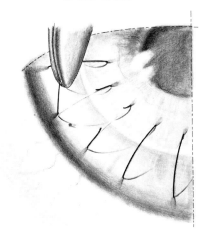

C. Removing the knot from the donor needle tract.

D. Knot alternatively being pulled through the suture tract from the recipient side.

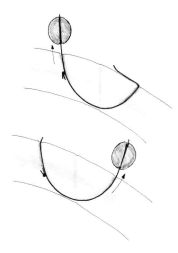

E. Cut thread ends of knot directed away from direction of forceps traction.

Then, using the same maneuver as for cutting the thread loops adjacent to the knot, the point of the razor knife is used to cut in sequence the anterior thread connecting every other loop of the continuous suture. Each intact intermediate subepithelial thread is then elevated into a loose externalized loop. The point of the knife, with the sharp edge of the blade held toward the cornea, is slipped through the epithelium under the suture loop. The dull back edge of the blade (Plate 14-3) is moved up to elevate the thread loop. Each elevated thread loop, in turn, is grasped, and the free thread ends are pulled easily from their tracts.

The thread may be cut or broken accidentally as the loop is isolated or pulled out. It will be necessary then to remove the two pieces of suture material separately. During the removal of the sutures, care is taken to disturb the epithelium as little as possible.

Plate 14-3

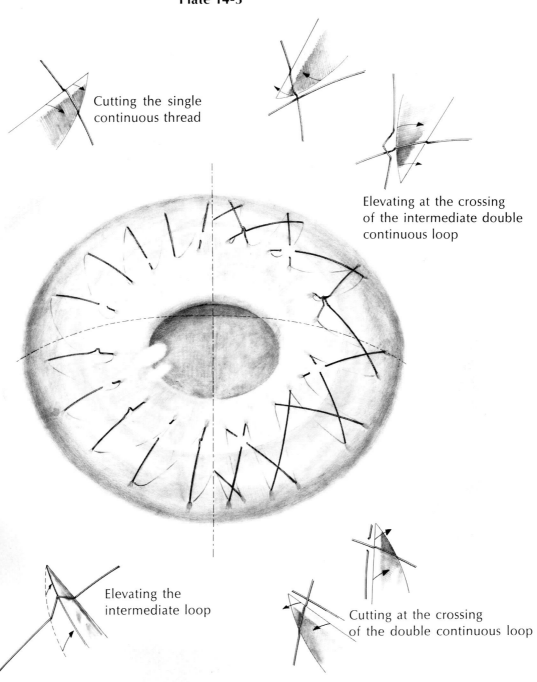

Cutting the single continuous thread

Elevating at the crossing of the intermediate double continuous loop

Elevating the intermediate loop

Cutting at the crossing of the double continuous loop

Cutting and elevating a continuous suture loop in preparation for removal

On occasion, some stromal overgrowth will be seen to emerge from and to extend subepithelially adjacent to the tracts of the exiting suture loops. This appears as a gray haze at the level of, and sometimes partially obscuring, the anterior suture loop and may continue across the incision (Plate 14-4). Since it usually lies on top of Bowman's membrane, this tissue may be removed easily with the flat of the razor knife by stroking away first the epithelium and then the underlying stromal overgrowth.

If the apparent overgrowth is very thick and edematous, this maneuver must be performed cautiously, especially if the incision line also is covered by the overgrowth. This more extensive stromal overgrowth originates from the wound rather than from the suture tracts and is caused by a malapposed incision or an untreated wound elevation. With a poorly apposed incision, the removal of the reinforcing overgrowth can result in wound separation. Removal of this overgrown tissue should be delayed until the edema has subsided, at which time the integrity of the wound will be better ensured than immediately after suture removal.

Plate 14-4

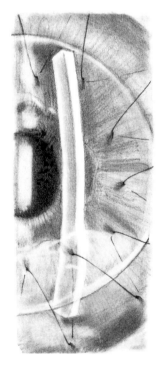

Slit-lamp appearance of stromal overgrowth.

Biomicroscopy is done and keratometer readings are taken just prior to, immediately after, and 15 minutes and 1 hour following suture removal. Almost always there will be a moderate shift in astigmatic axis and amount, with an overall steepening of the corneal curvatures. A marked or continuing shift and steepening may signal an impending wound elevation or separation, which always occurs in the wound at the axis of the flatter meridian. A wound dehiscence, even if incomplete, is resutured (see Chapter 13) as soon as hospitalization and operating time can be arranged. In the interim, a therapeutic contact lens is used to close the wound temporarily and, thus, to allow the anterior chamber to reform or to prevent its loss.

If marked astigmatism occurs and persists during the late postoperative period, in the absence of obvious wound separation or elevation, the patient is a candidate for the Troutman corneal wedge-resection procedure. This must not be done for 3 to 6 months after corneal K is stabilized. The stress of a wedge resection done on one quadrant centered at the flatter meridian may pull the wound apart to the side opposite the resection, not only nullifying the optical result but complicating the eventual repair.

LATE POSTOPERATIVE PERIOD—AFTER THE SIXTH MONTH

Following suture removal, the eye need not be patched unless there has been extensive removal of epithelium or there is wound elevation or separation. An antibiotic ointment, such as chloramphenicol, is placed in the lower cul-de-sac prophylactically. The patient is instructed to use hydrocortisone (1%) eye drops three times daily for 1 week. Graft rejection is more likely to occur during the period immediately after suture removal. This probably is the result of endothelial disturbance from released wound compression and the subsequent shifting of the donor-recipient relationship as the graft takes on its final "set."

A final refraction may be done usually 2 or 3 weeks after suture removal; however, the patient is cautioned that there may be further changes requiring a change in spectacle correction during the first year. The possibility of late graft reaction is discussed with the patient, and signs and symptoms are reviewed, with the absolute necessity for early treatment being stressed. Because of the increased incidence of graft reaction that seems to occur with febrile viral infections, the patient is strongly advised, in the absence of medical contraindications, to have the current influenza immunizations.

SPECULAR MICROSCOPY AND PACHYMETRY

Specular microscopy of the (graft) endothelium is done at intervals between surgery and suture removal, 6 months after suture removal, and then yearly. These examinations can provide some early indications of an impending graft reaction or corneal decompensation, so that appropriate preventive measures can be taken early. It is important to do the specular microscopic examination of the endothelium just before and several weeks following suture removal and again later, especially should any ocular inflammatory signs or symptoms appear that could affect the cornea. Corneal thickness measurements can be taken with the specular microscope or with a corneal pachymeter attachment to the slit lamp. An increase in corneal thickness also may herald corneal decompensation or homograft reaction; conversely, thinning can indicate a resolution or positive response to therapy.

SUMMARY

The final result of the most exact surgical technique applied to the most ideal case will be compromised if not followed by meticulous postoperative care. Such follow-up care should include not only each medical but also every optical consideration, so that the patient will obtain maximum vision benefit within the shortest possible time. Success in corneal surgery is not only a clear graft but also an optically functional one. Painstaking postoperative management will ensure an optimal result.

EPILOGUE

Surgery of the cornea, more than any other surgery on the human body or on the eye, approaches an exact science. This has to do primarily with the fact that small alterations in the clarity or in the curvature of the cornea, which comprises the major optical system of the eye, can induce profound changes in the transmission of the surround to the retina. This volume is an attempt to present, in addition to the usual anatomic considerations, a more quantitative approach to the reparative surgery of these corneal optical alterations. Thus, it begins with a discussion of corneal optics rather than of surgical pathology. A major part of the text is devoted to detailed explanation of the optical, as well as the anatomic, principles involved in corneal surgical techniques. I am the first to recognize that my efforts, as well as current results, are only early and inadequate compared to what will occur as these principles and succeeding ones are applied by future generations of ophthalmic surgeons.

Ophthalmic surgeons have an advantage given to no other surgeon. The human eye, within reasonably precise limits, is an optically measurable organ with predictable optical effects from developmental, pathologic, or surgical tissue alterations. In consideration of things to come, I believe that Kelvin's dictum applies: "When you can measure what you are speaking about and express it in numbers you know something about it. But when you cannot (or do not) measure it, when you cannot express it in numbers, your knowledge is of meager and unsatisfactory kind."

We are at the threshhold of understanding how surgically to manipulate precisely the optics of the eye. We are able to measure the powers of its various components and to put these measurements into meaningful numbers that can then be translated readily into a precise optical surgical technique. Further advances in microsurgery and instrumentation will continue to refine the approach. It is my hope that this book will contribute, in a small way, not only toward the improvement of present techniques for anatomic restoration of the integrity of the human eye but also to the vast and new fields of optical surgery that will occupy an increasing amount of our attention in the future.

SELECTED READINGS

Barraquer, J., and Ruttlán, J.: Surgery of the anterior segment of the eye, vol. 2: Corneal surgery, Barcelona, 1971, Instituto Barraquer.

Barraquer, J., Ruttlán, J., and Troutman, R. C.: Surgery of the anterior segment of the eye, vol. 1: General considerations and intracapsular cataract extraction, New York, 1964, McGraw-Hill Book Co.

Barraquer, J. I.: Compilation of reprints, vol. 1: Refractive keratoplasty, Bogotá, Colombia, 1970, Instituto Barraquer de America.

Barraquer, J. I.: Compilation of reprints, vol. 2: Refractive keratoplasty, Bogotá, Colombia, 1975, Instituto Barraquer de America.

Castroviejo, R.: Atlas of keratectomy and keratoplasty, Philadelphia, 1966, W. B. Saunders Co.

Harms, H., and Mackensen, G.: Ocular surgery under the microscope, Chicago, 1967, Year Book Medical Publishers, Inc.

Kelly, S. E., Ehlers, J., Llovera, I., and Troutman, R. C.: Comparison of tissue reaction to nylon and prolene sutures in rabbit iris and cornea, Ophthalmic Surg. 6:105-110, 1975.

King, J. H., and Lemp, M.: Second Meeting of the World Congress of the Cornea, Washington, D.C., 1976 (in press).

King, J. H., and McTigue, J.: First Meeting of the World Congress of the Cornea, Washington, D.C., 1965.

Troutman, R. C.: Astigmatism and myopia in keratoplasty, South African J. Ophthal. 1:29-35, 1973.

Troutman, R. C.: Cataract surgery after keratoplasty (abstract), Datelines Ophthalmol., vol. 11, no. 1, 1974.

Troutman, R. C.: Cataract surgery combined with keratoplasty. Aphakic and combined grafts. In Emery, J. M., and Paton, D., editors: Current concepts in cataract surgery, St. Louis, 1976, The C. V. Mosby Co., pp. 160-161.

Troutman, R. C.: Cirugia del Segmento Anterior del Ojo, An. Inst. Barraquer, vol. 7, no. 7-8, July-Oct., 1967.

Troutman, R. C.: Control of corneal astigmatism in cataract and corneal surgery, Trans. Pac. Coast Otoophthalmol. Soc. 51: 217-231, 1970.

Troutman, R. C.: Induced astigmatism as a result of corneal surgery, Transactions of the First South African Ophthalmological Symposium, Johannesburg, South Africa, 1969.

Troutman, R. C.: Instrumentation. How to begin using the microscope. In Emery, J. M., and Paton, D., editors: Current concepts in cataract surgery, St. Louis, 1976, The C. V. Mosby Co., pp. 30-32.

Troutman, R. C.: International Symposium of Microsurgery of the Eye, Tübingen, Germany, Aug. 23-25, 1966, Am. J. Ophthalmol. 63:869-877, 1967.

Troutman, R. C.: Management of corneal astigmatism. Management of pre-existing corneal astigmatism. In Emery, J. M., and Paton, D., editors: Current concepts in cataract surgery, St. Louis, 1976, The C. V. Mosby Co., pp. 189-190.

Troutman, R. C.: Management of corneal astigmatism. Prevention of astigmatism at cataract surgery. In Emery, J. M., and Paton, D., editors: Current concepts in cataract surgery, St. Louis, 1976, The C. V. Mosby Co., pp. 179-180.

Troutman, R. C.: Microsurgery for keratoplasty, development and techniques, Int. Ophthalmol. Clin. 10:297-311, 1970.

Troutman, R. C.: Microsurgery of the anterior segment of the eye, vol. 1, St. Louis, 1974, The C. V. Mosby Co.

Troutman, R. C.: Microsurgery of the cornea, Bull. N.Y. Acad. Med. 45:53-58, 1969.

Troutman, R. C.: Microsurgery of the eye,

First Symposium of the Ophthalmic Microsurgery Study Group, Tübingen, Germany, 1966, Adv. Ophthal. 20:82-87, 1968.

Troutman, R. C.: Microsurgery of the eye, Science Writers Seminar, New York, 1969, Research to Prevent Blindness, Inc., pp. 32-33.

Troutman, R. C.: Microsurgery of keratoconus. In Turtz, A.: Proceedings of the Centennial Symposium, vol. 1, St. Louis, 1969, The C. V. Mosby Co., pp. 242; Adv. Ophthalmol. 22:217-227, 1970.

Troutman, R. C.: Microsurgery of keratoconus, Microsurgery in glaucoma. Second Symposium of the Ophthalmic Microsurgery Study Group, Burgenstock, Switzerland 1968, Av. Ophthal. 22:217-227, 1970.

Troutman, R. C.: Microsurgery of ocular injuries, Third Symposium of the Ophthalmic Microsurgery Study Group, Merida, Yucatan, Mexico, 1970, Adv. Ophthal. 1970.

Troutman, R. C.: Microsurgical control of corneal astigmatism in cataract and keratoplasty, Trans. Am. Acad. Ophthalmol. Otolaryngol. 77:563-572, 1973.

Troutman, R. C.: The operating microscope in ophthalmic surgery, Trans. Am. Ophthalmol. Soc. 63:335-348, 1965.

Troutman, R. C.: The operating microscope, past, present and future, Trans. Am. Acad. Ophthalmol. Soc. 87:205-218, 1967.

Troutman, R. C.: Personal interview: Microsurgery, Highlights Ophthalmol. 7:162-180, 1964.

Troutman, R. C.: Recent advances in cataract and corneal surgery presented at the Second South African International Ophthalmological Symposium, Johannesburg, South Africa, September, 1973.

Troutman, R. C.: Vitrectomy in cataract and corneal surgery, Trans. Pac. Coast Otoophthalmol. Soc. 51:157-173, 1970.

Troutman, R. C.: The weightless intraocular lens, Ophthalmic Surg. 8:153-155, 1977.

Troutman, R. C., and Barraquer, J., Ruttlán, J.: Surgery of the anterior segment of the eye, vol. 1: New York, 1964, McGraw-Hill Book Co.

Troutman, R. C., Binkhorst, R. D., Weinstein, G. W., and Baum, G.: Axial length of aphakic eye, Am. J. Ophthalmol., 62(6):1194-1201, Dec. 1966.

Troutman, R. C., and Eve, F. R.: Deep suturing of corneal incisions, Ophthalmic Surg. 4:16-22, 1973.

Troutman, R. C., Kelly, S., Kaye, D., and Clahane, A. C.: The use and preliminary results of the Troutman surgical keratometer in cataract and corneal surgery, Trans. Am. Acad. Ophthalmol. Otolaryngol. 83:OP232-OP238, 1977.

Troutman, R. C., King, J. H., Jr., and McTigue, J. W.: The operating microscope in corneal surgery, The Cornea World Congress, Woburn, Mass., 1965, Butterworth (Publishers) Inc., pp. 424-434.

Troutman, R. C., and Meltzer, M.: Astigmatism and myopia in keratoconus, Trans. Am. Ophthalmol. Soc. 70:265-277, 1972.

Troutman, R. C., and Stuart, J.: Optical considerations in penetrating keratoplasty (abstract), Datelines in Ophthalmol., vol. 10, no. 4, 1973.

Troutman, R. C., and Stuart, J.: Optical considerations in penetrating keratoplasty, Ann. Inst. Barraquer, 12:229-237, 1975.

INDEX

A

Abscess, stitch, 319
Acetazolamide, 324
Acetylcholine, 230, 242
Acquired dystrophy, excessively flat recipient cornea in, 14
Active infection and corneal surgery, 35
Active inflammation and corneal surgery, 35
Adenine arabinoside, 319
Air in anterior chamber, 172, 230, 231, 236, 240, 256, 257, 300
Alcon needle, 106
Allergies, 312
Alpha chymotrypsin, 224-225
Amblyopia, functional, 35
Ametropia
  axial, 7, 20
  corneal, 4, 23-24, 26
    effect of anatomic and optical diameters on, 23-24, 26-27
    effect of corneal optics on, 18-20
  corneal-induced
    astigmatic, mechanisms of, 16-17
    mechanisms of, in keratoconus, 8-9
  curvature, 7
  meridional, surgical keratometer in correction of, 32
  optical, 16
  posterior segment, 22
  surgical, correction of, 7-33
  surgically induced, 266
Amoils cryoextractor, 100, 226-229
Anastigmatic emmetropic schematic cornea, 10, 11
Anatomic diameter of cornea, 21, 23-24, 26
Anesthesia, 116
angle, 288, 291
  closure of, 144
Anisometropia, 46, 252
Anterior chamber, 14, 214, 230, 231, 256, 257, 288, 318, 333
  angle, 252
  loss of, 172
  reformed, 172, 173
Anterior segment
  extensive reconstruction of, in control of glaucoma, 288
  management of additional pathology of, 252-255
  reconstruction of, 108
  surgery of, use of fixation ring in, 120-127

Anterior segment—cont'd
  techniques for more extensive surgery of, 232
Anterior synechia, 144, 172
Antibiotics, 201, 300, 318, 324
  solution or ointment, 319
Antihistaminic medication, 311
Antitorque continuous suture; see Continuous suture, antitorque
Antiviral agents, 319
Aperture drape, 3M, 98, 100
Aphakia, hyperopic, 22
  and keratomileusis, 110
  and keratophakia, 110
Aphakic bullous keratopathy, 248
Aphakic glaucoma, 288
Aphakic hypermetropia, 14, 110
Aphakic hyperopia, 252
Aphakic keratoplasty, 95, 102, 142, 245-262, 287
  and Flieringa ring, 120
  general considerations for, 245
  and hyperopia, 46
  preparation for, 250
  recipient opening, cutting of, in, 252
  size of donor button in, 46
Aplanatic cornea, curvature of, 20
Application tube for chelation of corneal calcium deposits, 36-37
Aqueous leak, ii, 170, 174
Arc length, 268, 269, 270, 283
A-scan ultrasound tomography, 22
Astigmatic ametropia, corneal-induced, mechanisms of, 16-17
Astigmatic band, 26, 140
  axis of, 30
  compensation of, using secondary interrupted sutures, 170
  in donor cornea, 202
  following keratoplasty, 7, 44
Astigmatic cornea, projection of surgical keratometer on, 30-32
Astigmatic error, high, 317
  induced, 22
Astigmatic lens, pathologic, 22
Astigmatism, 4, 16, 24, 263, 274, 275, 319, 333
  circular button in wedge-resected recipient opening as cause of, 26-27
  compensation of, in recipient, by use of oval graft, 203, 203
  corneal, induced, 16
  correction of, Troutman wedge resection in, 263-286

Astigmatism—cont'd
  correction of—cont'd
    general considerations for, 263-265
  hyperopic, in familial dystrophy, 35
  iatrogenic, cause of, 24
  irregular or high, 217
    and contact lenses, 35
    following successful keratoplasty, 20, 22
  methods of eliminating, from grafts, 52
  mixed, induced, 16
  myopic, 26
  pathologic, cause of, 24
  physiologic, cause of, 24
  postoperative, 52
    "suture-in-place," 32
  preexisting, correction of, 206-211
  residual postoperative, correction of, 263-286
  with-the-rule, 18, 19
    correction of, 206-211
Atrophic optic cup, 288
Autograft, 50, 273
Axial ametropia, 7, 20
Axial myopia, 8, 14
Azathioprine, 313

B

Backing block; see Block, backing
Backing plate for trephine piston punch, 100
Bacterial superinfection, 319
Band, astigmatic, following keratoplasty, 7
Band keratopathy, calcium deposits in, 36
Barraquer, Joaquin, 1, 28, 264
Barraquer, José, 110, 198
Barraquer corneal optical lathe, 110
Barraquer cryolathe, 100
Barraquer lamellar microkeratome, 100, 110,
    132
Barraquer light-wire lid speculum, 98-99, 102,
    117, 182, 201, 232
  in combined keratoplasty and cataract extrac-
    tion, 219
  placement of, 117
  separation of lids by, in simple penetrating ker-
    atoplasty, 201
  in successive lamellar dissections, 182-184
Barraquer microkeratome, 110
Barraquer-de Wecker scissors, 98-99, 108
  midperipheral iridectomy with, 142-143
  in midperipheral iridectomy and radial sphinc-
    terotomy, 222
  in suturing of donor button to recipient cornea,
    162-163
  in trabeculectomy, 298
Barraquer-Mateus motor-driven trephine, 100,
    130-131
Basic salt solution, 172, 173, 230, 252, 298, 300
Beaulieu 16-mm cine camera unit, 112
Benoxinate drops, 326
Bias cutting of donor button, 92-93, 221
Binkhorst four-loop intraocular lens, 108, 236,
    240-241, 242
Binkhorst two-loop intraocular lens, 242, 243
Binocular zoom microscope for assistant, 112,
    113
Biomicroscope, 286, 326
Biomicroscopy, 333
Blade
  razor, for razor knife, 104, 109

Blade—cont'd
  trephine; see Trephine, blade for
Blade breaker, 103
  Troutman short-angled, 104
Bleb, conjunctival, 300
Blepharitis, 319
  proliferative, 319
Block, backing, 82-94
  aspheric or elliptical curve in, use of, 202, 203
  Cardona-Roskothen, groove, 90-94
  disposable, 84, 85, 86
    Troutman frame-and-piston assembly, 86-87
  double-curved concavity, 84, 85
  four-concavity, 84
  irregularities in, causing irregularities in donor
    button, 202-203
  meridian groove markings on, 88-89
  radius of curvature of, 82
  spherical, concave, 80
  stainless, for trephine piston punch, 98, 100
  Teflon, 82-85, 100, 148, 202-203, 252
  Troutman double-curved, 84
    disposable, 94
Blood clot in trabeculotomy, 304
Blood dyscrasia, rejection of donor eye from pa-
    tient with history of, 72
Blood staining, corneal graft, 318
Blunted iris hook, 236
Blurring as sign of homograft reaction, 310, 311
Bonn forceps
  dog-toothed, 103
  in suturing of donor button to recipient cornea,
    153
Bowman's membrane, 328, 332
  crater-like dehiscences extending through, in
    donor eye, 70-71
Box-hinged hemostat, 102
Box-hinged microhemostat, 98-99, 102
Brain-heart infusion broth for culture of donor
    eye, 72-73
Bronson B-scan ultrasound tomography, 48, 50,
    246-249
B-scan ultrasound tomography
  for aphakic keratoplasty indications, 246-249
  Bronson, 48, 50, 246-249
  detection of vitreous opacity by, 22, 48, 249
  determination of lens power by, 22
  of intravitreous foreign body, 249
  of morning glory (total) retinal detachment, 249,
    260
  normal, 249
  in postoperative management of keratoplasty,
    323
  of resolving intravitreous hemorrhage, 249
  of tumor in posterior segment, 249
  of vitreous opacifications, 249
  waterbath, 48
Bullae, corneal, 44
Bullous keratopathy, 44
  aphakic, 248
Burn, corneal, 44, 50, 310
Button
  circular, in wedge-resected recipient opening as
    cause of astigmatism, 26-27
  corneal, 10-15
  donor; see Donor button
  excised; see Recipient opening
  oval, in circular recipient 16, 17
  pathologic, 220, 240, 242, 250

339

C

Calcium, deposits of, on cornea
  in band kerotopathy, 36
  chelation of, 36-37
Cam-guided corneal knife, 100, 104-105, 132-133,
      204-205, 206-207
Canal, Schlemm's, 294, 296, 298, 302-303, 305
Capsule, anterior lens, 233, 234
Capsulectomy, anterior, 232-233
Capsulotomy, anterior, 234
Carbonic anhydrase inhibitor, 323, 324
Cardona-Roskothen cutting frame assembly with
      groove backing block, 90-94
Castroviejo, Ramón, 1
Cataract, 20, 22, 289, 312, 318
  extraction of
    combined with keratoplasty, 142, 218-219
      technique of, 219-232
    extracapsular, 111, 142, 217, 218, 232-235
      and intraocular lens implant, 236
    intracapsular, 217, 224-229
      and intraocular lens implant, 236
    simple, with or without intraocular implant,
        217
  microsurgery of, comparison of, with microsur-
      gery of cornea, 3-4
  minimal, keratoplasty in presence of, 218
  secondary, 216
  surgery
    combined with keratoplasty, 216-244
      general considerations of, 216-217
    and corneal opacification, 44
    following successful keratoplasty, 218
Cataract incision with diamond knife, 109
Cataract section scissors, use of, in preparation of
      corneoscleral segment of donor eye, 76-
      77
Cell, endothelial, in diagnosis of donor tissue fail-
      ure, 314-315
Cellulose sponge, 110; see also Weck-cel sponge
  in aphakic keratoplasty, 250, 261
  in intracapsular cataract extraction, 226
  moistened, in cutting of recipient cornea, 204-
      205
  in removal of loose epithelium from donor but-
      ton, 78-79
  in trabeculotomy, 300
Cephaloridine, 201, 219, 250, 300, 323
Chelation of corneal calcium deposits, 36-37
Chemical burns of cornea, 44, 50, 310
Chipping of donor button, 92-93
Chloramphenicol, 201, 215, 322, 324, 333
Chord length, 268, 269, 270, 283
Ciliary body, 291
Ciliary process, 298
Cine camera unit, Beaulieu 16-mm, 112
Circular lamellar graft, 38-39
  suturing of, 40-41
Circular penetrating graft for peripheral corneal
      defects, 46
Circular total corneal lamellar graft, 38
Circumferential lamellar graft combined with
      penetrating graft, 38-40
Clarity, loss of, corneal surgery for, 34
Clinical keratometer, 26, 28-29
Clinical keratometry, 26, 28-30, 32
Closure
  graft-to-recipient, in combined cataract extrac-
      tion and keratoplasty, 240-242

Closure—cont'd
  suturing donor button to recipient opening in
      penetrating keratoplasty, 150-172
  watertight, of eye, 172, 214, 230, 241
Coaxial illumination, 300-301
  system of surgical microscope, 22, 112-114
Colibri-handled corneal forceps, 103
Colibri-handled suture forceps, Troutman, 230,
      326
Coloboma, 144-147, 222, 254-255, 260
Combined cataract extraction and keratoplasty,
      216-244
Complications, postoperative; see Postoperative
      complications
Composite graft, flanged, 48
Concavo-convex lens, 20
Conjunctival flap, 292-293, 300-301, 304-305
Conjunctival remnants of donor eye, 74-75
Conjunctival scissors; see Scissors, conjunctival
Conjunctivitis, 319
Contact lenses, 22, 35, 36; see also Intraocular
      implant
  therapeutic, 319, 333
Continuity, loss of, of cornea, surgery for, 34, 38
Continuous suture, 230, 284
  adjustment of, 170, 171, 174
  antitorque, 41, 52, 53
    final adjustment of, 186-187
    in lamellar flanged penetrating graft, 196,
        197
    in penetrating keratoplasty, 172
    placement of, in lamellar graft, 184-185, 186-
        187
    in refractive lamellar keratoplasty, 186
    in repairing edge elevation, 284
    in suturing donor mushroom to recipient eye,
        194-195
  combined with interrupted sutures, 52, 53,
      170
  double, use of, in simple penetrating kerato-
      plasty, 50, 51, 52, 172, 212
  elasticity of, 174-175
  fixating the graft with, after intracapsular cata-
      ract extraction, 230-231
  fixation of MICRA-Pierse titanium ring with,
      102, 124-125, 182, 201
  fixation of scleral ring with, 124-125
  fixation, removal of, 176
  in keratoconus, 50, 51
  nylon, 319
  placement of, 168-172
  radially placed, 50
    torquing of, 40
  removal of, 52, 328-331
  with secondary interrupted sutures, 170, 172
  for semicircular lamellar graft, 40-41
  in suturing lamellar graft, 40
  in suturing penetrating graft, 50, 212-214
  tensioning of, 170, 171
  torquing effect of, 40, 172
  for vascularized recipient cornea, 52, 53
Coreoplasty, 144-147, 260-261
Coreoplasty needle, Troutman, 146-147
Cornea, 18-20, 23, 291
  anatomic diameter of, 21, 23-24, 26
  aplanatic, curvature of, 20
  astigmatic, projection of surgical keratometer
      on, 30-31

340

Cornea—cont'd
  calcium deposits on, chelation of, 36-37
  central, full-thickness, and superficial periph-
      eral pathology, repair of, 38-40
  central pathologic zone of, repair of, 38-39
  cloudy, 314
  conical, surgery of, with contact lens corneal
      cutter, 106
  curvatures of; see Curvature, corneal
  cutting of donor button to flatten cornea, 95
  debridement of, for calcium deposits on, 36
  defects of, peripheral
      circular penetrating graft for, 46-47
      lamellar graft for, 46-47
  diameter of, 21, 23, 268, 269, 270
  distortion of, and surgical keratometer, 102
  donor; see Donor eye
  emmetropic anastigmatic schematic, 10, 11
  excessively flat recipient, 14
  First World Congress on, 2
  flat, projection of surgical keratometer on, 30-
      31
  flattening of donor cornea due to graft-recipient
      disparity, 44
  folding of, with epithelial edema and dehis-
      cences in donor eye, 68-69
  graft of; see Graft
  inferior peripheral thinning of, repair of, 38,
      39
  introduction and general considerations of, 1-6
  keratoconic, 95
  measurement of, 26, 28, 30, 32
  membrane equation of, 266-272
  microsurgery of, comparison of, with microsur-
      gery of cataract, 3-4
  optical diameter of, effect of, on corneal ametro-
      pia, 23-24, 26
  optics of, effect of, on corneal ametropia, 18-20
  pathology of, 36-42
  peripheral vascular invasion of, 52
  physical structure of, 266-272
  power of, 23
  recipient; see Recipient cornea
  refraction of; see Refraction
  relationship of, to other ocular structures, 21
  repeat surgery, suturing of, 50
  Second World Congress on, 2
  standard, anterior curvature of, 23
  steep, projection of surgical keratometer on, 30-
      31
  steeper, use of
      to induce myopia, 95
      to reduce hyperopia, 95
  surgery of, 34-55
      and active infection, 35
      and active inflammation, 35
      general considerations of, 34-35
      indications for, 34-55
      for loss of clarity, 34
      for loss of continuity of cornea, 34
      operative plan of, 34-55, 288
      for optical irregularities, 34
      practice of, 3
      vision and condition of fellow eye and, 35
  topography of, measurement of, 30
  total anterior opacification of, repair of, 38-39
  vascularized, 50
      sutures in, 52, 53
  World Congress of, 2

Corneal ametropia; see Ametropia
Corneal bullae, 44
Corneal burns, 44, 46, 50, 310
Corneal cutter, contact lens, 106, 107
Corneal decompensation, 288, 344
Corneal degenerations, 36
  calcium deposits in, 36
Corneal dome, 266-267, 268
  distortion of, as cause of astigmatism, 24
Corneal dystrophy, 44
Corneal edema, 44
Corneal forceps, MICRA-Pierse, 103
Corneal graft punch, Polack, 94
Corneal guttata, 217
Corneal irregularities, 36
Corneal knife
  Lieberman single-point, cam-guided, 100, 104-
      105, 132-133, 204-205, 206-207
  MUDO oscillating, 106-107
Corneal lamellar splitter, Troutman; see Trout-
      man corneal lamellar splitter
Corneal limbus, 23, 60
Corneal margin, wedge-resected recipient, 26-27
Corneal meridian; see Meridian
Corneal optical lathe, Barraquer, 110
Corneal punch, 84
Corneal ring, 18-20, 23, 26; see also Limbal ring
  anatomic position of, 21
  definition of, 18
  distortion of, 26
      as cause of astigmatism, 24
  effect of altering shape of, 268-273
Corneal ring graft, half segment lamellar periph-
      eral, 38-39
Corneal scissors
  in combined keratoplasty and cataract extrac-
      tion, 220-221
  to complete incision of cam-guided corneal
      knife, 105
  to complete trephine cut, 210
  curved, in cutting donor button, 80-81
  Troutman, 106
      in cutting of internal corneal lamella, 136-
      141
      in excision of corneal button, 80-81
Corneal splitting and dissecting spatula knives,
      109
  Troutman No. 1, 47, 48
Corneal stroma, donor eye, 70-71
Corneal support ring, in simple penetrating kera-
      toplasty, 201
Corneal thinning, peripheral, lamellar graft for,
      38
Corneal trephine; see Trephine
Corneal-induced ametropia
  astigmatic, mechanisms of, 16-17
  mechanisms of, in keratoconus, 8-9
Corneoscleral junction, 272
Corneoscleral segment of donor eye, 74-77, 82-84
Corticosteroid drops, 311, 324
Crock, Gerard, 106
Cryo headpiece, microlathe with, 110
Cryoextractor, 100, 226-227, 228, 229, 235
Cryolathe, Barraquer, 100
Cryoprobe, retinal, in cyclocryothermy, 308-309
Cryoprobe tip of silicone sleeve, 226-239
Cul-de-sac, 250
Culture of donor eye, 72-73
Cupping of nerve, 248

Curettage, 319
Curette, use of, to remove calcium deposits on
	cornea, 36
Curvature
	anterior, of standard cornea, 23
	of aplanatic cornea, 20
	corneal
		alteration in, 319
		flattening of, resulting in hyperopia, 12-13,
			16, 17
		lengthening of axial length, resulting in myo-
			pia, 14-15
		shortening of axial length, resulting in hyper-
			opia, 12-13
		steepening of,
			resulting in myopia, 14-15, 16, 17
			in wedge-resected meridian, 26, 27
		variation of, expressed in radii and dioptric
			powers, 19
	radius of, 82, 84
Cutting
	bias, 221
	of donor button; see Donor button, cutting of
	of internal corneal lamella, 134-141
	irregularities of, of donor button, 92-93, 202-
		203
	of recipient cornea with trephine, 128-131
	of recipient opening; see Recipient opening, cut-
		ting of
	sloping, 221
	of wedge in wedge resection, 278-281
Cutting frame, 84
Cutting set, basic donor, of instruments, 98, 100
Cutting-frame, Cardona-Roskothen, 90-94
	cutting irregularities with, 92-93
CU-1 needle, Alcon, 106
CU-2 needle, Alcon, 106
CU-3 needle, Alcon, 106
Cyanoacrylatebutyrate lens, 35
Cyclocryothermy, 288, 306, 308, 309, 318
	retinal probe for, 100
Cyclodiathermy, 288
Cyclopentolate, 222
Cystotome, 234

D

Deep-to-Descement's suture
	for closure of keratoplasty wound, 150-151
	in suturing donor button to recipient cornea,
		160-162
Defect, corneal, peripheral
	circular penetrating graft for, 46-47
	lamellar graft for, 46-47
Dehiscence
	epithelial, with normal corneal stroma and en-
		dothelium in donor eye, 70-71
	folding of cornea with, in donor eye, 68-69
	wound, 316-317, 333
Deltasone, 219
Depo-Medrol; see Methylprednisolone acetate
Deposits, calcium, on cornea, chelation of, 36-37
Descemetocele, 46-47
Descemet's membrane, 240, 280-282
	of hypotensive donor eye, folding of, 66-67
Detachment, retinal, morning glory (total), B-scan
		of, 249
Dexamethasone (0.1%) drops, 312
Diameter of cornea, 21, 23, 268, 269, 270

Diamond knife
		in aphakic keratoplasty, 252-253
	in combined keratoplasty and cataract extrac-
		tion, 220
	in completion of trephine cut, 210
		in combined lamellar and penetrating kerato-
			plasty, 188, 189
	in correction of preexisting astigmatism, 210
	in preparation of recipient eye, 188
	with protective cover, 98-99, 109
	in repair of sector edge elevation, 284-285
	in successive lamellar dissections, 182-184
	in trabeculectomy, 292, 293, 298
	in trabeculotomy, 302
	in Troutman wedge resection, 278, 280-281
Dioptric powers, variation of corneal curvature
		expressed in, 18, 19
Dish, Petri, 88, 89, 100, 202, 220
Disodium ethylenediaminetetraacetate dihydrate
		(EDTA), 36
Disruption-aspiration device, lens, 100
Dissections, successive, lamellar, technique for,
		182-183
Distortion
	of corneal ring, 26
		as cause of astigmatism, 24
	of corneal tissue by trephine, 92-93
		avoidance of, 94
	optical, 140
Dog-toothed forceps
	Bonn, 103
	for enucleation of donor eye, 58-59
Dome, corneal; see Corneal dome
Donor button, 10-15
	on backing block, 88-89
	bias cutting of, 92-93, 221
	chipping of, 92-93
	and contact lens corneal cutting, 106
	cutting of, 202-203
		from anterior surface, 52, 78-81
		in aphakic keratoplasty, 252
		Cardona-Roskothen used in, 90-94
		in combined keratoplasty and cataract extrac-
			tion, 220, 224, 225, 230, 235, 236
		from endothelial surface, 44, 80
		free hand, 84
		irregularities of, 82, 92, 93, 220, 221
			with Cardona-Roskothen cutting-frame as-
				sembly, 92-93
		for phakic recipient eye, 202
		from posterior surface, 82-94, 95, 202
	excision of, 80-81
		on backing block, 82-83, 84, 85
		to prevent undercutting, 80
		for simple penetrating keratoplasty, 202-203
	fixation of, with interrupted suture, 222-223
	full-thickness, 46
		advantages of, 80
	ideal cut of, 92-93
	identification of 12 o'clock meridian of, 80-81
	and intraocular implant, 240, 242
	in lamellar graft, 38, 46
	lipping of, 92-93
	loose epithelium, removal of, by cellulose
		sponge, 78-79
	narrowing anterior diameter of, 92-93
	oval, 92-93, 202, 203
		in correction of preexisting astigmatism, 210-
			211

Donor button—cont'd
  oval—cont'd
    in refractive surgery, 200
    round, in correction of preexisting astigmatism, 206-207, 208-209, 210-211
  size of, 95
    in aphakia, 95
    to flatten recipient cornea, 95
    in keratoconus, 46
      to induce myopia, 46
    in keratoplasty
      aphakic, 46, 252
      lamellar, 44, 46, 95
      penetrating, 44, 46
    selection of, 95
    to steepen cornea, 95
  sloping cut of, 80, 220, 221
  suturing of, 95, 150-179
    to recipient opening in anterior segment pathology, 256
  transferring of, to recipient eye, 148-149
  trephining, 80-81
Donor cards for eye bank, 57
Donor cornea; see Donor eye
Donor cutting set of instruments, 98, 100
  Troutman, 94
Donor eye, 56-95
  anterior surface of, cutting of donor button from, 78-79
  Bowman's membrane, appearance of, precluding use of 70, 71
  conjunctival remnants of, 74-75
  containers for, 62-63
  corneal stroma of, 70-71
  corneoscleral segment of, preparation of, 74-77
  crater-like dehiscences extending through Bowman's membrane in, 70-71
  culture of, 72-73
    infusion broth for, 72-73
  diagnoses which preclude use of, 72
  endothelial surface of, precluding use of, 68, 69
  enucleation of, 57, 58-61
    instruments for, 58-59
  epithelial dehiscences with normal corneal stroma and endothelium in, 70-71
  epithelial edema of, 68, 69
  examination of
    external, 66
    by specular microscope, 70-71
  folding of cornea with epithelial edema and dehiscences in, 68-69
  folding of endothelium and Descemet's membrane in, 66-67
  K readings of, 80-81
  normal configuration and thickness of ideal cornea of, 66-67
  optic nerve of, cutting of, 60, 61
  orienting of, 60, 61
  and penicillin, 72
  peripheral lamellar dissection of, 188, 189
  peritomy of, 60-61
  posterior surface of
    cutting donor button from, 82-94
    folds in, precluding use of, 68, 69
  preparation of, 72-73
    for tissue-culture medium preservation, 74-77

Donor eye—cont'd
  rejection of, from patient with history of various diagnoses, 72
  removal of, from eye-bank container, 78-79
  scleral incision in, 76-77
  selection of, 64-71
  slit-lamp examination of, 64-71
  specular microscopy of, 64-71
  storage of, 62-63
  and streptomycin, 72
  suitable for keratoplasty, 70-71
  tissue-culture medium preservation of, preparation for, 74-77
  trephining of, 80-81
  ultraviolet light, use of, in preparation of, 74
  unsuitable, for keratoplasty, 68-69, 70-71
Donor mushroom
  preparation of, 188-191
  suturing of, to recipient eye, 192-195
Donor preparation cut from posterior surface, 202
Donor tissue, failure of, 307, 314, 315
  surgical management of, 314-315
Double continuous suture, use of; see also Continuous suture
  in keratoconus, 50, 52
  in simple penetrating keratoplasty, 50, 51, 172, 212
Doughnut-shaped lamellar graft, 38-39
  suturing of, 40-41
Douvas rotoextractor, 100, 109, 110, 111, 258-259, 318
Draeger motor-driven trephine, 100
Drape, 3M aperture, 98, 100
Draping, 116
Dressing
  firm pressure, 286
  monocular modified pressure, 186
  surgical, and fluorescein leak test, 232
  unilateral, 178-179, 214, 232, 300
Drug therapy, 313; see also individual drugs
Dyscrasia, blood, rejection of donor eye from patient with history of, 72
Dystrophy
  corneal, 44
  endothelial, 217
  endothelial-epithelial, 216, 289
  familial or acquired, excessively flat recipient cornea in, 14
    refraction in, 35
  marginal, repair of, 38-39

E
Early graft reaction, 313-314; see also Homograft reaction
Edema
  corneal, 44
    central, 216
  epithelial, 323, 324
    folding of cornea with, in donor eye, 68-69
EDTA; see Disodium ethylenediaminetetraacetate dihydrate
Elastic monofilament nylon suture; see Suture, nylon, elastic monofilament
Elastic theory of plates and shells, 266
Emmetropia, 206
  induction of, by graft in keratoconic cornea, 9
  spherical equivalent, 14, 206

Emmetropic anastigmatic schematic cornea, 10, 11
Endothelial cells in diagnosis of donor tissue failure, 314-315
Endothelial-epithelial dystrophy, 289, 325
Endothelium, 228, 311
  of donor eye unsuitable for keratoplasty, 70-71
  of hypotensive donor eye, folding of, 66-67
  normal, in donor eye, 70-71, 315
Enucleation of donor eye, 57, 58-61
Enucleation scissors, 58-59, 60-61
Envelope, scleral, 20
Epinephrine, 222
Epithelial dehiscences with normal corneal stroma and endothelium in donor eye, 70-71
Epithelial edema, folding of cornea with, in donor eye, 68-69
Epithelialization, 319
Epithelium, 330, 332
  loose, of donor eye, removal of, by cellulose sponge, 78-79
Erythromycin, 215
Escherichia coli, 201
Ethicon, 106
Ethicon needle
  GS-3, 98, 100, 102
  GS-9; *see* GS-9 Ethicon needle
  GS-14; *see* GS-14 Ethicon needle
  GS-15, 152-153
  GS-16, 106
  GS-17, 106
Ethylenediaminetetraacetate dihydrate, disodium, 36
Excised button; *see* Recipient opening
Expander, Girard scleral, 98-99, 101, 120, 250-251
Exposure and fixation
  in aphakic keratoplasty, 250-251
  in simple penetrating keratoplasty, 201
  using Troutman surgical keratometer, 219
Expression of lens nucleus, 235
Expulsive hemorrhage, 252
Extracapsular cataract extraction, 111, 142, 217, 218, 232-235, 236
  technique of intraocular implant after, 242-243
Extraction of cataract; *see* Cataract, extraction of
Eye
  anatomy of, and optical function, 18-20, 21
  donor; *see* Donor eye
  fellow, vision and condition of, in corneal surgery, 35
  perforated, use of trephine and scissors in, for penetrating keratoplasty, 46
  phakic, pars plana approach in removal of vitreous opacity in, 22
  soft, and penetrating keratoplasty, 46
Eye Bank for Sight Restoration, Incorporated, 56, 57-95, 318
Eye Bank Association of America, 56-57
Eye-bank, 56, 57
  containers, 62-63
    removal of intact globe from, 78-79
  operation, 57

F

Familial dystrophy
  corneal opacity, diffuse in, 44
  recipient cornea excessively flat in, 14

Familial dystrophy—cont'd
  flat cornea in, 35
Febrile viral infections, 333
Fiberoptic bundle of surgical keratometer, 28, 29
Filtering procedure, 288, 290
First World Congress on the Cornea, 2
Fixation and exposure; *see* Exposure and fixation
Fixation forceps, Troutman rectus, 98, 100, 101
Fixation rings
  Le Grand, 120, 121
  MICRA-Pierse titanium; *see* MICRA-Pierse titanium rings
  placement of, 120-127
  scleral, removal of, 176
  use of, 120, 121
Fixation sutures, inferior and superior rectus, 275
Flanged composite graft, 48, 188, 196-197
Flat cornea
  cutting of donor button to avoid, 95
  projection of surgical keratometer on, 30-32
Flattened cornea
  resulting in hyperopia, 12-13, 16-17
  resulting from wedge resected recipient, 26
Flieringa rings, 98-99, 100, 102, 103, 120, 121, 214
  in aphakic keratoplasty, 120, 250
  in combined keratoplasty and cataract extraction, 219
  in cutting of recipient opening, 204-205
  wire-circle, 120, 122-124
Fluorescein dye test, 174, 176, 194, 232, 256, 324
  in checking suture adjustment, 214
  in trabeculectomy, 300
Folding
  of cornea with epithelial edema and dehiscences in donor eye, 68-69
  of endothelium and Descemet's membrane in hypotensive donor eye, 66-67
Foot control of surgical microscope, 114-115
Forceps
  Bonn; *see* Bonn forceps
  colibri-handled, suture-removing, 230
  corneal, MICRA-Pierse, 103, 315
  dog-toothed, for enucleation of donor eye, 58-59
  fixation, rectus, 118
    Troutman, 98, 99, 100, 101
  MICRA-Pierse; *see* MICRA-Pierse forceps
  ring fixation, 103
  tissue
    MICRA-Pierse; *see* MICRA-Pierse titanium tissue forceps
    in placing continuous suture, 168, 169, 170, 171
  titanium; *see* MICRA-Pierse titanium tissue forceps
  toothed, in preparation of corneoscleral segment of donor eye, 76
  Troutman colibri-handled suture, 326
  Troutman rectus fixation, 98, 100, 101
  Troutman suture handling, pointed, with Barraquer-de Wecker handle, 98, 109
  Troutman suture removal, pointed, 328
  tying
    in adjustment of continuous suture, 170-171
    Harms; *see* Harms tying forceps
    in intracapsular cataract extraction, 226-227, 230

Forceps—cont'd
  tying—cont'd
    in removal of interrupted fixation suture, 170
    in suturing donor button to recipient cornea, 162
    Troutman, 98-99, 109
Foreign body, intravitreous, B-scan of, 249
Fornix of lens capsule, 234, 235, 242
Four-concavity block, 84
Four-loop intraocular lens, Binkhorst, 240-241, 242-243
Fox-type metal shield, 322
Frame for suction cutting, 132-133
Frame-to-piston assembly, Troutman; on disposable block, 86-87
Full-thickness donor button, 46, 80
Fundus contact lens, 22
Fungous infection, 319

G

Gambs keratometer, 26, 28
Garamycin; see Gentamicin
Gentamicin, 201, 250
Girard lens disruption-aspiration device, 100
Girard scleral expander, 101, 120, 250-251
Glaucoma, 216, 248, 250, 252, 318, 324
  aphakic, 250, 288
  indications for surgery for, 288-289
  phakic, 288
  as postoperative complication, surgical management of, 307-309
  steroid medication in, 287
  surgery for, and keratoplasty, 287-306
    general considerations for, 287
Graft
  autograft, 50, 273
  clouding of, 288
  corneal, optical considerations and cutting techniques of, to control and minimize ametropia, 7-33
  disparate-sized, and recipient opening, 22, 44, 46
    optical effects of, 10-15, 16, 17
  edge elevation, 275
  failure of
    and elastic monofilament nylon suture, 4
    major cause of, 4
  fixation of, with continuous suture, 230-231
  flanged composite, 48, 188, 196-197
  induction of emmetropia by, in keratoconus, 9
  lamellar; see Lamellar graft
  methods of eliminating astigmatism from 52
  mushroom, 40; see also Donor mushroom
  oval, 26
    in round recipient opening, 16, 17, 210, 211
  penetrating; see Penetrating graft
  reaction, 44, 333, 334
  recipient cornea, suturing of penetrating, and 150, 171
  and reconstructive surgery, 38
  rejection of, 333
  repeat, 50
    and tectonic surgery, 38
  rotation of, in recipient bed, 40
  size of
    in keratoconus, 8-9
    in vascularized cornea, 48, 49, 50

Graft—cont'd
  successful postoperative management of, 321-334
    general considerations of, 321
  suturing of, 212-214
    to vascularize recipient cornea, 52-53
Graft punch, corneal, Polack, 94
Graft-recipient disparity, 22, 44, 46
  effects of, 16, 17
Graft-to-recipient closure in keratoplasty combined with intraocular lens implant
  after extracapsular extraction, 242, 243
  after intracapsular extraction, 240, 241
Grieshaber contact lens corneal knife, 106
Grieshaber MUDO oscillating knife, 106
Grieshaber rotoextractor, 100
GS-3 Ethicon needle, 98, 100, 102
GS-9 Ethicon needle, 98-99, 102, 106, 118, 124
  in combined keratoplasty and cataract extraction, 219
  in preparation of donor mushroom, 190-191
  in simple penetrating keratoplasty, 201
GS-10 Ethicon needle, 106
GS-14 Ethicon needle, 98-99, 106
  and Binkhorst four-loop intraocular lens, 240
  fixation of intracapsular cataract extraction graft with, 230
  for iris suturing, 146-147
  in placement of antitorque continuous suture, 186-187
  position of, in titanium needleholder, 166-167
  in suturing donor mushroom to recipient eye, 192-193
GS-15 Ethicon needle, 152--153
GS-16 Ethicon needle, 106
GS-17 Ethicon needle, 106
GS-19 Ethicon needle, 230

H

Haag-Streit keratometer, 26
Haptic of intraocular lens implant, 234, 236
Hard contact lenses, 35, 36
Harms, Heinrich, 1, 2
Harms tying forceps, 98-99, 109, 146
  in adjustment of continuous suture, 170, 171
  in iris suturing, 146
Hazy vision as sign of homograft reaction, 310, 311
Hematoma, 102, 118, 124
Hemorrhage
  expulsive, 252
  resolving intravitreous, B-scan of, 249
  subchoroidal, 252
  surgical management of, 318
Hemostat, box-hinged, 99, 102
Hepatitis, infectious, rejection of donor eye from patient with history of, 72
Herpetic keratitis, 48, 319
High-water content contact lenses, 35
Homograft, 50, 314, 315
  reaction of, 307, 310-313, 334
  repeat, 50
Hook, muscle, for enucleation of donor eye, 58-59, 60-61
Hyaloid face, 254
Hydrocortisone, 310, 311, 322, 333
Hypermetropia, aphakic, 14

Hyperopia, 14, 44, 286
  and aphakic keratoplasty, 46
  caused by flattening of corneal curvature, 12-13,
      16-17
  caused by shortening of axial length, 12-13
  circular button in wedge-resected recipient
      opening as cause of, 26-27
  compensated by graft-recipient disparity, 46
  and keratomileusis, 110
  spherical equivalent, 26
  steepening of cornea to reduce, 95
Hyperopic aphakia, 22
Hyperopic meridian, 17
Hypertension, transient ocular, 287-288
Hypertonia, 308
Hypotension, 288
Hypotensive donor eye, folding of endothelium
    and Descemet's membrane in, 66-67

I

Iatrogenic astigmatism, cause of, 24
Iatrogenic corneal edema, 44
Iatrogenic vitreous loss, 120
IBSM microscope, Weck, 112, 113
Idoxuridine, 319
Illumination system, coaxial, of surgical micro-
    scope, 112-114
Immunosuppressive agents, 250, 312
Implant, intraocular; see Intraocular implant
Incandescent light sources in surgical keratome-
    ter, 28-29
Incision
  scleral, in donor eye, 76-77
  Troutman relaxing, 286
Infection
  active, and corneal surgery, 35
  bacterial, 201
  fungous, 319
  large virus, rejection of donor eye from patient
      with history of, 72
  localized, rejection of donor eye from patient
      with history of, 72
  surgical management of, 307, 318-319
Infectious hepatitis, rejection of donor eye from
    patient with history of, 72
Inflammation, 201
  active and corneal surgery, 35
Influenza immunization, 333
Influenza vaccine, 310
Infusion broth, brain-heart, for culture of donor
    eye, 72-73
Infusion-aspiration unit, 233, 235
Instruments in microsurgical keratoplasty, 96-
    115; see also specific instruments
  basic donor cutting set of, 98, 100
  description of uses of, 100-109
  for enucleation of donor eye, 58-59
  for lamellar or penetrating keratoplasty, 96-
      100
  special or optional, 100, 109-111
  sterilization of, 97
  suction cutting frames for preparation of donor
      button, 132-133
  vitreous, sucking cutting; see Vitreous sucking-
      cutting instruments
Integral beam splitter microscope; see Weck IBSM
    microscope
International Eye Foundation, 57

International Ophthalmological Congress, 2
Interrupted fixation suture, placement of, in la-
    mellar graft, 184-185
Interrupted suture
  in closing graft, 213
  in closing incision of wedge resection, 282
  closing intracapsular cataract extraction inci-
      sion with, 230-231
  in closing wedge-resected sector, 213, 214
  in combined cataract surgery and keratoplasty,
      230, 231
  to fix wire Flieringa ring, 102, 122, 123
  fixation
    left in place, 170
    removal of, 176
  fixation of donor button with
    in intraocular lens implant, 242
    in midperipheral iridectomy and radial
        sphincterotomy, 222-223
  in lamellar flanged penetrating graft, 196, 197
  overlying, for square lamellar graft, 42-43
  placement of temporary, to fix donor button
      in keratoplasty, 150-163
  removal of, 52
  in repair of edge elevation, 284
  secondary, use of, 50, 170, 174
    removal of, 174
  for semicircular lamellar graft, 40-42
  in suturing of donor button to recipient cornea,
      162-163
  in suturing donor mushroom to recipient eye,
      194
  temporary
    placement of, 150-153
    removal of, 170-171, 176
      after placement of continuous suture, 230
  temporary fixation, 212, 214
  in trabeculectomy, 300, 301
  in trabeculotomy, 304, 305
  use of, to prevent torquing effect, 40
  for vascularized recipient cornea, 52-53
    time interval of removal of, 52
Intracapsular cataract extraction, 217, 224-225,
    236
Intracapsular surgery, 219
Intracorneal suture, 42
Intraocular contact lens, implantation of; see In-
    traocular lens implant
Intraocular lens implant, 106, 217, 218-219, 236,
    243
  Binkhorst four-loop, 108, 236, 240-241, 242
  Binkhorst two-loop, 242-243
  after extracapsular extraction, technique of,
      242-243
  intracapsular, technique of, 236-239
  power of, 22
  simple cataract extraction with or without, 217
  Worst, 108, 236-239
Intraocular pressure, 132, 266, 267, 287, 308, 318,
    323, 324
Intrascleral fixation suture, 118
Intrascleral interrupted suture to fix fixation ring,
    102
Intrascleral needle passage, 125
Intrascleral retraction suture, position of, 118,
    119
Intravitreous foreign body, B-scan of, 249
Intravitreous hemorrhage, resolving, B-scan of,
    249

Iridectomy, 217, 298, 299
  marginal, 108, 259
  midperipheral, 142-143, 190-198, 210, 222, 240,
      242, 304
  peripheral, 108, 142, 299
  sector, 108, 142
  superior, 144
Iridosphincterotomy, 144-147
Iridotomy, 108, 142, 217, 298
Iris, 20, 291
  atrophy of sphincter, 142
  attachment of, to corneal endothelial surface,
      252, 254
  diaphragm, 48, 144, 217, 230, 244
  disinsertion of, 146
  incarcerated, 172, 173
  necrosis of, 142
  needle catching, in suturing of donor button to
      recipient cornea, 158-161
  prolapse of, 317
  staphyloma involving, 49
  surgery for, 244
  suture of, 144-147, 254
    technique of, 146-147
  vision-obstructing, pathology of, 22-23
Iris coloboma, 144-147
Iris scissors
  Barraquer-de Wecker, 108
  MICRA-Pierse, 98-99
Iris suture, 222, 254-255, 260-261
Iris-vitreous spatula, 98-99, 108-109
  in trabeculectomy, 298-299
Irrigation needle, Troutman olive-tipped; see
      Troutman olive-tipped irrigation needle
Irrigation-aspiration needle, 31-gauge, angled, 98-
      99
Irrigator, Troutman olive-tipped, 98-99, 235

J

Jacob-Creutzfeldt syndrome, rejection of donor eye
      from patient with history of, 72
Javal principle of Haag-Streit keratometer, 26

K

K reading; see also Keratometer
  clinical, during postoperative management of
      successful keratoplasty, 323, 324, 333
  of donor eye, 80
  qualitative and quantitative, 275
  in repair of sector elevation, 284
Kaufman vitrector, 258-261
Kelman lens disruption-aspiration device, 100
Keratitis, 319
  herpetic, 48, 310
Keratoconjunctivitis, 319
Keratoconus
  central discrete corneal opacities in, 44
  double continuous suture pattern for, 50-52
  grafts in, size of, 8-9
  induction of emmetropia by graft in, 9
  induction of myopia by graft in, 9
  keratoplasty for, 46, 142
  mechanisms of corneal-induced ametropia in, 8-
      9
  penetrating keratoplasty for, myopia following,
      14
  posterior, 20

Keratoconus—cont'd
  refraction of cornea in, 8, 35
  size of donor button in, 46, 95
Keratocytic proliferation of cells, 321
Keratome, 106, 110
Keratometer, 7; see also Keratometry
  clinical, 26, 28, 219, 275, 323, 324
  Gambs, 26, 28
  Haag-Streit, 26
  surgical, 219, 230, 272, 316, 319
  Troutman surgical, 7, 10, 28-32, 40, 100, 102-
      103, 122, 125, 128, 172, 174, 176, 265,
      275
    in checking accuracy of graft, 212-214
    in correction of meridional ametropia, 32
    exposure and fixation of globe using, 219
    fiberoptic bundle of, 29-30
    in final adjustment of antitorque continuous
        suture, 186-187
    final suture adjustment using, 214, 230, 256-
        257
    incandescent light sources in, 28-29
    in management of anterior segment pathol-
        ogy, 256-257
    projection of, on cornea, 30-32
    in refractive lamellar keratoplasty, 186
    reticle of, 29-30
    in selection of sector in wedge resection, 275-
        277
    split-image prism, device of, 30
    suturing donor mushroom to recipient, use of
        in, 194-195
    in trabeculectomy, 300
    in Troutman wedge resection, 282-284
  Zeiss, 28
Keratometer reading; see K reading
Keratometry; see also Keratometer
  clinical, 28, 32, 35
  and refraction, 35
  surgical, 28-32
Keratometry reading; see K reading
Keratomileusis, 20, 110, 132, 180, 198, 264
Keratopathy
  aphakic bullous, 248
  band, calcium deposits in, 36
  bullous, 44
  striate, hypotensive donor eye resembling, 66
Keratophakia, 20, 110, 132, 180, 198, 264
Keratoplasty
  aphakic, 14, 46, 95, 245-262
    general considerations for, 245
    and hyperopia, 46
    size of donor button in, 44, 46
  astigmatic band following, 44
  cataract surgery combined with, 14, 20, 22, 142,
      216-244
    general considerations of, 216-217
  combined with cataract extraction, 142, 218-
      219
    technique of, 219-232
  common techniques of, 116-178
    general considerations of, 116
  and coreoplasty, 144
  deep-to-Descemet's suture in closure of, 150
  donor eye suitable for, 70-71
  donor eye unsuitable for, 68-69, 70-71
  and glaucoma surgery, 287-306
    general considerations for, 287
  instruments for, description of uses of, 100-109

Keratoplasty—cont'd
  lamellar; *see* Lamellar keratoplasty
  microsurgical
    astigmatic band following, 7
    axial ametropia following, 7
    optical considerations of, 7-33
    optical results of, relationship of cornea and
      ocular structures to, 20, 21
  penetrating; *see* Penetrating keratoplasty
  phakic, 102
  in presence of minimal cataract, 218
  refractive, lamellar, 186
  successful
    cataract surgery following, 218
    irregular or high astigmatism following, 20
    late postoperative period of, 333
    postoperative management of, 321-334
      general considerations of, 321
      from hospital discharge through sixth week,
        323-324
      immediate, 322-323
      sixth week through sixth month, 324-333
      suture removal in postoperative manage-
        ment of, 325-331
  through-and-through suture for closure of, 150-
    151
  and trabeculectomy, 290-301
  and trabeculotomy, 302, 305
  and wedge resection, suturing of, 151
Keratoplasty scissors, Troutman, 98-99, 106, 252
Keratoprosthesis, 50, 198
Keratoscope, 30
King, John Harry, Jr., 57
Kloti reciprocating vitreous sucking-cutting in-
    strument, 100, 110
Knife
  corneal, 100, 104-105, 132-133, 204-205, 206-
    207
    Lieberman single-point, cam-guided, 100,
      104-105
  corneal splitting
    and dissecting spatula, 109
    in preparation of recipient eye, 188
  diamond; *see* Diamond knife
  MUDO oscillating, 106, 107
  razor; *see* Razor knife
Knots
  in suture removal, 328-329
  uncovered, and vascularization, 48

L

Lamella
  internal, corneal, technique of cutting of, 134-
    141
  peripheral, purse string of, 190-191
Lamellar autograft, symmetrical, wedge resection
    used as, 273
Lamellar dissection
  peripheral, of donor eye, 189
  successive, technique for, 182-183
Lamellar donor button, 46
Lamellar excision
  depth of, 181
  shape of, 181
  size of, 181
  slit-lamp illumination for, 182
Lamellar flange, 190-191

Lamellar flanged penetrating keratoplasty, 196-
  198
Lamellar graft, 38; *see also* Lamellar kerato-
    plasty
  circular, 38-39, 184
    suturing of, 40-41
    total corneal, 38
  and contact lens corneal cutter, 106
  in descemetocele, 46
  donor button in, 38
  doughnut-shaped, 38-39
    suturing of, 40-41
  flanged, and penetrating keratoplasty, 196-198
  and interrupted fixation sutures, 184
  and penetrating graft, 38-40
    circumferential, 38-40
    sector, 38-40
  segmental, 42, 43
  semicircular, 38, 39
  size of, 184
  square, 38-39
    suturing of, 42-43
  suturing of, 40-43, 184-187
  triangular, 38-39
    suturing of, 42-43
Lamellar keratoplasty; *see also* Lamellar graft
  combined with penetrating keratoplasty, 188-
    195
    preparation of donor mushroom, 188, 189
    preparation of recipient, 188, 189
    suturing mushroom to recipient, 192-195
  general considerations of, 180
  instruments for, 96-100
  in keratomileusis, 198
  in keratophakia, 198
  and keratoprosthesis, 198
  refractive, 186
  size of donor button in, 44, 46, 95
  successive dissections in, 182, 183
  surgical plan, factors in, 180
  technique of, 180-199
  trephine, use of, in, 182, 183
Lamellar microkeratome, Barraquer, 100, 110,
  132
Lamellar peripheral corneal ring graft, half seg-
    ment, 38-39
Lamellar recipient bed, preparation of, 180-181
Lamellar scleral flap, 292, 293
Lamellar splitter, Troutman corneal; *see* Trout-
    man corneal lamellar splitter
Laminar flow hood, 74
Late graft reaction 313, 333
Lathe, Barraquer corneal optical, 110
LeGrand ring, 120, 121, 250
Lens, 20, 222
  astigmatic, pathologically, 22
  cataractous, 22
  concavo-convex, 20
  contact, 35, 36
  cortex, 233
  cyanoacrylate butyrate, 35
  high water content, 35
  intraocular implant; *see* Intraocular lens im-
    plant
  nucleus of, expression of, 235
  opacities of; *see* Opacification
  oxygen permeable, 35
  polymer, 35

Lens—cont'd
  power of, determination of, by A- and B-scan
      ultrasound tomography, 22
  silicone, 35
  subluxated, 22
  Troutman neutral buoyancy, 240
Lens disruption-aspiration device, 100
Leukemia, rejection of donor eye from patient
      with history of, 72
Leukoma, 48-49
Levator aponeurosis, tearing of, 102
Levator muscle, 102, 118
Lid speculum
  Barraquer light-wire; see Barraquer light-wire
      lid speculum
  caution in use of, 102
  meridional error induced in soft eye by, 177
  placing of, for keratoplasty, 117
  removal of, 178, 179
  solid-bladed, for enucleation of donor eye, 58-
      59
Lieberman single-point cam-guided corneal knife,
      100, 104-105, 132-133
  in correction of preexisting astigmatism, 206-
      207
  in cutting of recipient opening, 204-205
Light, incandescent, in surgical keratometer, 28-
      29
Limbal diameter, 84
Limbal ring, 266-267, 268, 269, 270, 272
Limbal zone, 44
Limbus, 252, 266-267, 292
  surgical, donor eye, 61
Lipping of donor button, 92-93

M

Machemer rotoextractor, 100, 109
Mackensen, Gunter, 1, 2
Mackensen trabeculotomy probe, 294-295, 302,
      303, 304, 305
Malbran, E., 181
Mannitol, 219, 220, 250
Manual depression, eye softened by, 219
Marginal dystrophy, repair of, 38-39
Mattress suture
  in lamellar flanged penetrating keratoplasty,
      196, 197
  for semicircular lamellar graft, 40-41
  for triangular lamellar graft, 42-43
McLean, John, 1
Measurement of cornea, 26, 28, 30, 32
Medallion lens, Worst, 108, 236-239
Melbourne University Department of Ophthalmo-
      logy, 106
Membrane
  Bowman's, 70-71
  Descemet's, 66-67
Membrane equation of cornea, 266-272
Meperidine, 322
Meridian, 268-269
  corneal, 88, 268, 269, 270, 271
    dimensions of, before and after wedge resec-
        tion, 270, 271
    flattened, 12, 13, 16, 17, 18, 26, 27, 268, 269,
        270, 271
    horizontal, 270
    of resection, surgical keratometer projection of,
        275, 276, 277

Meridian—cont'd
  steepened, 14, 15, 16, 17, 18, 26, 27, 270, 271
  12 o'clock
    marking of, of donor eye, 60-61
      identification of, 80-81
  wedge-resected, steepening of curvature in, 26,
      27
Meridian groove markings on backing block, 88-
      89
Meridional ametropia, surgical keratometer in
      correction of, 32
Meridional distortion, compensation of, 174, 175
Meridional error, 266
  compensation of, 206
  correction of, 105
  in donor cornea, 202
  in soft eye, induction of, by lid speculum, 177
Methylmethacrylate contact lenses, 35
Methylmethacrylate intraocular lens implant,
      236
Methylprednisolone acetate, 311
Methylprednisolone sodium succinate, 311
MICRA-Pierse forceps
  in completion of trephine cut, 210
  corneal, 103
  countertraction with, 141
  curved tip, 103, 315
  in cutting of recipient opening, 204-205
  in midperipheral iridectomy and radial sphinc-
      terotomy, 222
  open-cupped, 126, 140, 142, 152
    in combined keratoplasty and cataract extrac-
        tion, 220
  plain, 98-99, 109
  titanium cup-tipped, 103
  in trabeculectomy, 298
MICRA-Pierse iris and suture scissors, 98-99
MICRA-Pierse needleholder, 98-99, 103, 146-147,
      164-167
MICRA-Pierse razor knife, 98-99, 103; see also
      Razor knife
MICRA-Pierse suture scissors, 98-99
MICRA-Pierse tissue forceps, 98-99, 103
  in placement of antitorque continuous suture,
      186-187
  in suturing of donor mushroom to recipient eye,
      192-193
MICRA-Pierse titanium rings, 98-99, 100, 102,
      103, 104, 120, 121, 124-126
  in combined keratoplasty and cataract extrac-
      tion, 219
  in cutting of recipient opening, 204-205
  in phakic keratoplasty, 120
  in simple penetrating keratoplasty, 201
  in successive lamellar dissections, 182
MICRA-Pierse titanium tissue forceps, 98-99
  open-cupped, 126, 127, 220
    in cutting of internal corneal lamella, 140-
        141
    in iris suturing, 146-147
    in suturing donor button to recipient cornea,
        152-153
Microhemostat, box-hinged, 98-99, 102
Microkeratome, Barraquer lamellar, 100, 109
Microlathe with cryo headpiece, 110
Microscope
  Barraquer surgical, 28
  binocular zoom, for assistant, 112, 113

Microscope—cont'd
  examination of donor eye by, 70-71
  specular; *see* Microscopy, specular
  surgical, 100, 105
  Troutman surgical; 112-115
    cine camera unit, 112
    coaxial illumination system of, 112-114
    fiberoptic light source, 112, 113
    foot control of, 114-115
    magnification, range of, 114
    rheostat speed control of, 112, 113
    with surgical keratometer, 100, 112, 113, 114
    tilt control of, 114
    translation mechanism of, 112
  Weck IBSM, 112
  zoom magnification, 1
Microscopy, specular, 218, 318-324,
  in assessment of successful keratoplasty, 333-334
  in diagnosis of donor tissue failure, 314-315
  of donor eye, 70-71
    of endothelium of donor eye unsuitable for keratoplasty, 70-71
  endothelial, 323
  in homograft reaction, 311
Microsurgery; *see also* Surgery
  of the Anterior Segment of the Eye, Volume I, 1
  of cataract, comparison of, with microsurgery of cornea, 3-4
Microsurgery Study Group, 2
Miosis of pupil, 242
Miotic agent, 216
M-K tissue-culture fluid, 77, 88-89, 202, 252
Monocular modified pressure dressing, 186
Monofilament nylon suture, elastic; *see* Suture, nylon, elastic monofilament
Morning glory (total) retinal detachment, B-scan of, 249
Morphine, 322
MUDO, 106
MUDO corneal trephine, 106, 107
MUDO oscillating knife and corneal trephine, 106, 107
Muscle, oblique, location and cutting of, 60-61
Muscle hook for enucleation of donor eye, 58-59
Mushroom, donor; *see* Donor mushroom
Mushroom graft, 40; *see also* Donor mushroom
Mydriatic, 311, 322
Myopia, 20, 286
  axial, 8, 14, 35, 46
  caused by steepening of corneal curvatures, 14-15, 16
  corneal, following penetrating keratoplasty for keratoconus, 14
  high, and posterir segment ametropia, 22
  induced by graft in keratoconic cornea, 9
  induced by keratomileusis, 110
  posterior keratoconus, 20
  residual, 22
  size of donor button in, 46, 252
  spherical equivalent, 8, 52
  steeper cornea, use of, to induce, 95
Myopic astigmatism, 26
Myopic meridian, 17

N

Needle
  Alcon, 106

Needle—cont'd
  angled, 30-gauge, 172, 256
  BV-5, 146
  coreoplasty, 146, 147
  GS-3 Ethicon, 98, 100, 102
  GS-9 Ethicon; *see* GS-9 Ethicon needle
  GS-10 Ethicon, 106
  GS-14 Ethicon; *see* GS-14 Ethicon needle
  GS-15, 152-153
  GS-16, 106
  GS-17, 106
  intrascleral, 125
  irrigation-aspiration, 98-99
  reverse cutting, 118
  spatula, 102
  in suturing of donor button to recipient cornea, 152-163
  Troutman olive-tipped irrigation, 172-173, 224-225
Needleholder
  MICRA-Pierse, 98-99, 103
    titanium, 164-167
      in iris suturing, 146-147
  microsurgical, 102
  Troutman, 98-99, 103, 164
Nodal point, 217
Nucleus of lens, expression of, 235
Nylon suture; *see* Suture, nylon

O

Oblique muscle, location and cutting of, 60
Ocular hypertension, transient, 287-288
Ocular hypotonia, 287
Ocular structures, 18-20
  of secondary optical importance, 20-23
  having secondary influence on optical results of keratoplasty, relationship of, to cornea, 20, 21
Olive-tipped irrigation needle, Troutman, 172-173, 224-225
Olive-tipped irrigator, Troutman, 98-99, 235
Olive-tipped needle, Troutman, 172-173
One-eyed patient; *see* Patient, one-eyed
Opacification
  calcium, removal of, 36-37
  central discrete, 44
  corneal, 20, 42, 44
    paracentral, 217
    total
      anterior, lamellar graft for, 38
      penetrating graft for, 50
  of lens, 20, 22; *see also* Cataract
    removal of, by vitrous sucking-cutting instruments, 22
  in staphyloma, 48
  total anterior corneal, repair of, 38-39
  vitreous, 48
    detection of, by B-scan ultrasound tomography, 22, 249
    pars plana approach in removal of, 22
Opening, recipient; *see* Recipient opening
Operative plan, cornea, surgery of, 34-55
Operculum, 222, 223, 224
Optic nerve, 287
  cupping of, 50
Optical aberrations, cause of, in healed graft, 82
Optical ametropia, 16
Optical axis and penetrating graft, 44, 45, 128

Optical considerations of microsurgical kerato-
    plasty, 7-33
Optical diameter of cornea, 21, 23-24, 26
Optical effects of disparate-sized graft and reci-
    pient opening, 10-15, 16, 17
Optical irregularities, corneal surgery for, 34
Optical lathe, Barraquer corneal, 110
Optical zone of cornea, 20, 44
Optics, corneal, effect of, on corneal ametropia, 18-
    20
Oscillating knife, MUDO, 106, 107
Oval cut, of donor button, 92-93, 202, 203
Ovaling of recipient opening by wedge resection,
    268
Overgrowth, stromal, slit-lamp view of, 332
Overlying interrupted suture, 42-43
Overrefraction, 35
Oxygen-permeable lens, 35

P

Pachymeter
    in assessment of successful keratoplasty, 333-
        334
    corneal
        attachment to slit lamp, 334
        in diagnosis of donor tissue failure, 314-315
Pachymetry, 325, 333
Paracentesis, 184-185, 280, 282, 304
Pars plana approach in removal of vitreous opacity
    in phakic eye, 22
Pathologic astigmatism, cause of, 24
Pathology, corneal, 42, 44, 45, 46
Patient with history of various diagnoses, rejec-
    tion of donor eye from, 72
    one-eyed
        avoidance of unnecessary aphakic kerato-
            plasty surgery in, 248
        chelation of corneal calcium deposits in, 36
        poor surgical risk, chelation of corneal calcium
            deposits in, 36
    preparation of, preoperative
        for combined keratoplasty and cataract ex-
            traction, 219
        for simple keratoplasty, 200, 201
        surgical, 116
Paton, R. Townley, 1, 56
Paton transfer spatula, 100, 148-149
Paufique, Louis, 1, 180
Penetrating graft, 42, 44-54; see also Penetrating
        keratoplasty
    circular, 42, 44
        for peripheral corneal defects, 46-47
    contact lens corneal cutter used for, 106
    discrete corneal pathology and, 44
    and high astigmatic band, 44
    and lamellar graft, 38-40
    for peripheral corneal defects, 46-47
    for peripheral corneal perforation secondary to
        ulceration, 46
    size of, 44
    suturing of, 50-53, 150
        to vascularized recipient corneas, 52-53
    use of trephine for cutting donor button in, 44-
        46
    in vascularized cornea, 50
Penetrating keratoplasty, 2, 32, 44, 275, 320; see
        also Penetrating graft
    combined with lamellar keratoplasty, 188-195
    donor button for, preparation of, 48

Penetrating keratoplasty—cont'd
    instruments for, 96-100
        special, 109-111
    lamellar flanged, 196-198
    and peripheral corneal defects, 46
    simple, 200-215
        cutting the donor button for, 202-203
        exposure and fixation of the globe, 201
        general considerations of, 200
        preparation for surgical procedure of,
            200-201
        suture adjustment in, 214-215
        suturing of, 50-52, 150, 212, 214
    size of donor button in, 44, 46
    trephine cut, completing the, 210
Penicillin and donor eye, 72
Pentazocine lactate, 322
Perforation, peripheral corneal, 46
    secondary to ulceration, 46
Peripheral circumferential pathology. 38
Peripheral corneal thinning, 38
Peripheral vascular invasion, 50
Peritomy of donor eye, 60-61
Perlon 30-micron (9-0) monofilament elastic nylon
        suture, 2
Petri dish, 100
Peyman reciprocating vitreous sucking-cutting in-
        strument, 100, 110, 318
Phacoemulsification, 218, 318
    infusion-aspiration tip, 111
Phakic glaucoma, 288, 289
Phakic keratoplasty, 102
Phthisis bulbi, 288, 308
Physiologic astigmatism, cause of, 24
Pinhole, use of, to determine vision, 323
Piston, Troutman, universal design of, 86-87
Piston guide, 84, 86, 87, 100
    Teflon, 94
Piston punch
    Troutman-Amsler trephine, 98, 100
    universal, 98, 100
Polack corneal graft punch, 94
Polaroid reproductions of B-scans, 249
Polymer contact lenses, 35
Polypropylene, 42, 48, 98, 106, 108, 109, 212, 230,
        260, 310
    in Binkhorst four-loop intraocular lens, 240,
        241, 242
    for iris suture, 146
    in repair of sector edge elevation, 285
    22-micron monofilament, in iris suturing, 146
Posterior capsule, 217
Posterior keratoconus, 20
Posterior pigment layer of the iris, 298-299
Posterior segment, structures of
    B-scan tomography of, 48, 50
    pathology of, 48, 50
    visualization of, 48, 50
Postkeratoplasty intraocular hypertension, 287-
        288
Postoperative astigmatism, "suture-in-place," 32
Postoperative complications
    glaucoma as, 307-309
    surgical management of, 307-320
        general considerations of, 307
Postoperative management, 321
    follow-up, time periods of, 321
Power
    of intraocular lens, 22

Power—cont'd
of lens, determination of, by A- and B-scan ultrasound tomography, 22
radii and dioptric, variation of corneal curvature expression in, 19
Practice of corneal surgery, 3
Prednisolone, 323
Prednisone, 201, 219, 250, 300, 312, 323
Preoperative preparation of patient
for combined keratoplasty and cataract extraction, 219
for simple keratoplasty, 200, 201
Pressure, intraocular, 132, 266-267, 287, 308, 318, 323, 324
Pressure dressing, monocular modified, 186
Probe
Mackensen trabeculotomy, 294-295, 302, 303, 304, 305,
retinal, 100
Procedure, Troutman wedge-resection; see Troutman wedge-resection procedure
Prolaspse
iris, 307, 317
lens, 307
uvea, 196, 316
vitreous, 307
Prolene, 106
Protective dressing, unilateral, 178-179, 214, 232, 300
Protective shield, 178-179
Pseudomonas, 201
Pterygium, resection of, 38-39
Ptosis, postoperative, 102, 180
Punch
Polack corneal graft, 94
Troutman piston, in combined keratoplasty and cataract extraction, 220
Troutman-Amsler trephine piston, 98, 100
universal piston, 98, 100
Pupil
eccentric, 144
margin, 236
reconstruction of, 260, 261
size and centration of, variation in, 20
stenopeic, 20
Pupillary block, 142, 212
Purse-string suture in preparation of donor mushroom, 190-191

R

Radial iridosphincterotomy, 144
Radial sphincterotomy, 144, 145, 222
Radii powers, variation of corneal curvature expressed in, 18, 19
Radius, 269, 270, 272
of curvature, 82, 84
scleral, 84
Ratio, steepening-to-flattening, 18
Razor blade for razor knife, 104
superblade, 104, 109
Razor knife, 104
in aphakic keratoplasty, 252-253
in combined keratoplasty and cataract extraction, 220, 230
to complete incision of cam-guided corneal knife, 105
in completion of trephine cut, 210
in combined lamellar and penetrating keratoplasty, 188, 189

Razor knife—cont'd
dissection of conjunctival remnants of donor eye with, 74-75
in donor tissue failure, 314, 315
MICRA-Pierse, 98-99, 103
in preparation of recipient eye, 188
in preparation of sector lamellar graft, 188
razor blades for, 104
in removal
of calcium deposits from cornea, 36
of interrupted sutures, 230
fixation, 170
of sutures in postoperative management of successful keratoplasty, 326-331
for scleral incision in donor eye, 76-77
in successive lamellar dissections, 182-183
in trabeculectomy, 292
in trabeculotomy, 302
Troutman angled, 98-99, 104
use of, to vary recipient shape, to correct meridional errors, 105
Reaction, homograft, 310-313, 314
tissue, and suture knob, 50
Recipient bed, lamellar, preparation of, 180-182
Recipient cornea
cutting of, with trephine, 128-131
excessively flat, 14
suturing of donor button to, 150, 172
adjustment of sutures 174-175
suturing of graft to, 150-151
vascularized, suturing of, 52-53
Recipient corneal button, 220
Recipient eye
preparation of, in combined lamellar and penetrating keratoplasty, 188
protection of, during preparation of donor button, 204, 205
suturing of donor mushroom to, 192-195
transferring donor button to, 148-149
Recipient opening
cutting of, 204-205
in aphakic keratoplasty, 252
in combined keratoplasty and cataract extraction, 220-221
in penetrating graft, 44
and disparate-sized graft, optical effects of, 10-15
oval, in correction of preexisting astigmatism, 206-207
ovalling of, in refractive surgery, 200
round, in correction of preexisting astigmatism, 208-209, 210-211
shelving of, 210
size of, 95
suturing of donor button to, in anterior segment pathology, 256-257
wedge resection of, 26
Recipient-graft disparity effects, 10-15, 16, 17
Reconstructive corneal surgery, 38, 180
Rectus fixation forceps, 118
Rectus fixation suture, 102
Rectus muscle, 100, 118
Rectus suture, 100
placement of, 118-119
removal of, 214
Red fundus reflex, 142, 300-301
Refraction, 323
of cornea in keratoconus, 8, 35
in familial dystrophy, 35

Refraction—cont'd
  and keratometry, 35
  subjective, 35
Refractive surgery, 200
Refractive vision, 324
Rejection, graft, 333
Relaxing incision, Troutman, 286
Removal of suture; see Suture, removal of
Repair
  of marginal dystrophy, 38-39
  of total anterior corneal opacification, 38-39
Resection, suturing edges of, in Troutman wedge
    resection; see Troutman wedge-resection
    procedure
Residual astigmatism, 286
Reticle of surgical keratometer, 29-30
Retinal cryoprobe in cyclocryothermy, 308-309
Retinal detachment, 48
  morning glory (total), 248
    B-scan of, 249
Retinal probe for cyclocryothermy, 100
Retraction suture, 102
  intrascleral, placement of, 118, 119
Rheostat speed control of Troutman surgical mi-
    croscope, 112, 113
Ring
  corneal; see Corneal ring
  fixation, placement of, 120-127
    forceps, 103
  Flieringa; see Flieringa rings
  LeGrand, 120, 121, 250
  scleral fixation, 120, 121
    removal of, 176
  titanium, MICRA-Pierse; see MICRA-Pierse ti-
    tanium rings
Rotoextractor, 260, 298
  in coreoplasty, 260
  Douvas, 100, 110, 111, 258, 259
  Grieshaber, 100
  Machemer, 100, 109, 110
  in trabeculectomy, 300
Running suture; see Continuous suture

S

Sato, 264
Schlemm's canal, 294, 296, 298, 302-303, 304,
    305
Scissors
  Barraquer-de Wecker; see Barraquer-de Wecker
    scissors
  cataract section, for scleral incision in donor eye,
    76-77
  conjunctival
    blunt-pointed, for enucleation of donor eye,
      58-59
    for peritomy of donor eye, 60-61
  corneal; see Corneal scissors
  enucleation, 58-59, 60-61
  iris
    Barraquer-de Wecker, 108
    MICRA-Pierse, 98-99
  keratoplasty, right and left, 252
  removal of donor eye conjunctival remnants
    with, 74-75
  suture, MICRA-Pierse, 98-99
  Troutman corneal, in excision of corneal button,
    80-81
  Troutman keratoplasty, 98-99, 106

Scissors—cont'd
  use of, with trephine, in keratoplasty of per-
    forated eye, 46
  Vannas; see Vannas scissors
Sclera, 266-267
Scleral envelope, 20
Scleral expander, Girard, 98-99, 101, 250-251
Scleral fixation ring, removal of, 176-178
Scleral flap, 292, 293, 296, 300, 301
Scleral radius, 84
Scleral segment, 20
Scleral spur, 20, 23
Scleral staphyloma, 196-197
Scleral support ring, 230, 292
Second International Corneal Congress, 57
Second World Congress on the Cornea, 2
Sector
  crescent-shaped, 278
  selection of, for wedge resection, 276-277
Sector edge elevation, repair of, 284-285
Sector lamellar graft, 188
  combined with penetrating graft, 38-40
Segmental lamellar graft, 42-43
  continuous suture of, 42-43
Semicircular lamellar graft, 38-39
  suturing of, 40-41
Septicemia, rejection of donor eye from patient
    with history of, 72
Serrated knife; see Troutman corneal splitting
    knife
Shield
  metal, Fox-type, 322
  protective, 320
Shoch lens disruption-aspiration device, 100
Shortening of axial length resulting in hyperopia,
    12-13, 16-17
Silicone
  lens, 35
  sleeve, of Amoils cryoprobe tip, 226, 227
Silk suture, 98, 100, 102, 124, 182, 190, 196, 201
  6-0 traction, 219
  7-0, 98
16-Micron nylon suture; see Suture, nylon, elastic
    monofilament, 16-micron
Slit-lamp, 319, 322, 324
  pachymeter attachment to, 334
Slit-lamp examination
  of donor eye, 64-71
  following keratoplasty, 174, 176
  in graft reaction, 312, 313
  in successive lamellar dissections, 182-183
Slit-lamp aperture, use of, in trabeculotomy, 300,
    304
Sloping cut, 80, 220, 221
Soft contact lenses, 35, 36
Solid-bladed lid speculum for enucleation of donor
    eye, 58-59
Solu-Medrol; see Methylprednisolone sodium suc-
    cinate
Spatula
  iris, 98-99, 108, 172, 173, 237, 298-299
  no. 1, use of, in preparation of donor mushroom,
    188
  1-mm, 222, 223, 260, 261
  Paton transfer, 100, 148-149
Spatual knife, corneal dissecting, 109
Spatula needle, use of, in lamellar dissections,
    182
Spectacle, protective, 320

Spectacle correction following debridement of cornea, 35, 36
Spectacle lens, 217
Specular microscope; *see* Microscopy, specular
Speculum, 230
    Barraquer light-wire lid; *see* Barraquer light-wire lid speculum lid; *see* Lid speculum
Sphere, effect of peripheral distorting force on, 24-26
Spherical equivalent emmetropia, 14
Spherical equivalent hyperopia, 26
Spherical equivalent myopia, 52, 264
Sphincterectomy, 144-145
Sphincterotomy, radial, 144-147, 222
Split ring of Troutman piston, 86, 87
Split-image prism device in surgical keratometer, 30
Splitter, Troutman corneal lamellar; *see* Troutman corneal lamellar splitter
Sponge
    cellulose; *see* Cellulose sponge
    Weck-cel, 300
Spur, scleral, 20, 23, 294
Square lamellar graft, 38-39
    suturing of, 42-43
Staphyloma, 48-49
    scleral, 196-197
Steep cornea
    projection of surgical keratometer on, 30-31
    size of donor button to steepen cornea, 95
Steepening
    of corneal curvatures resulting in myopia, 14-15, 16-17
    of curvature in wedge-resected meridian, 26, 27
Steepening-to-flattening ratio in Troutman wedge-resection procedure, 18
Stenopeic pupil, 20
Sterilization of instruments, 97
Steroid medication in glaucoma, 287
Steroids, 216, 218, 311, 312, 319, 323, 324
    systemic, 312, 318
Stitch abscess, 319
Streptomycin and donor eye, 72
Stroma, corneal, 230, 328
    in donor eye, 70-71
Stromal overgrowth, slit-lamp view of, 332
Subchoroidal hemorrhage, 252
Subluxated lens, 22
Sub-Tenon's capsule, injection of, 250
Sucking-cutting instrument, vitreous; *see* Vitreous sucking-cutting instruments
Suction cutting frames and instrumentation, technique of, 132-133
Superblade, 104, 109
Superinfection, bacterial, 319
Surgery
    anterior segment; *see* Anterior segment
    cataract; *see* Cataract, surgery for
    corneal; *see* Cornea, surgery of
    iris, 144-147, 244
    preparation for, 116, 250
    reconstructive corneal, 38
    tectonic corneal, 38
    vitreous, 244
Surgical ametropia; *see* Ametropia
Surgical keratometer; *see* Keratometer, Troutman surgical

Surgical microscope; *see* Microscope, Troutman, surgical
Surgical plan; *see* Cornea, surgery of, optical plan
Suture
    adjustment of, with Troutman surgical keratometer, 256
    antitorque, 172
    continuous; *see* Continuous suture
    deep-to-Descemet's; *see* Deep-to-Descemet's suture
    double-continuous, in suturing graft
        for keratoconus, 50, 51, 52
        in simple penetrating keratoplasty, 214
    final adjustment of, using Troutman surgical keratometer, 214, 230
    fixation, 212
    globe retraction, 102
    interrupted; *see* Interrupted suture
    interrupted fixation, 184-185
    intracorneal, 18, 42
    intrascleral, to fix fixation ring, 102
    intrascleral retraction, position of, 118, 119
    mattress; *see* Mattress suture
    nylon, elastic monofilament, 1-2, 42, 106, 108, 109, 310
        and graft failure, 4
        for simple penetrating keratoplasty, 50-51
        16-micron, 48, 50-51, 53, 106, 230, 250
            for continuous when combined with interrupted, 52, 53
            for iris suturing, 146-147
            knots of, 50
            in suturing graft, 212, 213
            for total corneal opacity, 50
        30-micron (9-0) (Perlon), 2
        22-micron, 50-53, 98-99, 106, 222, 230, 240, 250, 300, 305
            for interrupted when combined with continuous, 52, 53
            for iris suturing, 146-147
            in suturing graft, 212-213
    opposing (double) continuous, in keratoconus, 50
    polypropylene, 42, 48, 98, 106, 108, 109, 212, 230, 260, 310
    preplaced, use of, in lamellar keratoplasty, 184, 185
Prolene (Ethicon), 106
purse string, 190-191
rectus
    placement of, 118-119
    removal of, 176, 214
rectus fixation, 100, 102
removal of
    knots in, 326, 327, 328
    in postoperative management of successful keratoplasty, 325-331
ring fixation, 124
running, 300-301; *see also* Continuous suture
silk, 98, 100, 102, 124, 182, 190, 196, 201
    3-0, 98, 99
    6-0 traction, 219
    7-0, 98
single continuous, removal of, 331
through-and-through; *see* Through-and-through suture
torquing effect of continuous, 40

Suture—cont'd
  and vascularization, 48
Suture bites
  diagonally placed, 40
  malpositioned, 40
Suture forceps, Troutman colibri-handled, 326
Suture handling forceps, 109
  Troutman pointed, with Barraquer-de Wecker handle, 98, 109
Suture loop tension, 40, 44
Suture scissors, MICRA-Pierse, 98-99
Suture tract, 328
"Suture-in-place" postoperative astigmatism, 32
Suturing
  of donor mushroom to recipient eye, 192-195
  of graft in keratoconus, 52
  of iris, 144-147
    technique of, 146-147
  of lamellar graft, 40-43, 184-187
  of penetrating graft, 50-53
  of simple penetrating keratoplasty, 50-52
  of vascularized cornea, 52, 53
Symblepharon, resection of, 38-39
Synechiae, 222, 260-261, 288, 290, 316
Systemic immunosuppressive agent, 300
Systemic medication, 324

T
Technique
  of iris suturing, 144-147
  of keratoplasty
    combined with cataract extraction, 219-232
    intraocular implant after extracapsular extraction, 242-243
    intraocular implant after intracapsular extraction, 236-241
    preparation for surgical procedure of, 219
    common, 116-178
    for successive, lamellar dissections 182-183
  of lamellar keratoplasty, 180-199
  of midperipheral iridectomy, 142-143, 145
  for more extensive anterior segment surgery, 232
  for suction-cutting frames and instrumentation, 132-133
  of Troutman edge-resection procedure, 276-283
Tectonic purpose of keratoplasty, 180
Teflon backing block, 82-85, 100, 148, 202-203, 252
Teflon piston guide, 94
Template, use of, in preparations of sector lamellar graft, 188
Tenon's capsule, donor eye, 60-61
30-Micron (9-0) monofilament elastic nylon (Perlon) suture, 2
3M aperture drape, 98, 100
3-0 Silk suture, 98-99
Through-and-through suture
  for closure of keratoplasty wound, 50, 51, 150-151, 154, 155, 156, 157
  in mushroom graft, 192-195
  in suturing donor button to recipient cornea, 162
  interrupted in combined cataract and keratoplasty, 222
Tilt control of surgical keratometer, 114
Tilted lens, 22

Timing in Troutman wedge-resection procedure, 276
Tissue forceps
  MICRA-Pierse; see MICRA-Pierse tissue forceps
  MICRA-Pierse titanium; see MICRA-Pierse titanium tissue forceps
Tissue-culture fluid, 220
  M-K, 77, 88-89, 202, 252
Tissue-culture medium preservation of donor eye, preparation of, 74-77
Tissue-culture preserved cornea, 188
Titanium cup-tipped forceps, MICRA-Pierse, 103
Titanium needleholder, MICRA-Pierse, 146-147
Titanium rings, MICRA-Pierse; see MICRA-Pierse titanium rings
Titanium tissue forceps, MICRA-Pierse; see MICRA-Pierse titanium tissue forceps
Tomography
  A-scan ultrasound, 22
  B-scan ultrasound; see B-scan ultrasound tomography
Tonometry in postoperative management of keratoplasty, 323
Topography, corneal, measurement of, 30
Torquing of continuous sutures
  cause of, 214
  effect of, 40, 316
Trabecular meshwork, 291, 294, 296, 304
Trabeculectomy, 288, 290-301
Trabeculotomy, 288, 302-305
Trabeculotomy probe, Mackensen, 294-295, 302, 305
Tract, needle or suture, 328, 329, 332
Transfer spatula, Paton, 100, 148-149
Transient ocular hypertension, 287-288
Translation mechanism of surgical microscope, 112, 113, 114, 115
Trauma, 318
  surgical management of, 319-320
Traumatic corneal edema, 44
Trephine
  Barraquer-Mateus motor-driven, 100, 130-131
  blade for, 220
    damaged, 129
    disposable, 82, 86, 98-99, 100, 104
      Troutman piston fitted with, 86-87
      used to penetrate corneoscleral segment, 82-83
    inspection of, 128, 129
    measurement of diameter of, 95
    used to outline pathology in lamellar keratoplasty, 182
  in combined penetrating and lamellar keratoplasty, 188, 189
  to cut oval donor button, 202, 203
  in cutting of donor button and recipient opening in aphakic keratoplasty, 252
  cutting recipient cornea with, 128-131
  distortion of corneal tissue by, 92-93
    avoided, 94
  Draeger motor-driven, 100
  effect on soft eye of excessive vertical pressure of, 220, 221
  handle of, 98-99
  microscopic examination of cutting edge of, 128, 129, 204
  motor-driven, 100, 104, 130-131, 132, 204

Trephine—cont'd
  MUDO, 106, 107
  obturator of, 104, 128, 129, 204
  in preparation of recipient eye, 188, 189, 204
  in repair of edge elevations, 284
  size of
    to cut donor button, 95
    discrepancy in, 104
  Troutman guided-piston, 202
  use of
    in lamellar flanged penetrating graft, 196,
      197
    in lamellar keratoplasty, 182
    in mushroom graft, preparation of, 188-191
    in penetrating graft, 44-46
    and scissors, in perforated eye, 46
  wedge resection, 270
Trephine cut, completion of, 210
Trephine diameters, 45, 46
Trephine piston punch set, Troutman-Amsler, 98,
  100
Trephining of donor eye, 80-83
Triangular lamellar graft, 38-39
  peripheral, 38-39
  suturing of, 42-43
Troutman angled razor knife, 98-99, 104
Troutman colibri-handled suture forceps, 326
Troutman coreoplasty needle, 146-147
Troutman corneal lamellar splitter, 46, 47, 98
  in combined lamellar and penetrating kerato-
    plasty, 188
  in successive lamellar dissections, 182-183
  in trabeculectomy, 292-293
Troutman corneal scissors; see Corneal scissors,
  Troutman
Troutman corneal splitting knives, 46, 47, 98, 182,
  183, 196
Troutman corneal wedge resection, 263, 333
Troutman donor cutting instrument, 94
Troutman double-curved disposable backing block,
  94
Troutman frame-and-piston assembly on dispos-
  able block, 86-87
Troutman guided-piston trephine, 86, 87, 202
Troutman keratoplasty scissors, 98-99, 106, 252
Troutman needleholder, 98-99, 103, 164
Troutman neutral buoyancy lens, 236, 240
Troutman olive-tipped irrigation needle, 172-173,
  224-225
Troutman olive-tipped irrigator, 98-99, 235
Troutman olive-tipped needle, 172-173
Troutman piston
  fitted with disposable blade, 86-87
  split ring of, 86-87
  Troutman piston punch, 220
  Troutman razor knife, 99, 104
  Troutman rectus fixation forceps, 98, 99, 100,
    101
  Troutman relaxing incision, 286
  Troutman short-angled blade breaker, 104
  Troutman spherical double-curve Teflon back-
    ing block, 202
  Troutman surgical keratometer; see Keratom-
    eter, Troutman surgical
  Troutman suture handling forceps, pointed, on
    Barraquer-de Wecker handle, 98, 109
  Troutman tying forceps, 98-99, 109
  Troutman universal piston, design of, 86-87

Troutman piston—cont'd
  Troutman wedge-resection procedure, 26, 27, 52,
    108, 109, 263-286, 333
  clinical application of, 274-275
  for correction of astigmatism, 263-286
  cutting of wedge in, 278-281
  in high astigmatism, 22, 26
  postoperative care in, 284-286
  practical application of theoretic considerations
    of, 274
  preparation for, 275
  principle of, 266
  and refractive surgery, 200
  selection of sector in, 275-277
  single, or double, of recipient margin, in correc-
    tion of preexisting astigmatism, 208-209,
    210-211
  steepening-to-flattening ratio in, 18
  surgical technique of, 275-283
  suturing edge of resection in, 282-284
  technique of, summary of, 282
  timing in, 275
Troutman-Amsler trephine piston punch set, 98,
  100
Tumor in posterior segment, B-scan of, 249
12 O'clock meridian; see Meridian, 12 o'clock
22-Micron nylon suture; see Suture, nylon, elastic
  monofilament, 22-micron
Two-loop intraocular lens, Binkhorst, 242-243
Tying forceps; see Forceps, tying

U
Ulceration, 310
  central discrete corneal opacities, 44
  peripheral corneal perforation secondary to, 46
Ultrasound tomography
  A-scan, 22
  B-scan, 22; see also B-scan ultrasound tomogra-
    phy
Ultrasound unit for sterilization, 97
Unilateral protective dressing, 178-179, 214, 232,
  300
Universal piston punch, Troutman-Amsler, 98,
  100
Urrets-Zavalia, 142
Uvea, 120
  atrophy of, 318
  prolapse, 196
Uveitis, 250, 323

V
Vannas scissors, 98, 99, 108
  in aphakic keratoplasty, 254-255
  in combined keratoplasty and cataract extrac-
    tion, 220
  in completion of trephine cut, 210
  in coreoplasty, 260-261
  in correction of preexisting astigmatism, 210
  for iris suture, 146
  for radial sphincterotomy or sphincterectomy,
    144-146
  for trabeculotomy, 302-303
  in Troutman wedge-resection procedure, 280-
    281
Vascularization, corneal, 42, 250, 310
  and leukoma, 48
  sector peripheral, 212
  superficial, 48

Vascularized recipient cornea, suturing of, 52-53
Virus infections, large, rejection of donor eye from patient with history of, 72
Vision
    of fellow eye, corneal surgery and, 35
    hazy, as sign of homograft reaction, 310
Visual field loss, 287
Vitrectomy, 108, 244, 318
    anterior, 298
        shallow, 258-261
    in control of glaucoma, 288, 300
Vitrector, Kaufman, 258
Vitreitis, 250, 311, 323
Vitreous, 20, 217, 250, 252-254, 259, 260
    adherent strands, 260, 261
    attachment to corneal endothelial surface, 252
    loss of, 120, 196, 258-259
    opacity of; see Opacification
    pathology of, 22-23, 48, 50
    prolapse of, 172
    spatula, iris, 108-109
    surgery of, 120, 244
Vitreous sucking-cutting instruments, 100, 110, 111, 132, 253, 258, 318
    in aphakic keratoplasty, 252-254
    reciprocating, 100
    removal of lens opacity by, 22
    rotoextractor, 100
    in shallow anterior vitrectomy, 258-259
    in trabeculectomy, 298

W

Waterbath B-scan tomography, 48
Watertight wound closure, 172, 214

Weck IBSM (integral beam splitter) microscope, 112
Weck-cel sponge, 108, 300
Wedge, cutting of, in wedge resection, 278-281
Wedge resection; see Troutman wedge-resection procedure
Wedge-resected meridian, steepening of curvature in, 26, 27
Wedge-resected recipient corneal margin, 26-27
Wire lid speculum, Barraquer, 98, 99
Wire-circle Flieringa ring, 98, 99, 102, 120
With-the-rule astigmatism, 18, 19
    correction of, 206-211
World Congress of the Cornea, First, Second, 2
Worst medallion lens, 108, 236-239
Wound
    closure of, watertight, 172, 214
    dehiscence of, 333
    elevation of, 333
    leaks in, 172
        control of, 50
    posterior, 140
    separation of 275, 333
    surgical management of, 316-317
    testing integrity of, 172-175

Z

Zeigler-type knife, 252
Zeiss keratometer, 28
Zone, optical, 20
Zonules, 226
Zoom magnification opthalmic surgical microscope, 1, 2
Zoom microscope, binocular, for assistant, 112, 113